Postgraduate Paediatric Orthopaedics

The Candidate's Guide to the FRCS (Tr & Orth) Examination

Postgraduate Paediatric Orthopaedics

The Candidate's Guide to the FRCS (Tr & Orth) Examination

Edited by

Sattar Alshryda MRCS SICOT EBOT FRCS (Tr & Orth) MSc PhD
Consultant Paediatric Orthopaedic Surgeon
Royal Manchester Children's Hospital, UK

Stan Jones FRCS MBChB MSc Bio Eng FRCS (Tr & Orth)
Consultant Orthopaedic Surgeon
Sheffield Children's Hospital, UK
Honorary Senior Lecturer, University of Sheffield

Paul A. Banaszkiewicz FRCS (Glas) FRCS (Ed) FRCS (Eng) FRCS (Tr & Orth) MClinEd FAcadMEd FHEA
Consultant Orthopaedic Surgeon
Queen Elizabeth Hospital and North East NHS Surgical Centre, Gateshead
Visiting Professor, Northumbria University

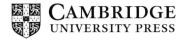
CAMBRIDGE
UNIVERSITY PRESS

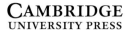

University Printing House, Cambridge CB2 8BS, United Kingdom

Cambridge University Press is part of the University of Cambridge.

It furthers the University's mission by disseminating knowledge in the pursuit of education, learning and research at the highest international levels of excellence.

www.cambridge.org
Information on this title: www.cambridge.org/9781107644588

First published 2014

Printed in the United Kingdom by TJ International Ltd. Padstow Cornwall

A catalogue record for this publication is available from the British Library

Library of Congress Cataloguing in Publication data
Postgraduate paediatric orthopaedics : the candidate's guide to the FRCS (Tr & Orth) examination / [edited by] Sattar Alshryda, Stan Jones, Paul A. Banaszkiewicz.
    p. ; cm.
Includes bibliographical references and index.
ISBN 978-1-107-64458-8 (Paperback)
I. Alshryda, Sattar, 1970– editor of compilation.   II. Jones, Stan (Orthopaedic surgeon), editor of compilation.   III. Banaszkiewicz, Paul A., editor of compilation.
[DNLM: 1. Bone Diseases–Examination Questions.   2. Adolescent.
3. Child.   4. Infant.   5. Musculoskeletal Abnormalities–Examination Questions.   6. Orthopedic Procedures–Examination Questions. WS 18.2]
RD82.3
617.9076–dc23   2013040354

ISBN 978-1-107-64458-8 Paperback

....

Every effort has been made in preparing this book to provide accurate and up-to-date information that is in accord with accepted standards and practice at the time of publication. Although case histories are drawn from actual cases, every effort has been made to disguise the identities of the individuals involved. Nevertheless, the authors, editors and publishers can make no warranties that the information contained herein is totally free from error, not least because clinical standards are constantly changing through research and regulation. The authors, editors and publishers therefore disclaim all liability for direct or consequential damages resulting from the use of material contained in this book. Readers are strongly advised to pay careful attention to information provided by the manufacturer of any drugs or equipment that they plan to use.

Contents

Contributors

Alwyn Abraham BSc MB ChB FRCS (Tr & Orth)
University Hospitals of Leicester NHS Trust

Akinwanda Adedapo MBBS FRCS (Eng) FRCS (Glas) FRCS(C)
James Cook University Hospital, Middlesbrough, UK

Mubashshar Ahmad MBBS FRCS (Tr & Orth)
Royal Manchester Children's Hospital, UK

Farhan Ali FRCS (Tr & Orth)
Royal Manchester Children's Hospital, UK

Fazal Ali MBBS MRCS FRCS (Tr & Orth)
Chesterfield Royal Hospital, UK

Sattar Alshryda MRCS SICOT EBOT FRCS (Tr & Orth) MSc PhD
Royal Manchester Children's Hospital, UK

Paul A. Banaszkiewicz FRCS (Glas) FRCS (Ed) FRCS (Eng) FRCS (Tr & Orth) MClinEd FAcadMEd FHEA
Queen Elizabeth Hospital, Gateshead, UK

Simon L. Barker BSc MD FRCSEd (Tr & Orth)
Royal Aberdeen Children's Hospital, Aberdeen, UK

Dean E. Boyce MB BCh FRCS FRCSEd FRCS (Plast) MD
The Welsh Centre for Burns and Plastic Surgery, Swansea, UK

Lee M. Breakwell MSc FRCS (Tr & Orth)
Sheffield Children's Hospital, UK

Manish Changulani MBBS MS MRCS FRCS (Tr & Orth)
Royal Hospital for Sick Children, Glasgow, UK

Ashley A. Cole BMedSci BMBS FRCS (Tr & Orth)
Sheffield Children's Hospital, UK

Anthony Cooper BSc MBChB MRCS FRCS (Tr & Orth)
British Columbia Children's Hospital, Vancouver, Canada

Gavin De Kiewiet MBChB FRCS RCPS (Glas) FRCS (Ed) FRCS (Orth)
Sunderland Royal Infirmary, UK

James A. Fernandes MS (Orth) DNB (Orth) MCh (Orth) FRCS (Tr & Orth)
Sheffield Children's Hospital, UK

Richard O.E. Gardner MBBS MRCS FRCS (Tr & Orth)
CURE Ethiopia Children's Hospital, Addis Ababa, Ethiopia

Sevan Hopyan MD PhD FRCS (C)
The Hospital for Sick Children, Toronto, Canada

Stan Jones FRCS MB ChB MSc Bio Eng FRCS (Tr & Orth)
Sheffield Children's Hospital, UK

Simon P. Kelley MBChB FRCS (Tr & Orth)
The Hospital for Sick Children, Toronto, Canada

Mohamed O. Kenawey MBBCh MSc MRCS PhD
The Hospital for Sick Children, Toronto, Canada

Om Lahoti MS (Orth) Dip N B (Orth) FRCS (Orth) FRCS(C)
King's College Hospital, London, UK

Matt Nixon MD FRCS (Tr & Orth)
Royal Manchester Children's Hospital, UK

Tim Nunn MRCS (Ed) FRCS (Tr & Orth)
Sheffield Children's Hospital, UK

Kathryn Price BMBS MRCS (Ed) MMedSci FRCS (Tr & Orth)
Queen's Medical Centre, Nottingham, UK

Anish P. Sanghrajka MBBS MRCS FRCS (Tr & Orth)
Norfolk and Norwich University Hospitals, Norwich, UK

Gino R. Somers MBBS PhD FRCPA
The Hospital for Sick Children, Toronto, Canada

Jeremy Yarrow MB BCh MRCS FRCSPlast
The Welsh Centre for Burns and Plastic Surgery, Swansea, UK

Foreword

Since 1998, I have convened an annual core curriculum lecture course in paediatric orthopaedics at Alder Hey Children's Hospital. Over the years, we have frequently been asked to recommend books that succinctly cover all of the necessary information and I now believe that we have found such a book in *Postgraduate Paediatric Orthopaedics: The Candidate's Guide to the FRCS (Tr & Orth) Examination*. As the title suggests, the text is targeted toward trainees sitting the FRCS (Tr & Orth) examination but the book would also be useful for those who seek to enhance or maintain their paediatric orthopaedic knowledge base, including practicing orthopaedic surgeons, GPs, paediatricians and specialist physiotherapists. The text is much more than lecture notes and covers all of the major subjects with sufficient information to keep the reader interested, while still delivering the required facts to an examination candidate as quickly as possible. I congratulate the editors and the authors for producing such as useful text.

Colin E. Bruce
Consultant Children's Orthopaedic Surgeon
Alder Hey Children's Hospital
Liverpool, UK

Preface

Why another exam-related FRCS (Tr & Orth) book? Don't we cover paediatrics in the chapters of the other *Postgraduate Orthopaedics* books?

We always felt the need for a more definitive guide to the paediatric component of the FRCS exam.

We were never entirely happy that the FRCS (Tr & Orth) paediatric syllabus was particularly well covered or developed in a number of orthopaedic books. Most lacked the specific subject focus that candidates needed to pass the FRCS (Tr & Orth) exam.

General orthopaedic books tended to scratch the surface of a difficult area of orthopaedics that needs to be learnt well for the exam. Specialized books on paediatrics meant you could lose all focus of the subject's relevance and end up not extracting the relevant or specific detail required to pass the exam. Moreover, you could find yourself spending a lot of unnecessary time and effort drowning in these specialized textbooks and not have enough time left to read the basic science, trauma or hands sections.

Our aim with this book is to make it all-encompassing, so that it covers everything you need to know to pass the FRCS (Tr & Orth) section of the exam without having to cross-reference from other larger textbooks. A tall order but one, we hope, that we manage to fulfil.

We were careful not to make the book too detailed, so it ends up being like a subspecialty book in paediatrics. At the same time, we didn't want it to become too flimsy, such that you felt you were missing something and you repeatedly needed to go to the larger specialized textbooks of paediatric orthopaedics.

We decided to include in detail all components of the exam; therefore, we have added multiple-choice and extended matching questions. There really should not be an artificial separation between Parts I and II of the exam.

As with all the books in the *Postgraduate Orthopaedics* series, we make no claim for the originality of the material contained in the text. This material is widely available in the larger orthopaedic community. We have simply distilled and focused this knowledge into something that will hopefully get you through the exam.

We hope you find this book useful in preparing for the exam and wish you every success. We hope that in some small (or large) way the book will make the difference between you passing and failing the exam.

Sattar Alshryda
Stan Jones and
Paul A. Banaszkiewicz

Acknowledgements

We would like to thank all people who helped through various stages of writing this book. We are particularly grateful to:

- Ania Milkowski, for her immense help in producing the book's figures and graphs,

- The staff of the Hospital for Sick Children in Toronto,
- The staff of the Royal Hospital for Sick Children in Glasgow.

Interactive website

www.postgraduateorthopaedics.com

This website accompanies the textbook series *Postgraduate Orthopaedics*, which includes:

- *Postgraduate Orthopaedics: The Candidate's Guide to the FRCS (Tr & Orth) Examination*, 2nd edition,
- *Postgraduate Orthopaedics: Viva Guide for the FRCS (Tr & Orth) Examination*,
- *Postgraduate Paediatric Orthopaedics: The Candidate's Guide to the FRCS (Tr & Orth) Examination*.

The aim is to provide additional information and resources, so as to maximize the learning potential of each book.

Additional areas of the website provide supplementary orthopaedic material, updates and web links. *Meet the Editorial Team* provides a profile of authors who were involved in writing the books. Details of forthcoming courses are provided, as are details of the next exam dates.

There is a link to additional orthopaedic websites that are particularly exam-focused.

It is very important that our readers give us feedback. Please email us if you have found any errors in the text that we can correct. In addition, if we haven't included an area of orthopaedics that you feel we should cover please let us know. Likewise, any constructive suggestions for improvement would be most welcome.

Abbreviations

AAI atlantoaxial instability

ABC aneurysmal bone cysts

ACL anterior cruciate ligament

ADI anterior atlantodens index

ADM abductor digiti minimi

AER apical epidermal ridge

AI acetabular index

AIIS anterior inferior iliac spine

AP anteroposterior

ASIS anterior superior iliac spine

ATD articulotrochanteric distance

AVN avascular necrosis (see also ON)

BMP bone morphogenic protein

CAPTA Child Abuse Prevention and Treatment Act

CAVE cavus, abduction, varus and equinus

CCV congenital coxa vara

CEA centre edge angle

CMCJ carpometacarpal joint

CML classical metaphyseal lesions

CMT Charcot–Marie–Tooth disease

CNS central nervous system

CORA centre of rotation of angulation

CRP C-reactive protein

CSL central sacral line

CT computed tomography

CTEV congenital talipes equinovarus (club foot)

CV coxa vara

CVS cardiovascular system

DCV developmental coxa vara

DDH developmental dysplasia of the hip

DEXA dual-energy X-ray absorptiometry

EDF elongation, derotation and flexion

EEC ectrodactyly–ectodermal dysplasia–clefting

EF external fixation

EMA epiphyseal–metaphyseal angle

EMQ extended matching question

ESR erythrocyte sedimentation rate

FAV femoral anteversion

FDS flexor digitorum superficialis

FFD focal fibrocartilaginous dysplasia

FIN flexible intramedullary nailing

FPA foot progression angle

g gram

GHJ glenohumeral joint

GMFCS Gross Motor Functional Classification System

GP general practitioner

HEA Hilgenreiner epiphyseal angle

IGHL inferior glenohumeral ligament

IJO idiopathic juvenile osteoporosis

IU International Unit

JLCA joint line convergence angle

kg kilogram

LCL lateral collateral ligament

LCPD Legg–Calvé–Perthes disease

LLD leg length discrepancy

m metre

MACS Manual Ability Classification System

MBD metabolic bone diseases

MCL medial collateral ligament

MCPJ metacarpophalangeal joint

MCQ multiple-choice question

MDA metaphyseal–diaphyseal angle

mLDFA mechanical lateral distal femoral angle

mLDTA mechanical lateral distal tibial angle

mLPFA mechanical lateral proximal femoral angle

MED multiple epiphyseal dysplasia

MGHL middle glenohumeral ligament

MPFL medial patella-femoral ligament

MPTA medial proximal tibial angle

MRI magnetic resonance imaging

MRSA methicillin-resistant *Staphylococcus aureus*

MTPJ metatarsophalangeal joint

NAI non-accidental injury

NF neurofibromatosis

NICE National Institute for Health and Care Excellence

NSA neck–shaft angle

NSAID non-steroidal anti-inflammatory drug

OA osteoarthritis

OBPI obstetric brachial plexus birth injury

OI osteogenesis imperfecta

ON osteonecrosis (see also AVN)

P *P* value

PCL posterior cruciate ligament

PFFD proximal femoral focal deficiency

PH Pavlik harness

PHHA posterior humeral head articulation

PHV peak height velocity

PIPJ proximal interphalangeal joint

PIS pinning *in situ*

PMNST peripheral malignant nerve sheath tumour

POP plaster-of-Paris

PPA patellar progression angle

PSA posterior slip angle

PSACH pseudoachondroplasia

PTH parathyroid hormone

RANK receptor activator of nuclear factor κB

RCT randomized controlled trial

RMI Reimer's migration index

ROM range of motion

RVAD rib–vertebra angle difference

SAC space available to the cord

SAPHO synovitis, acne, pustulosis, hyperostosis and osteitis

SD standard deviation

SED spondyloepiphyseal dysplasia

SPNBF subperiosteal new bone formation

SUFE slipped upper femoral epiphysis

TAR thrombocytopaenia absent radii

TFA tibiofemoral angle

TMA transmalleolar thigh angle; tarsometatarsal angle

UCL ulnar collateral ligament

VACTERL vertebral defects, anal atresia, cardiac defects, tracheo-esophageal fistula, renal anomalies and limb abnormalities

vs versus

VMO vastus medialis obliquus

WCC white cell count

ZPA zone of polarizing activity

°C degree Celsius

Chapter

1

Introduction and general preparation

Paul A. Banaszkiewicz

Introduction

We can almost hear you sigh and exclaim, 'Not another chapter on general FRCS (Tr & Orth) exam guidance!' There are so many 'candidate's exam experiences' out there for everybody to read and digest. What new spin can they add to the same old story?

It is still necessary to include this chapter, as it neatly sets the scene for the exam. Perhaps more importantly, the exam focus regularly changes and you definitely want to keep ahead with the latest developments.

Finally, the nature of the book means that it is necessary to consider how the paediatric section of the exam fits together within the wider FRCS (Tr & Orth) exam.

A lot of this general advice can be found elsewhere, as we alluded to, in the various candidate accounts floating round the internet. The problem is that most of these 'candidate experiences' are in a very similar vein and after reading the first two or three very little extra new material is then uncovered. While the general exam guidance advice in the general and viva-focused *Postgraduate Orthopaedics* books contains few surprises, both books cover the material to a greater depth and sophistication than elsewhere. Candidates may want to search out the relevant book chapters for this information.

This general FRCS (Tr & Orth) exam guidance material can become a little dull and recurring to most candidates. Therefore, we have tried to avoid any unnecessary repetition of material, concentrating on the important details vital for exam success.

The aims of the exam are to see if you have enough knowledge to practice safely as a day-one orthopaedic consultant in a District General Hospital. The exam is not set out to test you in microscopic detail about trivial irrelevancies. The exam is not even designed to test for subspecialty interest.

The first day you are on call as a consultant, your registrar may phone you up about a child with a painful hip in casualty. A child with knock knees may have been wrongly referred to your adult knee clinic. Your trauma practice may cover children and you may worry about risks of growth arrest with particular fracture patterns.

The history of the FRCS (Tr & Orth) exam

In the late 1970s, the old-style FRCS had long ceased to mark the end of training and had become your entry into higher surgical training. The only exam in Britain devoted exclusively to orthopaedics was the MChOrth from the University of Liverpool. To take this exam, you generally had to work in or around the Mersey Deanery.

The situation was clearly unsatisfactory and, under the guidance of the Royal College of Surgeons in Edinburgh, a Specialty Fellowship exam in orthopaedics was introduced in 1979. This exam was optional but soon became established as a benchmark of completion of training and a quality assurance measure. It was an entirely clinical exam with a viva voce format. The standard was high and the pass mark variable. It was not an easy exam to pass but it became accepted that recognition of the standard of higher surgical training by assessment in the form of an exam was essential in orthopaedics. This is, in fact, applicable to all surgical specialties, not just orthopaedics.

In time, the exam was accepted by all four Royal Colleges, and in 1990 a new intercollegiate exam was introduced. This originally took place twice a year in each of the colleges in turn. This exam was also initially voluntary but in 1991 it became a requirement for accreditation, together with the satisfactory completion of training in an approved programme that had been inspected and approved by the Specialist Advisory Committee.

For many years, it was difficult to get hold of any valuable exam guidance. The exam appeared to be surrounded in secrecy. Despite a curriculum and syllabus, many candidates entered the exam not really knowing what to expect. The usual line was that if you had undertaken good clinical work, read the appropriate literature and had a sound grasp of the basic sciences you would be OK and would be expected to pass.

It was also difficult to get useful information and tips from previous candidates, such as the expected standard or the questions likely to be asked. Another fact – now easily forgotten – was that the internet was in its infancy and there simply wasn't the candidate support network that there is today.

Postgraduate Paediatric Orthopaedics, ed. Sattar Alshryda, Stan Jones and Paul A. Banaszkiewicz. Published by Cambridge University Press.
© Cambridge University Press 2014.

In time, the pass rate began to fall and candidates hoping to avoid failure wanted to be better informed about what to expect.

There weren't a large number of courses available to guide a candidate on the expected standard. Some courses set the level far too high. The idea was that you were panicked into hitting the books, as you perceived that your knowledge wasn't up to the required standard. This was fine if you had a year to go before the exam and you could plan a more intensive schedule of revision but not so good if your exam was in 3 weeks' time.

The situation began to change around the turn of the millennium. A number of candidates began writing down their own experiences as a revision tool for the next wave of candidates sitting the exam. A small select number of candidates in larger training programmes began to form study groups. These study groups acquired and circulated these candidate accounts among themselves to help with exam preparation. The deal was that once you had passed you wrote your own account for those candidates coming after you to use with their own preparation. In time, these candidate's experience reports began to circulate more freely in a wider domain, such that most candidates, with a bit of detective work, were able to get hold of them.

Today there are numerous websites containing significant numbers of candidates' exam experiences. These include the British Orthopaedic Trainees Association, various regional training programme sites and, lastly, individual accounts from successful candidates. The major problem with many candidate experiences is that they deal with specific viva or clinical questions in a rather superficial way, mainly with bullet point headings. Also, we have yet to see an unsuccessful candidate's experience posted on the internet. Candidates generally learn more from what went wrong than if only successful accounts are presented.

The standard of FRCS (Tr & Orth) exam courses has, by and large, significantly improved and, in general, candidates are much more informed and have a better idea of what types of question tend to get asked regularly. So one of the most major changes with the FRCS (Tr & Orth) exam in the last 10 years is that the mystery surrounding it has evaporated away.

The old-style viva with a variable number of questions is definitely a thing of the past. The viva is now standardized for candidates, with similar questions being asked for each topic covered. This leads to a much fairer exam, with much less potential for any discrimination.

Exam format

The current FRCS (Tr & Orth) exam encompasses two sections: Part I is a written exam and Part II the clinical and oral exam. For further information, and to make sure that your information is up to date, we suggest that you carefully review the Intercollegiate Speciality Board website (http://www.jcie.org.uk).

Part I

This section consists of two separate papers; essentially, a multiple-choice question (MCQ) paper and an extended matching question (EMQ) paper. Part I was generally regarded as the easier section of exam to pass but since 2013 the pass mark has been raised by the Examination Board. This is to make sure that candidates entering Part II are more likely to pass. A number of candidates may be OK learning for an MCQ/EMI paper but be a long way off the standard for a clinical and viva exam.

The statistical analysis of a paper that was contained in the MCQ paper is likely to be scrapped by mid-2014.

Part II

Clinical cases

This section comprises clinical cases and structured oral interviews. The clinical component is divided into three short cases each for the upper and lower limbs, each of 5 minutes duration (30 minutes in total) and two intermediate cases of 15 minutes duration (which may be upper limb, lower limb or spine) The examiners are fairly strict with time allowance in the intermediate cases, with 5 minutes for history, 5 minutes for clinical examination and 5 minutes at the end for discussion.

Orals

The oral component is divided into four 30-minute viva sections:

- Basic science,
- Trauma, including spine,
- Adult elective orthopaedics including spine,
- Paediatric orthopaedics and hand surgery, including shoulder and elbow.

Paediatric section

The paediatric oral or viva section is combined with the hands and upper-limb section. The examiners now have to introduce themselves to the candidate and remind the candidate which oral he or she is about to be examined on, to allow the candidate time to settle. Feedback is given where appropriate, such as, 'OK, let's move on; we have covered this area, let's go on.' Examiners are encouraged to avoid such remarks as, 'Excellent, well done, that's great, fantastic.'

Props, such as radiographs, pictures, charts, are usually used to lead into a question.

Three paediatric topics are discussed: these usually cover a trauma-type question, one big (A-list) topic and a less-obvious clinical topic.

Hammering on when a candidate could not answer a question used to be a common candidate complaint but examiners are now actively dissuaded from this practice.

All candidates are treated in exactly the same manner and marks are based on performance only. Examiners are instructed to allow for candidates' nervousness and are told not to respond to inappropriate behaviour by a candidate. Inappropriate behaviour would include rudeness or sarcastic remarks to the examiners, impoliteness and bad mannered or derogatory comments about facilities or organization issues.

A significant change is that viva questions are now more clinically orientated and relevant to the types of situation that may present to a consultant orthopaedic surgeon in clinical practice. For this reason, potential exam questions are now significantly more scrutinized than previously before being approved by the exam committee for inclusion in the exam.

When to sit the exam

It is generally accepted that you will need about one full year of preparation before you will feel confident to sit the exam.

In theory, it should be relatively easy for you to decide if you have enough experience and have prepared in sufficient detail to sit the exam. In practice, a multitude of competing issues usually complicate this decision.

If you are a trainee, you will have been sitting the UK In-Training exam for the last 3 or 4 years and should know your annual scores. Many training programmes also have yearly 'mock' clinical and viva exams and will not let you sit the real exam unless you have achieved a good enough pass in these mock tests.

In the past you may have had a charitable training programme director who was willing to take a chance with you but this is now less likely, as it may have a direct bearing on the number of trainees allocated to a region.

Study groups

A key factor for your success will be the formation of a study group that meets regularly, discusses various topics and arranges practice viva sessions. There are a number of factors that will contribute to a study group's success and also some aspects that you should avoid. Essentially, the group should comprise three to five candidates, who all need to get on well with each other and should not be too far apart from each other in terms of knowledge. If there are significant rivalries and petty jealousies within the group, with people trying to score points off each other, the group is not going to work out. Be careful of candidates who think that they are too good for the group; they are likely to let you down near the end and do their own thing.

Also, be careful with the candidates who are unlikely to pass first time round and who are just too far behind with their studies to contribute significantly to group discussions. Give these candidates the benefit of the doubt, as surprises do happen, but be concerned if you draw repeated blanks with large gaps in core knowledge. Politely sideline such candidates if the extra input is significantly affecting the group's performance. In general, don't include candidates who are a few months or perhaps a year off sitting the exam. They are unlikely to have sufficient motivation and drive at this stage in their revision.

Last-minute preparation

In the last 2 to 3 weeks leading up to the exam try not to panic and attempt to go over all your revision again. This will not work and will just lead to you getting even more stressed and irrational. Use this time for quick focused revision.

Attending a last-minute revision course as a sort of dry run a couple of weeks before the real exam is becoming more popular these days. This only really works if you are not too far away from the required standard and the dry run is used to iron out, fine tune and rehearse your performance. Hoping to get lucky with a sort of quick revision before the real exam but with significant knowledge gaps is unlikely to be successful.

Exam tactics

Dress sensibly: no loud ties, short shirts or Vivienne Westwood high heels. Don't stink of stale cigarettes, as this is very off-putting for most people. A bit of cologne is OK, but unless you have a body odour problem, be careful not to use too much, as this may also be off-putting to examiners.

If you are one of a small number of candidates who are significantly affected with exam stress it may be reasonable to get some professional help. The scenario during the exam would be extreme nervousness, wet armpits and sweat pouring off your face. This situation is very uncomfortable and will affect your performance. A beta-blocker will probably have no significant physiological affect but psychologically may help to calm you down and improve your overall exam performance. We would suggest speaking to your GP for advice.

Book a hotel fairly near the exam venue, preferably within walking distance, although this may not always be possible.

Allow plenty of time to arrive promptly at the exam hall. We know the arguments of turning up too early and getting freaked out by other candidates talking too much and winding you up. This is irritating but a fair amount less stressful than leaving your arrival to the last minute and risking that you get caught up in traffic and turn up late.

Keep your distance

A piece of advice that we keep repeating is to get away from other exam candidates as quickly as possible after completing the various exam sections. It is extremely questionable whether anything useful can be gained by hanging around to chat to other candidates after completing the clinical or vivas.

At best, this will unnerve you and can make you feel uncomfortable; at worst, it will put you off for the remaining parts of the exam. Even worse, you may end up in a bar afterward, drinking too much alcohol in drowning the sorrows of a perceived poor performance and ruin any chances of that last-minute brush up of key topics you had planned for later that evening.

Stay focused during the exam period; don't let your guard down, don't relax and don't be fooled into a false sense of security.

At the same time, and in equal measure, don't get paranoid, edgy, nervy and uptight, as this is just as counterproductive. You need to come across as relaxed, professional, someone who is in control and who can be relied on. This mindset is much easier to achieve if you stay clear of other candidates. Perhaps the only exception should be the other candidates in your study group; you could chat to them for a few minutes after each exam section.

Recommended reading

Which orthopaedic paediatric books to use for preparation for the paediatric section of the FRCS (Tr & Orth) exam is very much a matter of personal preference and choice. However some books are more suited and better to use than others.

Staheli's *Practice of Pediatric Orthopaedics* [1]

The illustrations are first class and the book has excellent recommendations and reviews. It is easy to read and fairly comprehensive.

Joseph's *Paediatric Orthopaedics* [2]

This book is a tad disappointing as it promises a lot but doesn't quite deliver the goods. This is not to say that it isn't a good book; it is just that the contents don't quite match up to the hype.

The book is targeted at higher surgical trainees and younger consultants. It is written by paediatric orthopaedic surgeons from four different continents. However, although this gives the book a truly international flavour, in the highly focused world of FRCS (Tr & Orth) exams, this is probably a drawback.

The book discusses in depth the treatment options for particular paediatric conditions, hopefully allowing trainee orthopaedic surgeons to speak confidently about the approach to individual patients during their specialty exams.

Pediatric Orthopaedic Secrets, 3rd edition [3]

We are not great fans of the *Secrets* series. Some of the material does not particularly match the FRCS (Tr & Orth) syllabus and the format is only loosely applicable to the exam. That said, we have come across a number of candidates who swear by the *Secrets* series. We advise that you borrow one from the library before buying. It has good reviews.

Oxford Textbook of Trauma and Orthopaedics, 2nd edition [4]

This is more of a reference book with a fairly detailed paediatric section. Reducing the three-volume first edition into a single volume in the second edition was a masterstroke and makes the book much easier to read.

Miller's *Review of Orthopaedics* [5]

This has a reasonably good paediatric section. As the text is list led, the section is probably best suited for revision for Part I of the FRCS (Tr & Orth) exam.

AAOS Comprehensive Orthopaedic Review [6]

This book is similar in style to Miller but more comprehensive. It has excellent reviews and is recommended for FRCS (Orth) exam preparation. The biggest drawback is the price.

References

1. Staheli L (2011) *Practice of Pediatric Orthopaedics*. Philadelphia: Lippincott Williams & Wilkins.

2. Joseph B, Nayagam S, Loder R and Torode I (2009) *Paediatric Orthopaedics: A System of Decision-Making*. Boca Raton, FL: CRC Press.

3. Staheli LT and Song KM (2007) *Pediatric Orthopaedic Secrets*, 3rd edition. Philadelphia: Elsevier Saunders.

4. Bulstrode C, Wilson-MacDonald J, Eastwood DM *et al.* (2011) *Oxford Textbook of Trauma and Orthopaedics*, 2nd edition. Oxford: Oxford University Press.

5. Miller MD (2012) *Review of Orthopaedics*, 6th edition. Philadelphia: Saunders.

6. Lieberman JR (2009) *AAOS Comprehensive Orthopaedic Review*. Rosemont, IL: American Academy of Orthopaedic Surgeons.

History and examination of the paediatric patient

Stan Jones and Sattar Alshryda

History and examination

The assessment of a child presenting with a musculoskeletal complaint requires a thorough history and full clinical examination and should be carried out in a child-friendly environment. If this is done properly, a diagnosis can be made in the majority of cases.

The initial contact with the child and family involves introducing oneself to all the family members, including the child. This should be carried out in a professional yet friendly manner. The cultural background of the family should be considered and it is important to conform to gender order for introductions.

The next stage of the assessment should aim to allay the anxiety or fear of the child. This can be done in a variety of ways and depends on the age of the child. In a younger child an introduction to toys may be all that is required, while in the older child this may involve talking about friends, sports, school or a piece of clothing.

History
Presenting complaint

Common complaints include deformity, gait abnormalities, altered function and pain.

The duration of symptoms, mode of onset, history of any injury, frequency and timing of symptoms, aggravating or relieving factors, any functional impairment, previous investigations or treatment received should be noted. An older child should be involved in the discussion about presenting complaints.

It is also important to consider the presenting complaints in relation to the age of the child, e.g. Perthes disease has to be considered a differential in a young child (4 to 8 years of age) with a history of hip and knee pain, while in an adolescent with similar complaints one has to think of slipped upper femoral epiphysis (SUFE).

Deformities

In-toeing, out-toeing, bow legs, knock knees and flat feet are common reasons for attendance at the paediatric orthopaedic clinic. In the majority of patients, the deformities are normal variants and require no treatment other than parental reassurance. A history of progressive deformity or deformities that are asymmetrical or unilateral requires further assessment, to exclude a pathological cause.

Birth history and developmental milestones

A history of bleeding during pregnancy, maternal diabetes and reduced fetal movements during late pregnancy can be associated with abnormalities at birth. Breech presentation, premature birth and jaundice at birth are also significant factors to be enquired about.

Enquire about developmental milestones, e.g. when the child first sat and walked. In one-third of late walkers, the cause is pathological, e.g. cerebral palsy [1] (Table 2.1).

Family history

It is useful to enquire whether other members of the family have similar problems. A number of orthopaedic clinical conditions run in families, e.g. pes cavus. Details of past illnesses and hospitalizations complete the history.

Examination

The examination of a child commences as soon as the child and the family enter the consulting room. The child must continue to be observed while taking the history, as valuable clues can be gained.

The child should be undressed appropriately but with its cooperation and must be kept warm at all times. The modesty of the older child should always be respected, e.g. by providing a gown.

The infant can be examined on a parent's lap.
Examination involves:

- Screening and general assessment,
- Specific thorough musculoskeletal examination undertaken with the presenting complaint in mind.

Table 2.1 Normal developmental milestones

Age	Motor skills	Social skills
3 months	Lifts head up when prone	Smiles when spoken to
6 months	Sits with support, head steady when sitting	Laughs and smiles spontaneously
9 months	Sits without support	Waves 'bye-bye', vocalizes 'ma-ma' or 'da-da'
1 year	Walks with one hand support	Starts cooperating with dressing
2 years	Runs forward	Uses three-word sentences, matches colours
3 years	Jumps in place	Dresses self, puts own shoes on
5 years	Hops	Names four colours, counts ten objects correctly
6 years	Skips	Does small buttons on shirt, ties bows on shoes

Screening examination

1. Inspection of the child's face may reveal:
   - Dysmorphic features suggestive of a syndrome or skeletal dysplasia,
   - Blue eyes – a parent with blue eyes may clinch a diagnosis of osteogenesis imperfecta,
   - Mongoloid features (flat face with upward and slanted palpebral fissures or epicanthic folds, high-arched palate), in keeping with Down's syndrome,
   - Large tongue, suggestive of Beckwith–Wiedemann syndrome (Figure 2.1).
2. The height of the child should be noted, as well as the heights of the parents.
3. Asymmetry in body proportions, e.g. disproportion between the truncal height and limb lengths, may suggest a skeletal dysplasia.
4. Evidence of generalized ligamentous laxity (the Beighton score, Table 2.2). Excessive generalized joint laxity is associated with such conditions as Ehlers–Danlos syndrome and Marfan syndrome.

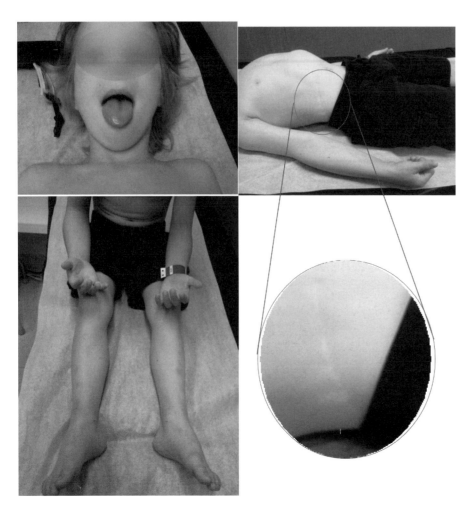

Figure 2.1 Beckwith–Wiedemann syndrome. There is a hemihypertrophy of the right side of the body including the tongue. There is a right loin scar from a previous nephrectomy.

Table 2.2 The Beighton score

Criteria	Note
Little finger dorsiflexion	1 if >90°, 2 if bilateral
Thumb to forearm (wrist flexion)	1 if thumb tips touch the forearm skin, 2 if bilateral
Elbow extension	1 if hyperextension >10°, 2 if bilateral
Knee extension	1 if hyperextension >10°, 2 if bilateral
Trunk flexion with knees full extended	1 if palms can rest flat on the floor

The Beighton score is a nine-point score: the higher the score, the greater the laxity. The threshold for joint laxity in a young adult ranges from 4 to 6.

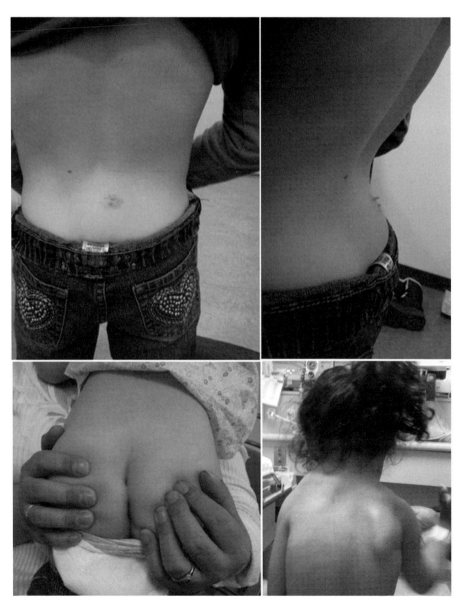

Figure 2.2 Useful signs on general inspection of the back. Top pictures: Skin tag and fatty swelling in a patient with lipomeningocele (see also Figure 10.8, which shows the feet of the same patient). Bottom left: Sacral dimple in an infant with developmental dysplasia of the hip. Bottom right: A patient with Klippel–Trénaunay–Weber syndrome and Sprengel's shoulder, which is associated with several orthopaedic abnormalities.

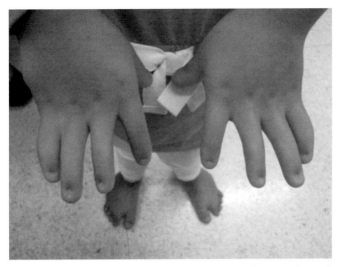

Figure 2.3 Absent nails. Nail abnormalities can be a manifestation of several orthopaedic problems, such as nail-patella syndrome and ectodermal dysplasia.

5. Café au lait spots (Figure 12.5), axillary freckling (Figure 17.8) and neurofibromas are suggestive of neurofibromatosis; vascular marking (haemangiomas) may suggest Klippel–Trénaunay–Weber syndrome; hairy patches, skin tags or sacral dimples may indicate underlying spinal pathology (Figure 2.2); nail abnormalities may indicate ectodermal dysplasia or nail-patella syndrome (Figure 2.3).

Specific examination

With the child standing, inspection is carried out from the front, sides and back, assessing:

- The standing posture and curvature of the spine,
- The level and contour of the shoulders,
- The level of the anterior superior iliac spines,
- For any evidence of genu valgum or varus (intermalleolar and intercondylar distance),
- For calf hypertrophy (myopathy) or muscular wasting,
- For surgical or other scars,
- For hindfoot alignment, valgus or varus,
- For evidence of tiptoeing, flat feet or cavus deformity.

Gowers' test is carried out if a myopathy is suspected. Gowers' sign is positive if, on rising from sitting on the floor, a child climbs his hands up his thighs for support.

Gait

The child is then asked to walk in a straight line. While doing so observe:

- For abnormal upper-limb movements, i.e. spasticity (cerebral palsy),

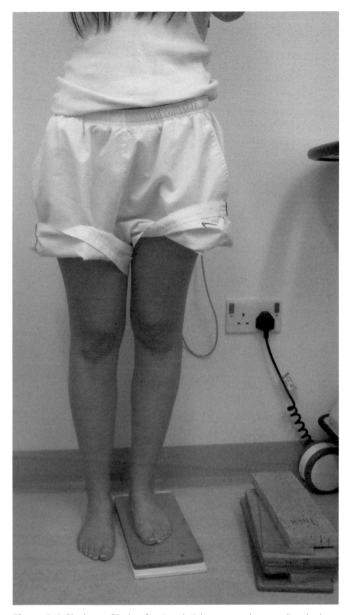

Figure 2.4 Block test. Blocks of various heights are used to equalize the legs and level the pelvis. This is a better way to estimate the height required for a shoe raise or insole.

- The knee and foot progression; these indicate in- or out-toeing, if present,
- Knee extension on heel strike and knee flexion in swing,
- For any evidence of a limp (asymmetrical movement of the lower limbs).

The different kinds of gait include:

1. Antalgic,
2. Trendelenburg,
3. Short limb,

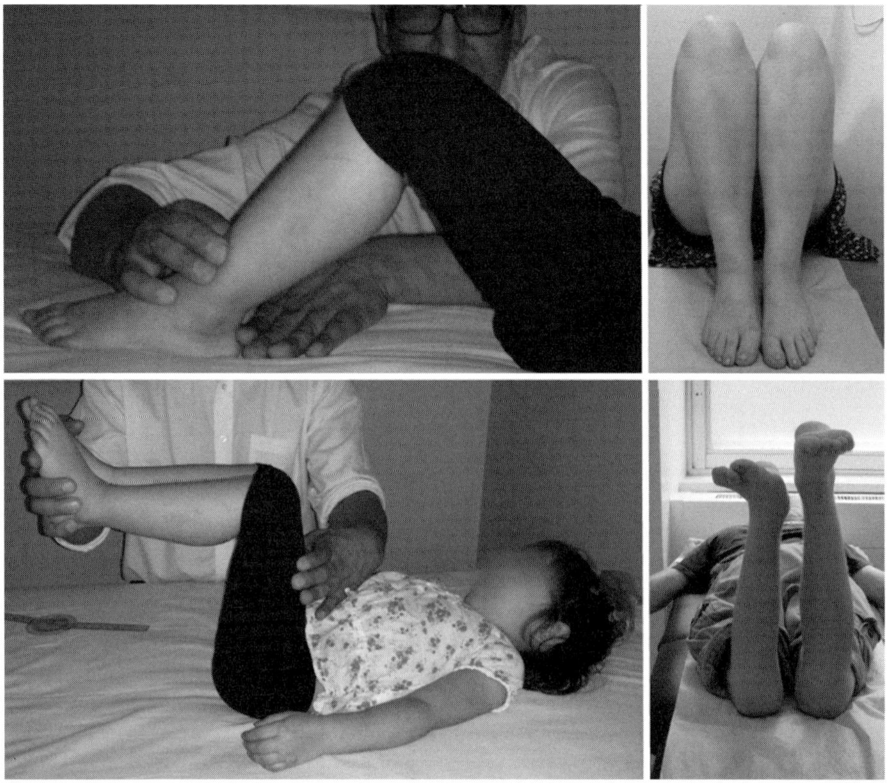

Figure 2.5 Galeazzi's test. These clinical photographs show various modification of Galeazzi's test to identify the site of the LLD, i.e. whether it is in the femur or the tibia.

4. High stepping,
5. Toe walking,
6. Ataxic.

Antalgic gait

This type of gait is the result of pain in the affected limb. The stance phase of the affected limb is hurried, with a quick swing phase of the opposite limb.

Trendelenburg gait

A failure of the hip abductor mechanism produces this type of gait pattern. The hemipelvis on the affected side dips during the stance phase of gait and there is a compensatory lurch of the ipsilateral shoulder to the opposite side, e.g. developmental hip dysplasia.

Short-limb gait

As the name implies, this gait is observed in children with a longitudinal limb deficiency, e.g. fibular hemimelia. The shoulder on the side of the short lower limb dips during the stance phase.

High stepping gait

This gait pattern is usually observed in children with hereditary sensory motor neuropathy. A lack of sufficient ankle dorsiflexion during the swing phase results in increased knee flexion to facilitate clearance of the foot.

Toe walking gait

This is observed when the child's initial contact is with the forefoot and not the hindfoot.

Ataxic gait

This gait pattern is of a broad base.

Limb length discrepancy

Limb length discrepancy can be assessed using a tape measure or by the block test. The block test is the preferred method.

The child is made to stand with the short leg on blocks of varying heights until the posterior superior or anterior superior iliac spines appear level to the examiner's eye (Figure 2.4). It is important that the hips and knees are kept extended.

In a child with a fixed flexion deformity of the hip or knee or an adduction or abduction deformity of a limb, the leg length discrepancy (LLD) assessment will have to be made with the child supine and the normal limb held in a position comparable to the deformed limb. Measurements are then made with a tape measure.

It is important to note that adduction deformities of the hip produce apparent shortening, while the opposite is true for abduction deformities.

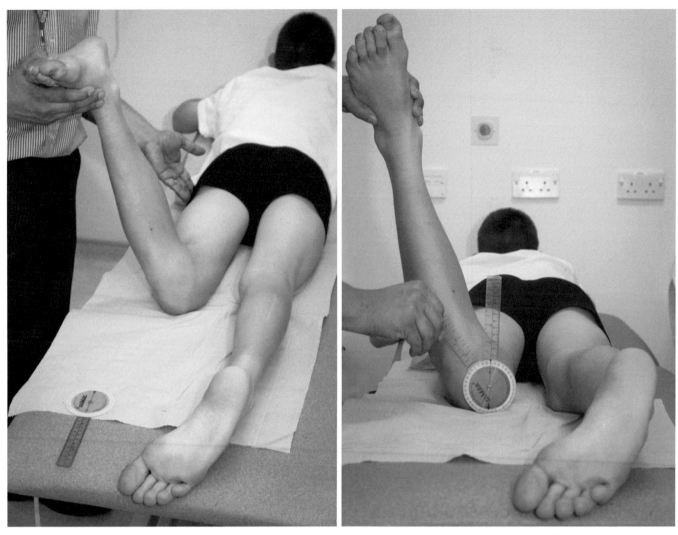

Figure 2.6 Gage test to estimate femoral anteversion. Left: Feel when the greater trochanter is most prominent and hold the leg. Right: Measure the angle between the long axis of the leg and an imaginary vertical line. Notice any rise in the ipsilateral hemipelvis on flexing the knee (Duncan–Ely test), which indicates a tight rectus femoris.

Once the LLD is established, *Galeazzi's test* is performed, to determine whether the shortening is above or below the knee (Figure 2.5).

Rotational profile

Deformities in the hip, femur, tibia or feet may lead to rotational malalignment. Hence it is important to examine all these segments when assessing the rotational profile of a lower limb.

The rotational profile assessment starts while assessing the gait, observing the foot progression angle (FPA) and the patellar progression angle (PPA). On the couch, rotational profile is best undertaken with the child lying prone (Staheli's rotational profile) [2], with the knee flexed and the examiner's palm applied to the back of the child to keep the pelvis level. The degree of internal and external rotation of the hip joint is noted (the normal range of external rotation is 45°–70°, and of internal rotation is 10°–45°). The presence of excessive internal rotation and limited external rotation would imply excessive femoral neck anteversion.

The Gage test (also known as Craig's test or Ryder's method) is then conducted, to confirm the degree of femoral anteversion (FAV). This is noted by measuring the angle between the long axis of the leg and an imaginary vertical line when the greater trochanter is most prominent (Figure 2.6). At birth, the femoral anteversion is about 40° and by age 16, it is approximately 16°. Figure 2.7 shows the relationship between the FPA and the FAV.

Tibial torsion is assessed by measuring the thigh–foot angle and the transmalleolar thigh angle (TMA). The thigh–foot

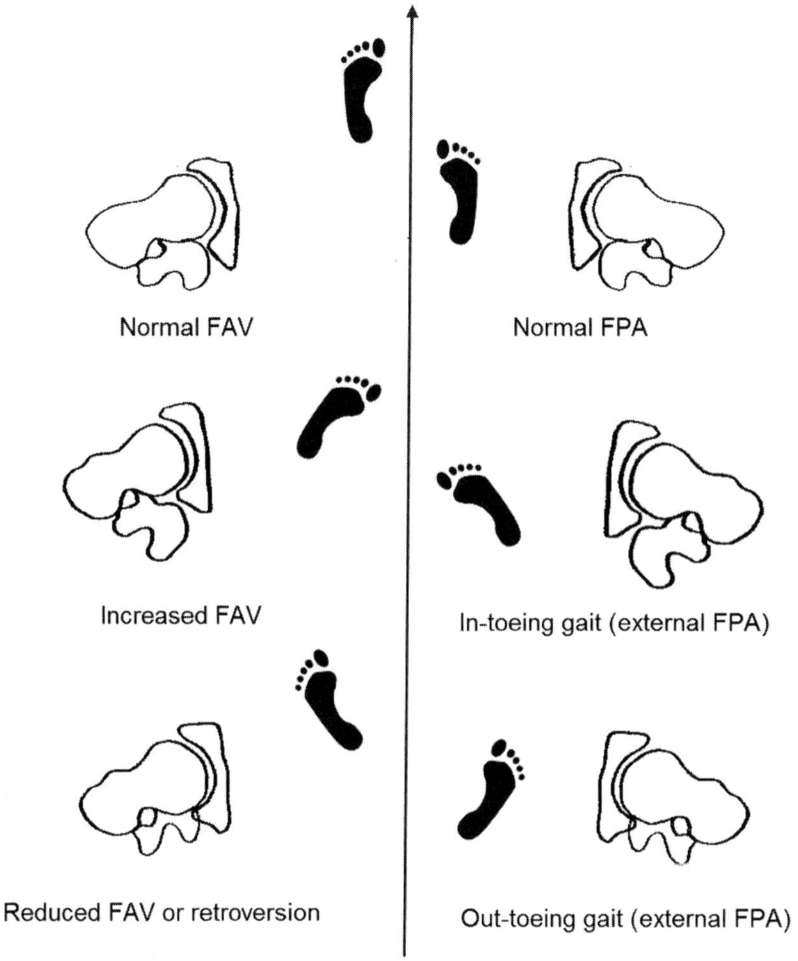

Figure 2.7 Relationship between the FPA (foot progression angle) and FAV (femoral anteversion).

Normal FAV

Normal FPA

Increased FAV

In-toeing gait (external FPA)

Reduced FAV or retroversion

Out-toeing gait (external FPA)

angle is the angle between the long axis of the thigh and a line bisecting the sole of the foot in its resting position (Figure 2.8). A normal angle is 10°–15° of external rotation. The TMA is the angle formed by the thigh axis and the line perpendicular to the transmalleolar line. Because the lateral malleolus is normally posterior to the medial malleolus, the TMA is more externally rotated than the thigh–foot angle (normally about 15°–20°).

Foot contribution to the rotational profile abnormalities are assessed using either the heel bisector line or the lateral border. These are both addressed in Chapter 4 (Figure 4.4).

Hip joint examination

The general rule for examination of joints; i.e. 'look, feel, move', applies.

Looking and feeling may not yield much information, as the hip is a deep-seated joint, though scars may be observed.

It is good practice to assess the active range of joint motion before the passive and to compare movement of the abnormal joint with that of the normal joint.

Abduction and adduction movements of the hip joint are assessed with the child supine while rotation is best assessed with the child prone. It is imperative to stabilize the pelvis with one hand while assessing abduction and adduction.

Any fixed flexion of the hip joint will be noted using *Thomas' test*. The child is instructed to flex both hips maximally with the knees flexed. The examiner places a hand under the lumbar region to obliterate the lumbar lordosis. The child is then asked to extend the hip being examined gently, while the contralateral hip is kept flexed (Figure 2.9).

Knee examination

Swelling around the knee may be localized or generalized. Localized swelling may be:

1. Anterior over the tibial tubercle (Osgood–Schlatter disease),
2. Posterior medial (semimembranosus bursa),
3. To the sides (bony exostosis).

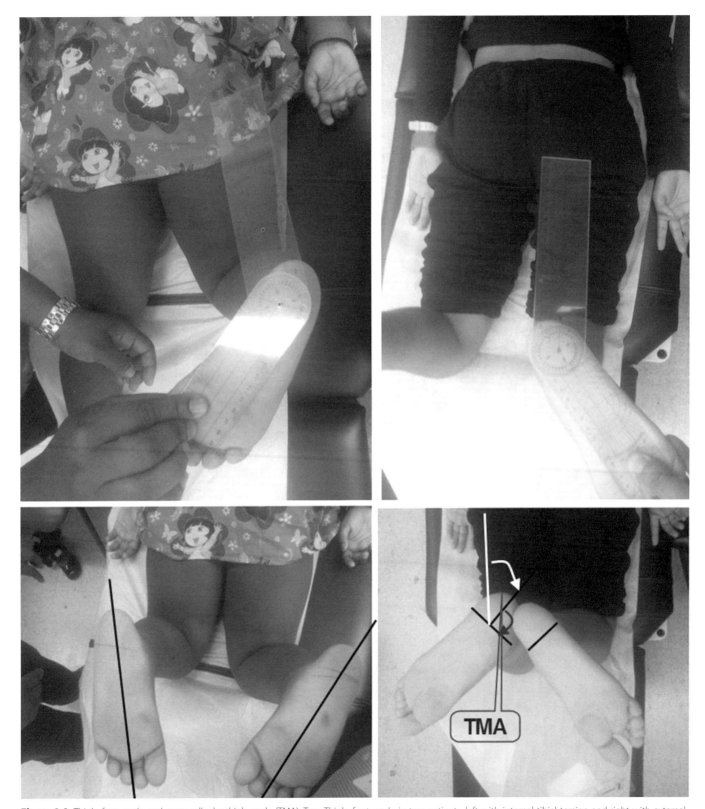

Figure 2.8 Thigh–foot angle and transmalleolar thigh angle (TMA). Top: Thigh–foot angle in two patients, left with internal tibial torsion and right with external tibial torsion. Bottom left: Heel bisector line. Bottom right: Transmalleolar angle.

Generalized swelling may be due to a large effusion or inflammatory synovitis.

While the child is seated on a couch with the limbs hanging freely, the position of the patella (alta or baja) and the way it tracks should be noted.

Knee ligament assessment is undertaken after assessing the range of motion and stability. The medial and lateral collateral ligaments are assessed by applying a valgus and varus stress, respectively, with the knee in extension and 30° of flexion.

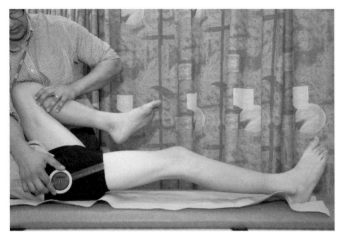

Figure 2.9 Thomas' test. The angle between the long axis of the thigh and the couch is the degree of fixed flexion. In the presence of a fixed flexion deformity of the knee it is advisable to allow the limb to extend over the side of the couch thus enabling a true measurement of the hip flexion deformity.

Foot and ankle examination

Examination of the feet should be undertaken while seated, standing and walking. Any scars, swellings or deformities should be evaluated.

In flat feet, the hindfoot may be in valgus and the medial arch absent while standing.

In a flexible flat foot, on tiptoeing, the hindfoot adopts a neutral or varus position and the medial arch forms (Figure 4.8).

Jack's test will also reproduce the medial arch (Figure 2.10). This will not be the case in an adolescent with flat feet who has a tarsal coalition or peroneal spastic flatfeet. In addition, in these cases the movement of the subtalar joint is reduced or absent.

In pes cavus, the medial arch is high, and clawing of the lesser toes may be observed. In addition, the hindfoot may be in varus. In the presence of hindfoot varus, the *Coleman block test* is required to ascertain whether the varus corrects, as this influences the surgical treatment options (Figure 2.11). Examination of the spine is necessary in pes cavus.

Localized tenderness may be observed over the second or third metatarsophalangeal joint (MTPJ) (Freiberg's disease) and the calcaneum (Sever's disease).

Joint range of motion should be assessed systematically, i.e. ankle, subtalar, midtarsal, metatarsophalangeal and interphalangeal joints.

A full neuromuscular examination completes the examination of any joint.

Additional tests

Several tests are used to assess patients with cerebral palsy. These are summarized in Table 2.3.

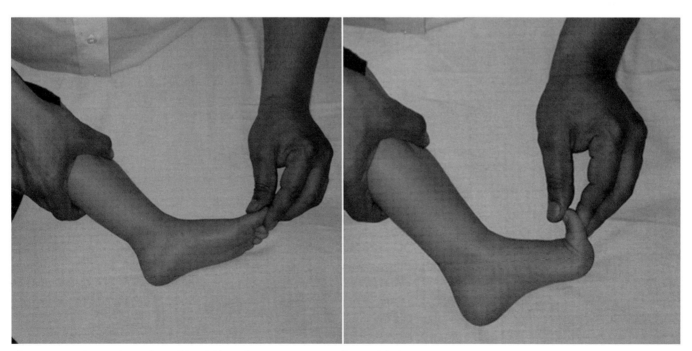

Figure 2.10 Jack's test. This can be useful in children who cannot tiptoe. Dorsiflexion of the big toe reconstitutes the medial arch. In children who can stand, this can be performed in a standing position.

Table 2.3 Tests to assess joint contractures in cerebral palsy [3]

Joint	Test	Description
Hip	Thomas' test (flexion contracture)	Child is supine, the contralateral hip flexed to flatten out the lumbar spine. The hip is extended and the angle between the tabletop and the femur is the degree of flexion contracture (Figure 2.9).
	Staheli test (flexion contracture)	Child is prone with the pelvis on the edge of the table and the contralateral hip is flexed. The angle between the horizontal line and the thigh is the degree of hip flexion contracture. Thomas' test is easier to perform; however, it cannot measure the amount of extension (which is less relevant) and it needs adjustment if there is a concomitant knee flexion contracture. Normally, hip extension is 10°–20°.
	Adductor contracture	Child is supine and the degree of hip abduction is measured with the hip and knee in extension (normal = 45°). Adductor contracture <45° indicates a risk of progressive hip subluxation. Repeat the test with the knee flexed to exclude the medial hamstring, which crosses both joints. If there is no medial hamstring tightness, the values should be similar (Phelp's test) (Figure 2.12).
	Ober's test (abductor contracture)	Child is on the side with the spine straight. The hip to be tested (the upper most) is then flexed to 90° (with the knee flexed to a right angle through the test), fully abducted, and brought into full hyperextension and allowed to adduct maximally. The angle of the thigh and a horizontal line parallel to the examination table represents the degree of abduction contracture. A normal limb will drop well below this horizontal line. If there is abduction contracture, the hip cannot be adducted to the neutral position.
	Duncan–Ely test (rectus femoris contracture)	Child is prone and the knee is gradually flexed. The examiner feels the spasticity and resistance of the rectus muscle and observes the elevation of the ipsilateral hemipelvis. A tight rectus femoris may contribute to a stiff knee gait (Figure 2.6). The elevation of the hemipelvis is usually subjectively graded into +, ++ and +++.
Knee	Range of motion, popliteal angle, hamstring shift and straight leg raise tests	The normal knee range of motion (ROM) is 0°–150°. The knee extension should be measured with the hip extended (which relaxes the hamstring muscles). This gives the fixed flexion deformity of the knee, which is usually caused by a capsular or bony deformity. The popliteal angle is measured with the child supine and the hip flexed at 90°, with the contralateral hip extended. The knee is then extended. The angle between the vertical line and the tibia is the popliteal angle (normal <20°) (Figure 2.13). Some practitioners measure the angle between the femur and tibia as the popliteal angle. Others flex the ipsilateral hip to 45° rather than 90° (mimicking the hip flexion in normal gait) and measure the angle. This latter is called the modified popliteal angle and is probably more relevant clinically. The difference between the measurements with the contralateral hip extended and those with the hip flexed is the hamstring shift. Flexing the hip beyond the hip fixed flexion deformity ensures that the pelvis is not anteriorly tilted and gives a more representative measure of hamstring tightness. The straight leg raise is another way to measure the degree of hamstring contracture: the limb is raised, keeping the knee in full extension (as in spine examination). The angle between the extremity and the table is measured (normal <70°).
Ankle	Silfverskiöld test	Child is supine, the heel inverted to lock the subtalar joint (prevent any dorsiflexion through the midfoot). The degree of dorsiflexion is measured with the knee flexed and extended. Flexing the knee relaxes the gastrocnemius and tests the tightness in the soleus. Extending the knee tests tightness in both muscles. If the tightness involves the gastrocnemius only it can be released selectively (Figure 2.14).
Foot		Evaluate the relationship between the hindfoot, midfoot and forefoot, the range of motion and spasticity.

It is important to differentiate between 'shortened muscle-static' and 'contracted muscle-dynamic' spasticity. The range of motion after a fast stretch is called R1, whereas the maximum range of motion with gentle and slow stretching is called R2. A large difference between R2 and R1 indicates greater spasticity and vice versa.

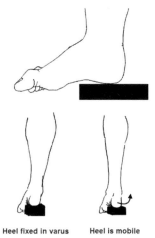
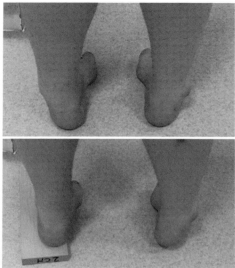

Heel fixed in varus   Heel is mobile

Figure 2.11 Coleman's block test. The rationale of Coleman's test is that the heel is in varus in a cavovarus foot, either as a primary pathology or because it is forced into varus to accommodate for fixed planter flexion of the first ray. Thus, if the first ray is allowed to drop over the edge of a block, this would remove its effect on the heel. If the heel corrects to neutral, this means that there is no fixed varus deformity of the heel and corrective osteotomy of the calcaneum is not required.

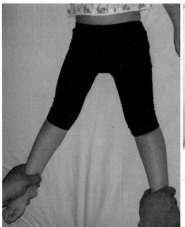
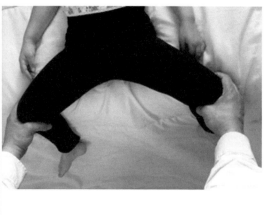

Figure 2.12 Phelp's test. Medial hamstring tightens with knee extension, reducing hip abduction. The difference in hip abduction with the knee flexed and extended indicates the tightness of this muscle group: the bigger the difference, the more tightness.

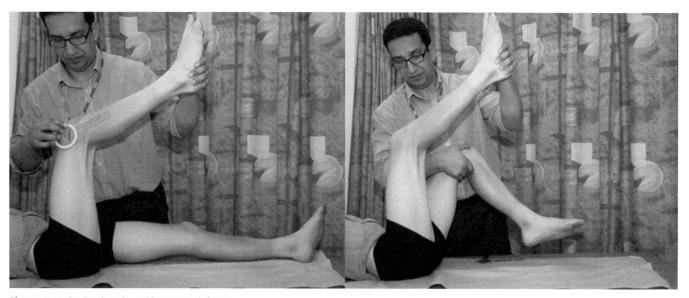

Figure 2.13 Popliteal angle and hamstring shift test.

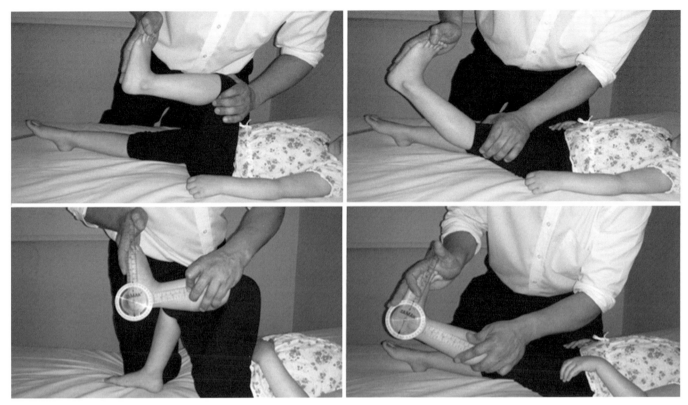

Figure 2.14 Silfverskiöld test. Flexing the knee relaxes the gastrocnemius and tests the tightness in the soleus. If there is no difference in ankle dorsiflexion with the knee flexed or extended, both muscle and Achilles tendon are tight. If the ankle dorsiflexion is reduced with the knee extended, a tight gastrocnemius is indicated and this needs selective lengthening.

References

1. Herring JA (2008) *Tachdjian's Pediatric Orthopaedics*, 4th edition, volume 1. Philadelphia: Saunders Elsevier.

2. Staheli L (2008) *Fundamentals of Pediatric Orthopaedics*, 4th edition. Philadelphia: Lippincott Williams & Wilkins.

3. Dormans JP (2005) *Pediatric Orthopaedics. Core Knowledge in Orthopaedics*. Philadelphia: Elsevier Mosby.

Chapter 3

The hip

Sattar Alshryda and Paul A. Banaszkiewicz

3.1 Slipped upper femoral epiphysis (SUFE)

Background

Although a rare condition (2:100 000), slipped upper femoral epiphysis (SUFE) is one of the most common types of paediatric and adolescent hip disorder. The incidence of SUFE varies with:

1. Sex: SUFE is more common in boys (75% of cases) with the peak incidence occurring at 12 to 15 years compared with 10 to 13 years in girls. Thus, boys tend to have their slip 2 years older than girls. SUFE is rarely reported after the age of 20 years [1].
2. Race [2]: SUFE is more common in those of African and Polynesian descent.
3. Laterality: SUFE is more common on the left side (as is developmental dysplasia of the hip (DDH)). The reason is unknown; it may be related to the sitting posture of right-handed children while writing. The incidence of bilaterality has been reported to be as high as 50%, although the generally accepted incidence is 20%. In children with bilateral involvement, 50–60% present with simultaneous SUFEs and those who present with a unilateral SUFE and subsequently develop a contralateral SUFE do so within 18 months. Younger patients and those with endocrine or metabolic abnormalities are at much higher risk of bilateral involvement.
4. Seasonal variations: this is debatable; some studies have suggested that SUFE is more common in June and July.

Aetiology

Although, the cause is poorly understood, it is believed that increased shear forces or a weak growth plate (the physis) in adolescence predisposes to SUFE. This results in the head of the femur staying in the acetabulum and the neck slipping forward and outward.

The following features lead to increased shear forces across the physis and set the stage for developing SUFE:

1. Increased weight (>80th centile),
2. Femoral retroversion (>10°),
3. Increased physis height due to a widened hypertrophic zone,
4. A more vertical slope of the physis,
5. Trauma.

Weakness of the physis may be due to:

1. Renal failure osteodystrophy (95% bilateral),
2. Previous radiation therapy,
3. Endocrine disorders (65% bilateral):

   a. Hypothyroidism (usually SUFE is the first presenting feature),
   b. Growth hormone deficiency,
   c. Growth hormone excess,
   d. Panhypopituitarism,
   e. Craniopharyngioma,
   f. Hypogonadism,
   g. Hyperparathyroidism,
   h. Multiple endocrine neoplasias,
   i. Turner's syndrome.

Although rare, endocrine disorders must be considered in every patient with SUFE. Loder and Greenfield [3] described the age–weight test to assist in the differentiation between idiopathic and atypical SUFE.

The test is defined as negative for age <16 years and weight ≥50th percentile and positive when beyond these boundaries. Multiple logistic regression analysis demonstrated that age and weight were predictors for an atypical SUFE. For two patients of equal weight, those younger than 10 or older than 16 were 4.2 times more likely to have an atypical SUFE; for two patients of equal age, those below the 50th percentile weight were 8.4 times more likely. The probability of a child with a negative test result having an idiopathic SUFE was 93%, and the probability of a child with a positive test result having an atypical SUFE was 52%.

Postgraduate Paediatric Orthopaedics, ed. Sattar Alshryda, Stan Jones and Paul A. Banaszkiewicz. Published by Cambridge University Press. © Cambridge University Press 2014.

Clinical presentation

The classical presentation of SUFE is in an overweight child who has poorly localized groin, thigh or knee pain (referred pain, obturator nerve) and is limping. There may be a history of minor trauma. The usual age is between 11 and 14 years. With a stable slip, a child is able to bear weight, with or without crutches. With an unstable slip, a child has severe pain, such that walking is not possible, even with crutches.

On examination, the leg is shortened and externally rotated (Figure 3.1.1). There is usually restricted flexion, abduction and internal rotation of the affected hip. Moreover, there is an obligatory additional external rotation when the hip is flexed further.

Investigation

Plain radiography (AP and true lateral views)

The diagnosis is usually confirmed on an anteroposterior (AP) radiograph of the pelvis. A frog lateral view is not recommended, as it may displace the slip further; it is less precise in assessing the severity of slip due to variations in positioning the limbs. The hallmarks of SUFE are (Figure 3.1.2):

1. Trethowan's sign is positive; a line (often referred to as Klein's line) drawn along the superior border of the femoral neck on the AP view should pass through the femoral head. In SUFE, the line passes superior to the head rather than through the head.
2. Decreased epiphyseal height, as the head is slipped posteriorly.
3. Increased distance between the teardrop and the femoral neck metaphysis.
4. Capener's sign: on AP pelvic radiographs, in a normal hip the posterior acetabular margin cuts across the medial corner of the upper femoral metaphysis. In SUFE, the entire metaphysis is lateral to the posterior acetabular margin.
5. Widening and irregularity of the physeal line (early sign).
6. Metaphyseal blanch sign of Steel; this is a crescent-shaped dense area in the metaphysis due to superimposition of the neck and the head.
7. Remodelling changes with a sclerotic, smooth superior part of the neck and callus formation on the inferior border. This is observed in chronic slips.

Computed tomography (CT)

This is not essential to diagnose and treat SUFE; however, it is valuable in:

1. Assessing the anatomical features accurately (e.g. degree of slip, head–neck angle, retroversion and severity of residual deformity),
2. Ruling out penetration of the hip joint by metalware,
3. Confirming closure of the proximal femoral physis.

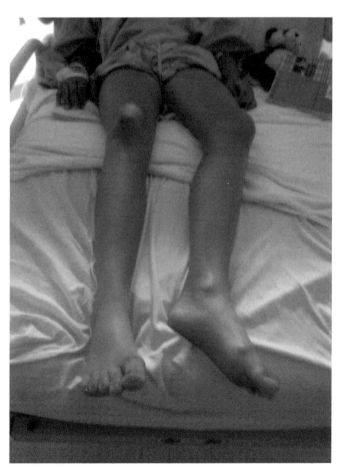

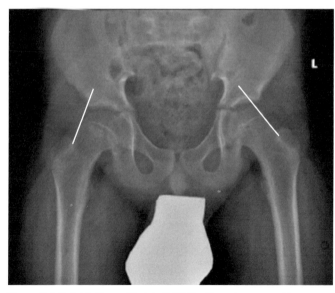

Figure 3.1.1 Child with SUFE. Notice the short and externally rotated left leg (mimic fracture neck of femur). The patient was not able to ambulate (unstable slip).

Figure 3.1.2 Pelvis X-ray with right SUFE. The X-ray shows a positive Trethowan's sign where the Klein's line passes above the femoral head. There is a widened physis with a positive Steel's blanch sign.

Ultrasound

This may be useful in diagnosing early slips by demonstrating a joint effusion and a step between the femoral neck and the epiphysis.

Magnetic resonance imaging (MRI)

This is valuable in detecting avascular necrosis (AVN); however, the metalware can affect the quality of the image and prevent an accurate diagnosis. An isotope bone scan is useful in this situation.

Classification

SUFE has been classified functionally, according to the patient's ability to bear weight (stable or unstable); chronologically, according to onset of symptoms (preslip, acute, chronic or acute-on-chronic); or morphologically, according to the direction of displacement of the femoral epiphysis relative to the neck (posterior or anterior slip).

Functional

This is done according to weight-bearing status after the acute event, as popularized by Loder:

Stable: The patient is able to ambulate and bear weight.

Unstable: The patient is in severe pain and is unable to ambulate with or without crutches.

In a multicentre study of 55 slips in 54 children, Loder *et al.* [4] reported that avascular necrosis (AVN) developed in 14 (47%) of unstable slips but in none of the stable hips. A reduction – either intentional or unintentional – occurred in 26 unstable slips (out of 30) and in two stable slips (out of 25). Loder's group demonstrated an association between early reduction (less than 48 hours) and the development of AVN. They found that the time from the onset of symptoms to the reduction of the slipped epiphysis was significantly less in patients in whom AVN developed (2 vs 6 days), suggesting that early reduction was unwise. There were concerns regarding a cause-and-effect relationship and it was postulated that children who had been internally fixed early had a more severe form of unstable slip that was associated with a higher rate of AVN. (See the section on timing of surgery.)

Chronological

SUFE has been classified chronologically, relating to the onset of symptoms:

Preslip: A patient has symptoms (limb pain following prolonged standing or walking) but with no anatomical displacement of the femoral head. There may be useful radiological evidence, such as widening and irregularity of the physis, or osteopaenia of the hemipelvis. This may represent a minimal slip not easily seen on plain radiographs.

Acute: There is an abrupt displacement through the proximal physis with symptoms and signs developing over a short period of time (<3 weeks). Acute slips account for 10% of all slips.

Chronic: Patients with a chronic slip present with pain in the groin, medial thigh and knee, occurring over a period >3 weeks (often months to years).

Acute-on-chronic: Patients have symptoms of >3 weeks duration but present with acute symptoms of sudden onset following a sudden increase in the degree of slip.

Morphological

1. In the majority of cases of SUFE, the epiphysis is displaced posteriorly and inferiorly (varus or posterior slip) relative to the femoral neck.

2. In rare cases, the displacement is either superior or posterior (valgus or anterior slip).

Grading

Grading is based on the severity of the slip on radiographs, either by proportion of slip (Wilson) or by angle of slip (Southwick) (Figures 3.1.3 and 3.1.4).

Wilson grades

Grade I (mild): The displacement of the physis as a proportion of neck width is less than one-third.

Grade II (moderate): The displacement is between one-third and two-thirds of the neck width.

Grade III (severe): The displacement is greater than two-thirds of the neck width.

Angular displacement

Angular displacement is measured by the Southwick angle [5]. This is measured on the lateral view of both hips. It is measured by drawing a line perpendicular to a line connecting the posterior and anterior tips of the epiphysis at the physis. The angle between the perpendicular line and the femoral shaft line forms an angle that is termed the lateral head–shaft angle. The Southwick angle is the difference between the slipped and the normal sides' angles. The lateral head–shaft angle is commonly misquoted (and accepted) as the Southwick angle.

Grade I (mild): An angle difference of less than 30°.

Grade II (moderate): An angle difference of between 30° and 50°.

Grade III (severe): A difference of over 50°.

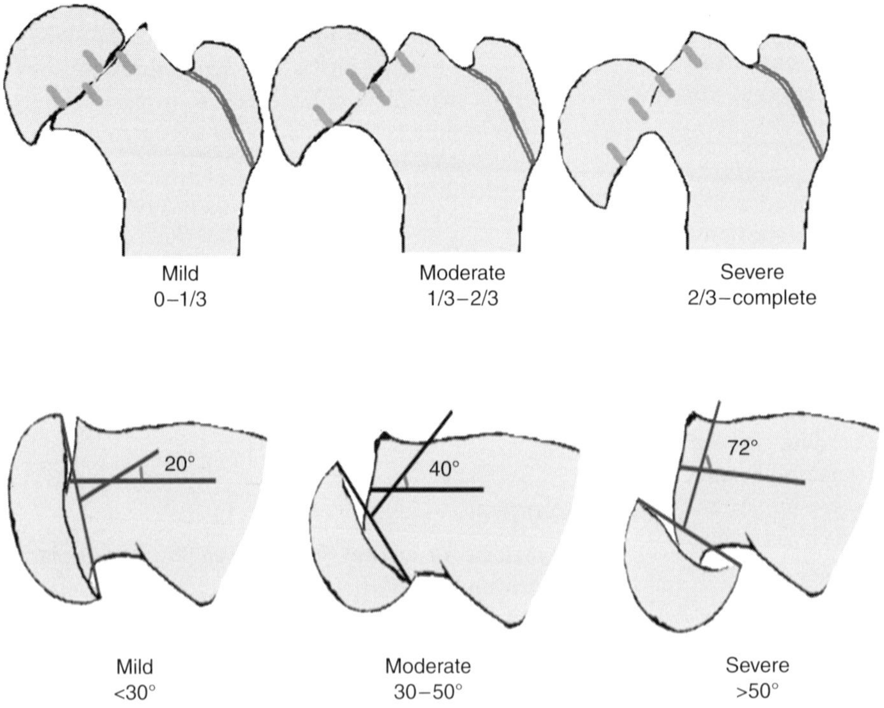

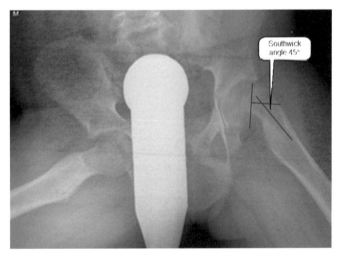

Figure 3.1.3 SUFE radiological grading.

Mild
0–1/3

Moderate
1/3–2/3

Severe
2/3–complete

Mild
<30°

Moderate
30–50°

Severe
>50°

Southwick
angle 45°

Figure 3.1.4 Lateral epiphyseal–shaft angle or Southwick angle.

In practice, most clinicians tend to use a combination of the Loder classification and one of the radiographic classifications. There is some crossover between classifications but severe slips are more likely to be unstable [6].

Treatment

The aim of the treatment is to prevent progression of the slip without complications. Although, it is logical to reduce the slip to near anatomical position; this desire has always been tempered by concerns about the potentially devastating complications of AVN and chondrolysis. The choice of treatment depends on the type of slip, its severity and surgical expertise. Figure 3.1.5 summarizes the authors' recommendations.

Treatment of stable SUFE

There is a reasonable clinical consensus that the treatment of mild and moderate slip should be by pinning *in situ* (PIS). This involves placing a single screw across the growth through a small incision on the thigh to prevent further slip until growth plate closure. Some authors advocate multiple smooth pins in very young affected children (younger than 8) to allow for growth. The screw must not be removed prior to physeal closure, otherwise progression of the slip may resume. The appropriateness of removal after physeal closure is contended.

If the slip is severe, pinning *in situ* can be technically very difficult. Fixation in this position gives poor stability. Forceful reduction is contraindicated, as this increases the risk of AVN. The options are either PIS (with a realignment procedure at a later date if remodelling is suboptimum) or primary corrective osteotomy. Avascular necrosis is uncommon in stable slips; this may explain why corrective osteotomy is not a popular choice in stable slips, even when they are severe. (*Primum non nocere!*)

Realignment procedures can be performed at one of three levels: subcapital, base of femoral neck and intertrochanteric (Figure 3.1.6). The ability to correct the deformity is greatest with a subcapital osteotomy, where the centre of rotation of angulation (CORA) is, least with a femoral neck osteotomy, and intermediate with an intertrochanteric osteotomy.

The risk of AVN is highest with subcapital and lowest with intertrochanteric osteotomy. The slip deformity correction involves flexion, valgus and internal rotation of the femur to

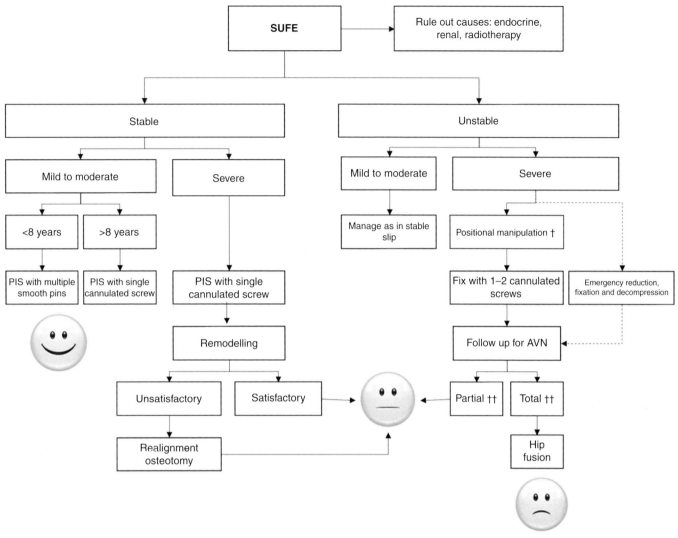

Figure 3.1.5 Flow chart of SUFE management. [†]There is some vagueness and controversy about the term 'positional manipulation'; some authors mean unintentional SUFE reduction during patient positioning, while others refer to gentle controlled reduction. [††]The choice between hip fusion and total hip replacement is controversial.

compensate for the SUFE deformity (extension, varus and external rotation).

Treatment of unstable SUFE

The treatment of an unstable slip is essentially the same as that of a stable slip but it is more controversial. There are three important issues to consider:

1. Being unstable, there is an opportunity for a spontaneous or unintentional reduction in the severity of the slip.
2. The high risk of AVN (47%). It is interesting how this high risk influences a surgeon's treatment decision. Some adopt a minimum intervention approach (such as PIS) to prevent the AVN risk from increasing. Others advocate an aggressive approach (open reduction of the slip) to reduce tension on the vessels in the posterior periosteum to lower the risk of AVN developing.

3. Aspiration of the hip joint has been recommended at the time of pinning to remove the haematoma and decompress the blood vessels.

The techniques for primary open reduction and fixation of the slip include the Fish osteotomy (1984) [7], Dunn's osteotomy (1978) [8] and Ganz surgical dislocation of the hip (2001) [9]. These techniques correct the slip at the subcapital level but they differ in their approach.

The Fish subcapital osteotomy involves an anterior approach to the hip and removal of an anterior-based wedge of bone from the metaphysis and physis. The epiphysis is then repositioned without tensioning or angulating the posterior retinacular vessels and is internally fixed with pins.

Dunn's osteotomy involves a trochanteric osteotomy through the growth plate with shortening of the neck to prevent the posterior retinacular vessels from stretching unacceptably at the time of reduction.

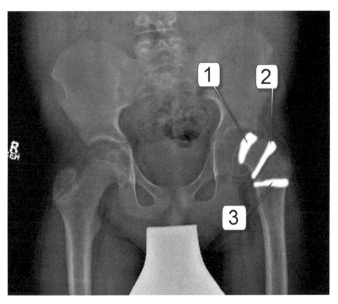

Figure 3.1.6 Sites of realignment procedures. 1: Subcapital osteotomy (Fish and Dunn). 2: Femoral neck (Kramer and Barmada). 3: Intertrochanteric (Southwick).

With the Ganz technique, the patient is positioned on one side, with the affected hip uppermost. A greater trochanter flip osteotomy is made and the greater trochanter retracted anteriorly along with the vastus lateralis and gluteus medius. The interval between the gluteus minimus and the piriformis is developed and the gluteus is retracted superiorly to expose the capsule.

The success of these approaches is closely related to protecting (or possibly restoring) the blood supply to the femoral head. The blood supply comes mainly from the posterior portion of the extracapsular anastomotic ring (Figure 3.1.7). This ring is formed by the medial and lateral femoral circumflex arteries from the profunda femoris artery. It gives rise to the ascending cervical branches, which are extracapsular, and these in turn give rise to the metaphyseal and epiphyseal branches.

The anterior portion of the extracapsular ring is formed primarily by the lateral femoral circumflex artery. The posterior, lateral and medial aspects of the ring are formed by the medial femoral circumflex artery. The greatest volume of blood flow to the femoral head comes through the lateral

Figure 3.1.7 Blood supply to the femoral head.

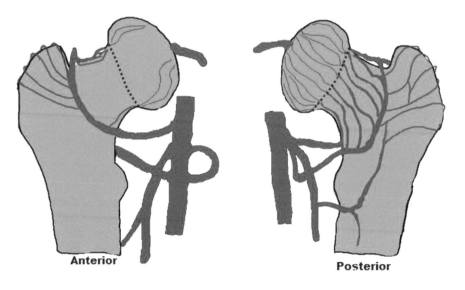

Anterior   Posterior

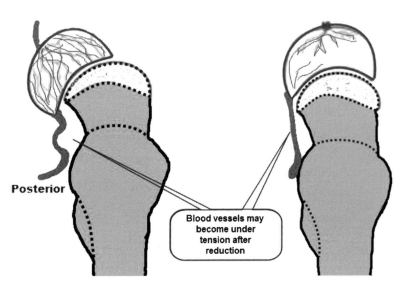

Posterior

Blood vessels may become under tension after reduction

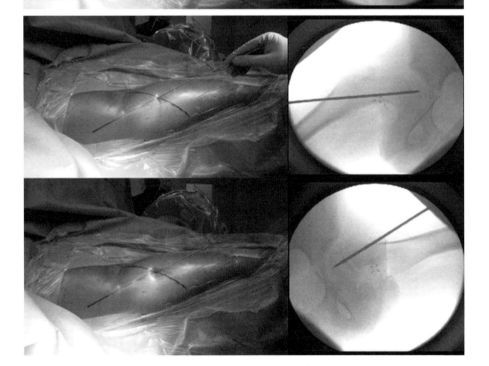

Figure 3.1.8 Main steps in pinning a SUFE.

ascending cervical vessel (the termination of the medial femoral circumflex artery), which crosses the capsule in the posterior trochanteric fossa, where it is vulnerable to injury by intramedullary nailing through the piriformis fossa or osteotomy of the greater trochanter (as in Dunn's osteotomy).

The Fish osteotomy does not violate the posterior capsule and blood vessels directly, but its visualization is suboptimal and may risk stretching these vessels.

The thickness (maximum 1.5 cm) and direction of the flip trochanteric osteotomy (in Ganz osteotomy) facilitates better visualization (and possibly protection) of these blood vessels.

How to undertake pinning *in situ*

This operation is performed under general anaesthetic. Intravenous antibiotics are given at induction. The patient is positioned supine on a fracture table with the patella facing anteriorly. No traction is applied to the affected leg. The other limb can be placed in traction and maximum abduction, or flexed and abducted on a stirrup to allow for imaging. Optimum visualization of the femoral head before the procedure is essential.

In bilateral stable slip, a radiolucent table is preferred over a fracture table because it reduces the chance of worsening the

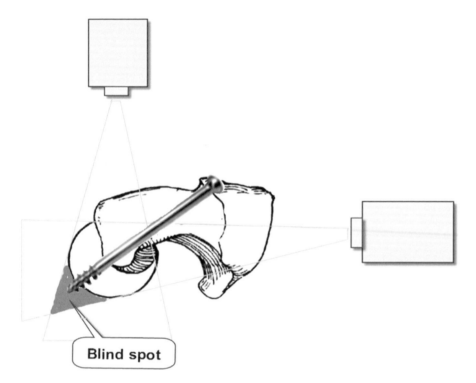

Figure 3.1.9 Main steps in pinning a SUFE (continued).

Blind spot

contralateral slip by overenthusiastic positioning and reduces the time needed for repositioning and re-draping the contralateral side.

The trajectory of the screw is identified and marked using a free guide wire placed on the skin overlying the proximal part of the femoral neck and head, crossing the physis in a perpendicular fashion in the AP and lateral views (Figure 3.1.8).

The guide pin is advanced freehand where the lines intersect through the soft tissues to engage the anterolateral femoral cortex. The position and angulations of the guide pin are adjusted under fluoroscopic guidance, to obtain the proper alignment before the guide pin is advanced into the bone. The entry point is usually quite anterior. It is essential to screen the hip to ensure that there is no protrusion of the guide pin in the joint; particularly in the blind spot (Figure 3.1.9). For unstable slips, one screw may not provide rigid fixation.

A second cannulated screw will give more rotational stability but will increase the risk of AVN and chondrolysis developing.

After the appropriate screw length has been determined, the femoral neck and epiphysis are drilled using the cannulated instruments while periodically checking the guide wire position to see that it is not advancing into the hip.

A 7.3 mm or 6.5 mm, fully threaded, reversed cutting cannulated screw is then inserted. The screw position should be carefully screened to ensure it does not violate the joint. It may be necessary to remove the foot from the stirrup to facilitate this. Alternatively an arthrogram may be obtained by injecting dye through the screw. For unstable slips, joint decompression can be done.

The patient is allowed partial weight-bearing with the use of crutches and gradually advances to full weight-bearing as tolerated. Follow-up is until physeal closure.

Timing of surgery

The timing of surgery is still controversial. Given the rarity of the condition (incidence, 2/100 000), most studies that have looked at the timing of surgery and outcome are suboptimal. Lowndes *et al.* [10] conducted a meta-analysis of five studies (130 unstable SUFEs; 56 treated within 24 hours and 74 treated after 24 hours of symptom onset). They found that the odds for developing AVN if treatment occurred within 24 hours might be halved, when compared with later treatment. Although the difference was large, it was not statistically significant ($P = 0.44$) and may have been a chance finding.

Peterson *et al.* [11] found that in 91 acute slips early stabilization within 24 hours was associated with less AVN (3/42 = 7%) in comparison with those slips stabilized after 24 hours (10/49 = 20%). Kalogrianitis *et al.* [12] reported that AVN developed in 50% (8/16) of unstable SUFE in their series. All patients but one were treated between 24 and 72 hours after symptom onset. Kalogrianitis *et al.* recommend immediate stabilization of unstable slips presenting within 24 hours. If this is not possible, they recommend delaying the operation until at least a week has elapsed. In contradiction, Loder *et al.* [4] noted that 87.5% (7/8) of patients treated within 48 hours of the onset of symptoms developed AVN but only 32% (7/22) did so if treated after 48 hours. However, Loder *et al.* have acknowledged that the true cause-and-effect relationship between the timing of intervention and the development of AVN cannot be determined.

Treatment of the contralateral non-slipped, asymptomatic side

This is controversial. The quoted risk of contralateral slip varies from 18 to 60%. Prophylactic PIS is not devoid of complications and benefits should be weighed against risks. Both proponents and opponents have some evidence to support their views [13].

Stasikelis *et al.* [14] performed a retrospective review of 50 children who presented with unilateral SUFE, to determine parameters that would predict the later development of a contralateral slip. They found that the modified Oxford bone age (a measure of physiological maturity) strongly correlated with the risk of development of a contralateral slip. A contralateral slip developed in 85% of patients with a score of 16, in 11% of patients with a score of 21, and in no patient with a score of 22 or more. The modified Oxford bone age is based on appearance and fusion of the iliac apophysis, femoral capital physis and greater and lesser trochanters.

Phillips *et al.* [15] examined the posterior slip angle (PSA) (Figure 3.1.10) in 132 patients as a predictor for developing a contralateral slip. The mean was $17.2° ± 5.6°$ in 42 patients who had subsequently developed a contralateral slip, which was significantly higher ($P = 0.001$) than that of $10.8° ± 4.2°$ for the 90 patients who had had a unilateral slip. If a posterior sloping angle of 14° had been used as an indication for prophylactic

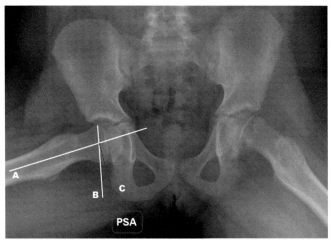

Figure 3.1.10 Posterior slip angle (PSA). A line (A) is drawn from the centre of the femoral shaft through the centre of the metaphysis. A second line (B) is drawn from one edge of the physis to the other, which represents the angle of the physis. Where lines A and B intersect, a line (C) is drawn perpendicular to line A. The PSA is the angle formed by lines B and C posteriorly, as illustrated.

fixation, 35 slips (of 42 = 83.3%) would have been prevented, and 19 (of 90 = 21.1%) would have been pinned unnecessarily.

The authors recommend adopting a pragmatic approach for contralateral pinning where the following factors play a role in decision making:

1. Age of the child (<10 years is associated with a higher risk of bilaterality).
2. The aetiology of the slip. Renal osteodystrophy and endocrine disorders have a high incidence of bilaterality.
3. Poor compliance of the child and family.
4. The nature of the current slip. A very severe slip occurring over a very short period of time may justify pinning the other side.

Hip spica and bone graft

In the past, a hip spica cast was used as the definitive management of SUFE. Advantages included avoiding complications associated with surgery and treatment of the contralateral hip. Difficulties include a high chondrolysis rate (53%), slip progression after removal of the spica (18%), pressure sores (12%) and casting difficulty in obese children. This method of treatment is outdated and rarely used today although there may be a role for hip spica as an adjunct to PIS, particularly if the bone quality is poor or the fixation suboptimal.

Bone graft (peg) epiphysiodesis avoids the complications associated with internal fixation, including unrecognized pin penetration and damage to the lateral epiphyseal vessels. Slippage is not prevented until the physis closes, so a spica cast is required.

However, PIS is a simpler procedure, with a smaller scar, decreased blood loss, shorter operative time, fewer postoperative complications and comparable clinical results. Bone graft epiphysiodesis may be used to support fixation when there is excessive osteolysis and the fixation is at risk of failure [16].

Potential complications

1. Avascular necrosis (AVN).
2. Chondrolysis: this is the rapid and progressive loss of articular cartilage, and is seen in some SUFEs. The cause is unknown; theories have postulated an autoimmune phenomenon or some interference with cartilage nutrition. Risk factors include immobilization in a cast, unrecognized pin penetration, severe SUFE, and rapid and progressive loss of articular cartilage after PIS. This may be due to pin penetration or a protruded screw, but it has also been reported in other situations. Clinically, the patient develops increasing pain and stiffness and radiographs demonstrate a decrease in the apparent joint space of >2 mm compared with the contralateral hip.
3. Residual deformity and femoro-acetabular impingement.
4. Osteoarthritis (OA).
5. Leg length discrepancy (LLD).

References

1. Kelsey JL, Keggi KJ and Southwick WO (1970) The incidence and distribution of slipped capital femoral epiphysis in Connecticut and Southwestern United States. *J Bone Joint Surg Am* **52**(6):1203–16.

2. Loder RT (1996) The demographics of slipped capital femoral epiphysis. An international multicenter study. *Clin Orthop Relat Res* **322**:8–27.

3. Loder RT and Greenfield ML (2001) Clinical characteristics of children with atypical and idiopathic slipped capital femoral epiphysis: description of the age-weight test and implications for further diagnostic investigation. *J Pediatr Orthop* **21**(4):481–7.

4. Loder RT, Richards BS, Shapiro PS, Reznick LR and Aronson DD (1993) Acute slipped capital femoral epiphysis: the importance of physeal stability. *J Bone Joint Surg Am* **75**(8):1134–40.

5. Southwick WO (1984) Slipped capital femoral epiphysis. *J Bone Joint Surg Am* **66**(8):1151–2.

6. Montgomery R (2009) (iv) Slipped upper femoral epiphysis. *Orthop Trauma* **23**(3):169–83.

7. Fish JB (1994) Cuneiform osteotomy of the femoral neck in the treatment of slipped capital femoral epiphysis. A follow-up note. *J Bone Joint Surg Am* **76**(1):46–59.

8. Dunn DM and Angel JC (1978) Replacement of the femoral head by open operation in severe adolescent slipping of the upper femoral epiphysis. *J Bone Joint Surg Br* **60-B**(3):394–403.

9. Ganz R, Gill TJ, Gautier E, Ganz K, Krügel N and Berlemann U (2001) Surgical dislocation of the adult hip a technique with full access to the femoral head and acetabulum without the risk of avascular necrosis. *J Bone Joint Surg Br* **83**(8):1119–24.

10. Lowndes S, Khanna A, Emery D, Sim J and Maffulli N (2009) Management of unstable slipped upper femoral epiphysis: a meta-analysis. *Br Med Bull* **90**:133–46.

11. Peterson MD, Weiner DS, Green NE and Terry CL (1997) Acute slipped capital femoral epiphysis: the value and safety of urgent manipulative reduction. *J Pediatr Orthop* **17**(5):648–54.

12. Kalogrianitis S, Tan CK, Kemp GJ, Bass A and Bruce C (2007) Does unstable slipped capital femoral epiphysis require urgent stabilization? *J Pediatr Orthop B* **16**(1):6–9.

13. Jerre R, Billing L, Hansson G and Wallin J (1994) The contralateral hip in patients primarily treated for unilateral slipped upper femoral epiphysis. Long-term follow-up of 61 hips. *J Bone Joint Surg Br* **76**(4):563–7.

14. Stasikelis PJ, Sullivan CM, Phillips WA and Polard JA (1996) Slipped capital femoral epiphysis. Prediction of contralateral involvement. *J Bone Joint Surg Am* **78**(8):1149–55.

15. Phillips PM, Phadnis J, Willoughby R and Hunt L (1996) Posterior sloping angle as a predictor of contralateral slip in slipped capital femoral epiphysis. *J Bone Joint Surg Am* **95**(2):146–50.

16. Herring JA (2008) *Tachdjian's Pediatric Orthopaedics*, 4th edition, volume 1. Philadelphia: Saunders Elsevier.

17. Beaule PE, Matta JM and Mast JW (2002) Hip arthrodesis: current indications and techniques. *J Am Acad Orthop Surg* **10**(4):249–58.

3.2 Perthes disease

Introduction

Perthes disease is an avascular necrosis of the femoral head in a growing child caused by interruption of its blood supply. The condition was first described by Waldenstorm, who attributed it to tuberculosis. It was then described more accurately, almost at the same time, by Arthur Legg, Jacques Calvé and George Perthes; hence the name Legg–Calvé–Perthes disease (LCPD).

It has an incidence of 1/10 000 and commonly affects children between 4 and 9 years old, who are often small with a delayed bone age. It is bilateral in 15% of cases but involvement is usually asymmetrical and, in contrast with multiple epiphyseal dysplasias, is never simultaneous.

Aetiology

The aetiology is unknown; however, several theories have been put forward:

The anatomical theory

The blood supply to the femoral head changes as a child grows (Table 3.2.1). At birth, it is supplied by the medial and lateral circumflex arteries, as well as the artery of the ligamentum teres. As the child grows, the contribution from the lateral circumflex artery diminishes, while that from the medial circumflex artery increases. This changeover to the adult pattern is thought to predispose ischaemic necrosis.

Hydrostatic pressure theory

This theory attributes the reduction in blood supply to the femoral head to an increase in intra-osseous venous pressure. Heikkinen et al. [1] studied the venous drainage of the femoral neck in 73 children with LCPD using intra-osseous venography films, using 55 contralateral symptomless hips as controls. They noted that the venous drainage was abnormal in 46/55 (82%) hips in the fragmentation phase and 7/18 (39%) hips in the re-ossification stage and normal in the healed stage. Two of the 55 symptomless hips showed pathological venous drainage. Heikkinen et al. found that the disturbances in the venous drainage of the femoral neck seemed to correlate with the stage of LCPD.

Thrombophilic theory

It is well known that children with hemoglobinopathies, such as sickle cell disease and thalassaemia, commonly have AVN of the femoral head. There is also some evidence of the association of LCPD with various forms of thrombophilia. In a study

by Balasa et al. [2], 72 patients with LCPD were compared with 197 matched healthy control subjects. The factor-V Leiden mutation was more common in the LCPD group (8/72) than in the control group (7/197) ($P = 0.017$). A high level of anticardiolipin antibodies was found in 19 of the 72 LCPD subjects compared with 22 of the 197 controls ($P = 0.002$). Some studies have shown an association of LCPD with protein S and C abnormalities [3, 4]. On the contrary, other studies [5, 6] have not shown such associations, and the role of coagulation abnormalities in the aetiology of LCPD is yet to be confirmed.

Other factors

There are other aetiological and associated factors but their exact roles remain unclear:

1. Trauma, hyperactivity and attention deficit disorder,
2. Susceptibility (abnormal growth and development):
   a. Low birth weight,
   b. Low socio-economic class,
   c. Bone maturation delays,
   d. Boys > girls (4/1),
3. Hereditary and familial factors,
4. Passive smoking,
5. Transient synovitis.

Presentation

Patients commonly present with an insidious onset of a limp and anterior thigh or knee pain. Usually, they have activity-related pain, which is relieved by rest. Some children may present with more acute onset of symptoms. There may be a history of minor trauma.

Examination usually reveals limited hip motion, particularly abduction and internal rotation. Gait is often antalgic and the Trendelenburg test is usually positive. There may be muscle spasm with evidence of thigh, calf and buttock atrophy from disuse. Leg length discrepancy indicates significant femoral head collapse. Evaluation of the patient's overall height, weight and bone age may be helpful, to exclude skeletal dysplasias or growth disorders.

Blood tests are helpful in ruling out other conditions (see differential diagnosis). In the majority of cases, plain radiographs (AP and frog-leg lateral) will confirm the diagnosis. However, in some early cases, radiographs may be normal and MRI or a bone scan is required. Radiological findings include widening of the joint space, a smaller capital femoral epiphysis, the crescent sign (denotes subchondral fracture) and flattening of the epiphysis.

A bone scan may be helpful in the early stages of the disease, when the diagnosis is in question, particularly if the differential diagnosis is between transient synovitis and LCPD.

The most accurate imaging modality for diagnosing early disease is MRI. Theissen et al. [7] reported a diagnostic

Table 3.2.1 Blood supply of the femoral head

Age	Birth to 4 years	4 years to adult	Adult
Source	Medial and lateral circumflex arteries (profunda femoris artery) Artery of ligamentum teres (posterior division of obturator artery)	Posterosuperior and posteroinferior retinacular from medial femoral circumflex artery Negligible lateral circumflex artery Minimum ligamentum teres	Medial femoral circumflex, which is the most important contributor to the lateral epiphyseal artery

accuracy of 97–99% for MRI, compared with 88–93% for plain X-rays and 88–91% for bone scans.

Differential diagnosis

Unilateral LCPD

1. Septic arthritis (usually the child is unwell, with a fever and elevated inflammatory markers),
2. Sickle cell disease (history, sickling test, Hb electrophoresis),
3. Eosinophilic granuloma (other lesions in the skull, radiological features, biopsy),
4. Transient synovitis (lack of characteristic radiographic changes).

Bilateral LCPD

This is not common and requires a skeletal survey and blood tests to exclude:

1. Hypothyroidism (thyroid function test).
2. Multiple epiphyseal dysplasia (usually bilateral simultaneously, with involvement from other joints epiphyses).
3. Spondyloepiphyseal dysplasia (involvement of the spine).
4. Meyer's dysplasia: delayed, irregular ossification of the femoral epiphyseal nucleus. This is more common in boys, usually occurs in the second year of life, is mostly bilateral and usually disappears by the end of the sixth year. Bone scans are normal.
5. Sickle cell disease.
6. Mucopolysaccharidoses.

Radiographic stages

The pathology is consistent with repeated infarction followed by pathological fractures. Waldenström classified the evolution of LCPD into four stages based on radiographic changes (Figure 3.2.1).

I. Initial (sclerotic or necrotic) stage

Ischaemia leads to subchondral bone necrosis (dead bone looks dense on a radiograph). There is joint space widening due to continuous cartilage growth (nutrients from synovial fluid) and hypertrophy of the synovium and ligamentum teres. This stage can be subdivided into 'early', if there is no loss in epiphysis height, and 'late', where there is some loss of epiphyseal height but the epiphysis is still in one piece. This stage usually lasts from 6 to 12 months.

II. Fragmentation (resorption) stage

In this stage, revascularization has started. Osteoclasts remove dead and necrotic bone causing radiolucent fissures among dead fragments. This stage usually lasts from 12 to 24 months and can be divided into 'early' (only one or two fissures) and 'late' (when the head is in several fragments). Most deformity occurs in this stage.

III. Re-ossification (healing) stage

Vascular regeneration by the process of creeping substitution leads to re-ossification of the femoral head. It starts peripherally and progresses centrally. This usually appears as a small and expanding fragment at the lateral part of the epiphysis marking. This stage usually lasts from 6 to 24 months.

IV. Remodelling (residual) stage

The head is considered to have healed when there is no avascular bone visible on radiographs (no changes in the density of the femoral head); however, the head continues to remodel until skeletal maturity. The head becomes large (coxa magna) and the neck wide. The acetabulum remodels, to match the femoral head deformity. The older the child, the less remodelling, and the poorer the outcome.

Radiographic classification

Various classifications have been described to assess the extent of involvement.

Catterall, 1971 [8]

Catterall proposed four groups based on the extent of head involvement at the fragmentation phase (Table 3.2.2).

Salter and Thompson, 1984 [9]

Salter and Thompson recognized that Catterall's first two groups and second two groups were distinct and therefore proposed a two-part classification:

Group A: Less than 50% head involved.

Group B: More than 50% head involved.

As in Catterall classification, the main difference between these two groups is the integrity of the lateral pillar.

Lateral pillar (Herring *et al.*), 1992 [10]

This is based on the integrity of the lateral pillar on the AP radiograph only, at the beginning of the fragmentation phase (Table 3.2.3 and Figure 3.2.2).

Classification addressing outcome

Mose classification

This system uses a concentric circle technique to compare and classify the final outcome in LCPD at the end of growth. The final shape of the head is compared with a perfect circle using a Mose template on both AP and lateral images (Figure 3.2.3 and Table 3.2.4).

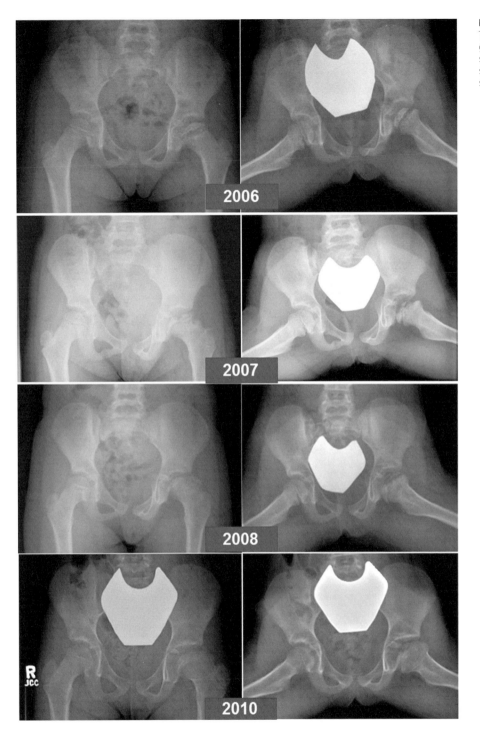

Figure 3.2.1 Waldenström radiographic stages. These pelvic X-radiographs (AP and lateral) are of a girl who presented with LCPD at 5 years old and show the four stages of the disease. 2006: Sclerotic stage. 2007: Fragmentation phase. 2008: Healing stage. 2010: Remodelling stage.

Given that a congruous but aspherical head can perform well, this suggests that Mose's criteria are too strict and also impractical to use.

Stulberg classification

Stulberg et al. [11] have demonstrated that a lack of sphericity and congruency are both predictors for poor outcome (symptomatic OA) (Table 3.2.5).

A modified version of Stulberg classification is becoming more popular and has a superior inter-observer agreement [12]. It consists of three groups: group A hips (Stulberg I and II) have a spherical femoral head, group B hips (Stulberg III) have an ovoid femoral head, and group C hips (Stulberg IV and V) have a flat femoral head.

Table 3.2.6 shows recognized clinical and radiological prognostic signs.

Table 3.2.2 Catterall classification of LCPD

Grade	Description	Diagram
Catterall I	0–25% head involvement Only anterior epiphysis (therefore seen only on frog lateral radiograph)	
Catterall II	25–50% head involvement Anterior and central segment: fragmentation (sequestrum) Lateral part, rim: intact (protects central involved area) Junction: clear Metaphyseal reaction present: anterior Subchondral fracture: anterior	
Catterall III	50–75% head involvement Anterior segment: involved Lateral head: also fragmented Only the medial portion is spared Loss of lateral part, support worsens the prognosis Junction: sclerotic Metaphyseal reaction present: anterior and lateral	
Catterall IV	>75% head involvement	

Table 3.2.3 Lateral pillar of LCPD (Herring *et al.*)

Group	Description
Group A	Normal height of the lateral 1/3 of the head is maintained
Group B	More than 50% of the original lateral pillar height is maintained There may be some lateral extrusion of the head
Group C	Less than 50% of the original lateral pillar height is maintained
Group B/C	Less than 50% of the original lateral pillar height is maintained The lateral pillar is higher than the central segment

Management

The management of LCPD is one of the most controversial topics in paediatric orthopaedics. The aims of treatment are to preserve range of movement and to maintain containment and coverage of the hip joint.

Various treatment modalities are used, including:

- Protected weight-bearing with crutches and physiotherapy,
- The use of abduction braces and orthosis,

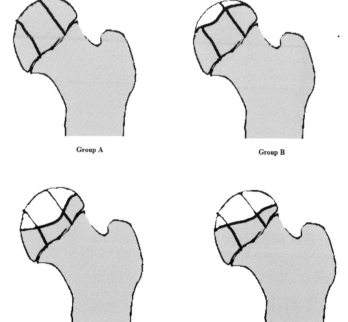

Figure 3.2.2 Herring classification.

Table 3.2.4 Mose grading of LCPD

Outcome	Description
Good outcome	Aspherical head contour is within 1 mm of a given circle on both views
Fair outcome	Aspherical head contour is 1–2 mm
Poor outcome	Aspherical head contour is >2 mm

Table 3.2.6 LCPD poor prognostic signs

Poor clinical prognostic signs (FOOBS)	Poor radiological prognostic signs
Female	Gage's sign (V shape lucency at lateral epiphysis (Figure 3.2.5)
Older age	Horizontal growth plate – implies a growth arrest phenomenon and deformity
Obesity	Lateral calcification (lateral to the epiphysis – implies loss of lateral support and head extrusion)
Bilateral	Lateral subluxation – implies loss of lateral support Uncovering of the femoral head >3 mm in excess of opposite side (measured as the horizontal distance between a vertical line through the outer lip of acetabulum and lateral edge of femoral head physis) or >20% of extrusion
Stiffness	Metaphyseal rarefaction or cyst

- Traction,
- Arthrodiastasis,
- Femoral or acetabular osteotomies,
- Acetabular shelf procedure.

Symptomatic management

This includes rest, analgesia, anti-inflammatory drugs, temporary non-weight-bearing with crutches and short periods of gentle traction. Physiotherapy plays an important role in improving range of motion. There is little evidence to suggest that prolonged non-weight-bearing is effective in preventing femoral head deformity.

Table 3.2.5 Stulberg grading of LCPD (see also Figure 3.2.4)

Head	Class	Description	Risk of future OA
Spherical and congruent	I	Normal spherical head	No increased risk of arthritis
	II	Spherical head, coxa magna/breva, steep acetabulum	
Aspherical but congruent	III	Ovoid or mushroom-shaped head	Mild to moderate arthritis develops in late adulthood
	IV	Flat head on flat acetabulum (may hinge on abduction)	
Aspherical and incongruent	V	Flat head but normal acetabulum	Severe arthritis before 50

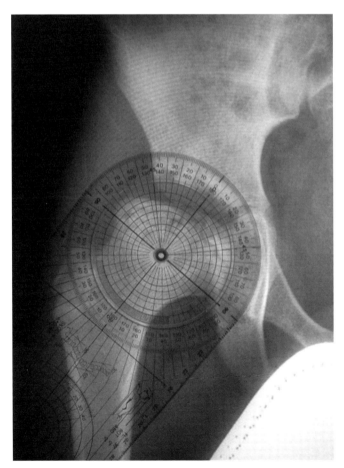

Figure 3.2.3 Mose grading of LCPD.

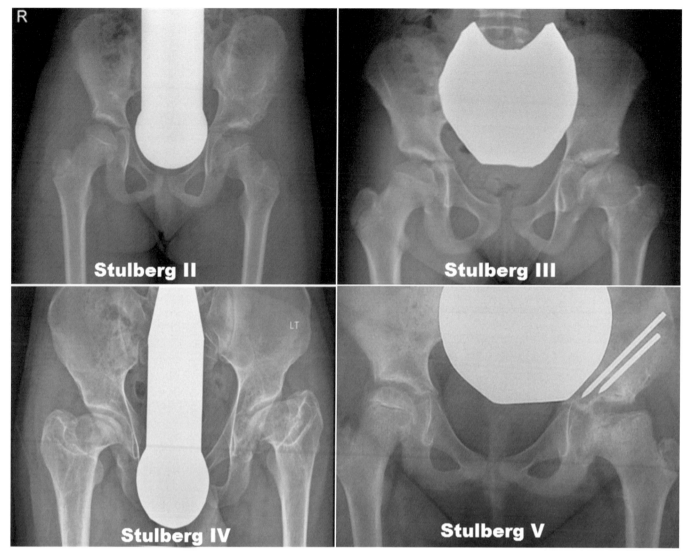

Figure 3.2.4 LCPD: Stulberg grading.

Casting and bracing

Several types of cast (Petri, broomstick) and brace (Scottish Rite, Birmingham, SWASH (standing, walking and sitting hip orthosis)) have been advocated to contain the femoral head within the acetabulum. They work by abducting and flexing (or internally rotating) the hip to reposition the femoral head deep in the acetabulum and protect it from collapse until re-ossification. This may take 2 years or more, which makes compliance a real issue in this age group. When there is a severe adduction deformity, a period of traction or an adductor tenotomy may be necessary before applying these casts or braces. Prolonged bracing is now less popular, as it appears to offer uncertain benefit over the long term.

Surgical management

Surgical containment

An arthrogram is advisable before undertaking bone surgery. This provides valuable information to guide the surgeon's decision making regarding surgery.

Containment can be achieved by undertaking a femoral varus osteotomy, which positions the hip into abduction and internal rotation. Epiphysiodesis of the greater trochanter may be required in the 7 to 12 year old, to prevent trochanteric overgrowth. In the presence of trochanteric overgrowth with an abductor lurch, a trochanteric advancement may help restore the abductor mechanism.

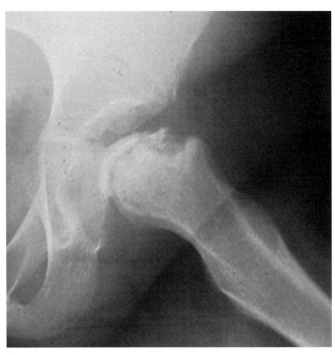

Figure 3.2.5 LCPD: Gage's sign.

Containment can also be achieved by pelvic surgery, i.e. a Salter's osteotomy, which redirects the acetabulum to provide more cover anteriorly and laterally.

Proximal femoral valgus osteotomy is beneficial in the presence of hinged abduction [13].

Several small studies have shown the benefit of acetabular shelf augmentation in cases with severe head involvement and lateral uncovering of the femoral head [14, 15].

Arthrodiastasis or hinged hip distraction is an alternative treatment for the older child in the Herring C group [16].

In a multicentre prospective study, Herring *et al.* [17] compared the success rate of achieving a spherical femoral head (Stulberg class I or II hips) after one of five treatments (no treatment, physiotherapy, Scottish Rite orthosis, femoral osteotomy or Salter's innominate osteotomy). They found that age, lateral pillar grading and treatment method were significantly related to outcome.

In patients with a lateral pillar classification of B or B/C who were older than 8 at the time of onset of LCPD, it was found that 73% of operated hips had a Stulberg I or II result compared with 44% of non-operated hips ($P = 0.02$). In group B hips with onset at 8 years or younger, no advantage was demonstrated for the surgical group. The group C hips were not shown to benefit from surgical or non-surgical treatment.

In a nationwide prospective study, Wiig [18] reported on the success rate of achieving a spherical femoral head after one of three treatment options (physiotherapy, Scottish Rite orthosis or femoral varus osteotomy). The success rate ranged from 46% to 53% in 168 patients with the onset of disease before the age of 6 years and from 20% to 43% in 146 patients with the onset of disease after the age of 6 years.

The study showed that the strongest predictor of poor outcome was femoral head involvement greater than 50% (modified Catterall classification) followed by age at diagnosis and lateral pillar grades. In children over 6 years at diagnosis with greater than 50% femoral head necrosis, proximal femoral varus osteotomy gave a significantly better outcome than orthoses or physiotherapy. There was no difference in outcome after any of the treatments in children under 6 years.

These two studies raise a question regarding why a femoral or Salter's innominate osteotomy produces good results in some patients but not in others. One theory is that while these osteotomies do provide some load-relieving effects on the necrotic femoral head, they do not specifically address the pathobiology of the disease and the impaired healing observed in the older children with LCPD [19].

In summary, patients older than 8 years at onset with lateral pillar B and B/C border involvement are likely to benefit from surgery. For the best result, surgery should be performed early in the course of the disease, perhaps even before it is possible to classify its severity. Probably, containment surgery is too late in the re-ossification (healing) stage (Stage III). On this basis, all children older than 8 with Perthes disease could be considered for early surgical treatment. Although group A and C hips are unlikely to benefit, these groups combined are represented in only 13% of children presenting at age older than 8 and therefore this non-selective approach may be justified [20].

Medical treatment

Medical treatment using bisphosphonate and bone morphogenic protein (BMP) may have a potential role in preventing or reducing head deformity in LCPD [21].

References

1. Heikkinen E, Koivisto E, Lanning P, Puranen J and Suramo I (1979) Venous drainage of the femoral neck in various stages of activity in Perthes' disease. *Röntgen-blätter* **32**(1):46–9.

2. Balasa VV, Gruppo RA, Glueck CJ et al. (2004) Legg–Calvé–Perthes disease and thrombophilia. *J Bone Joint Surg Am* **86-A**(12):2642–7.

3. Thomas DP, Morgan G and Tayton K (1999) Perthes' disease and the relevance of thrombophilia. *J Bone Joint Surg Br* **81**(4):691–5.

4. Hayek S, Kenet G, Lubetsky A, Rosenberg N, Gitel S and Wientroub S (1999) Does thrombophilia play an aetiological role in Legg–Calvé–Perthes disease? *J Bone Joint Surg Br* **81**(4): 686–90.

5. Hresko MT, McDougall PA, Gorlin JB, Vamvakas EC, Kasser JR and Neufeld EJ (2002) Prospective reevaluation of the association between thrombotic diathesis and Legg–Perthes disease. *J Bone Joint Surg Am* **84-A**(9):1613–18.

6. Gallistl S, Reitinger T, Linhart W and Muntean W (1999) The role of inherited thrombotic disorders in the etiology of Legg-Calvé-Perthes disease. *J Pediatr Orthop* **19**(1):82–3.

7. Theissen P, Rütt J, Linden A, Smolarz K, Voth E and Schicha H (1991) The early diagnosis of Perthes disease: the value of bone scintigraphy and magnetic resonance imaging in comparison with X-ray findings. *Nuklearmedizin* **30**(6):265–71.

8. Catterall A (1971) The natural history of Perthes' disease. *J Bone Joint Surg Br* **53**(1):37–53.

9. Salter RB and Thompson GH (1984) Legg-Calvé-Perthes disease. The prognostic significance of the subchondral fracture and a two-group classification of the femoral head involvement. *J Bone Joint Surg Am* **66**(4):479–89.

10. Herring JA, Neustadt JB, Williams JJ, Early JS and Browne RH (1992) The lateral pillar classification of Legg-Calvé-Perthes disease. *J Pediatr Orthop* **12**(2):143–50.

11. Stulberg SD, Cooperman DR and Wallensten R (1981) The natural history of Legg-Calvé-Perthes disease. *J Bone Joint Surg Am* **63**(7):1095–108.

12. Wiig O, Terjesen T and Svenningsen S (2007) Inter-observer reliability of the Stulberg classification in the assessment of Perthes disease. *J Child Orthop* **1**(2):101–5.

13. Bankes MJ, Catterall A and Hashemi-Nejad A (2000) Valgus extension osteotomy for 'hinge abduction' in Perthes' disease. Results at maturity and factors influencing the radiological outcome. *J Bone Joint Surg Br* **82**(4):548–54.

14. Daly K, Bruce C and Catterall A (1999) Lateral shelf acetabuloplasty in Perthes' disease. A review of the end of growth. *J Bone Joint Surg Br* **81**(3):380–4.

15. Domzalski ME, Glutting J, Bowen JR and Littleton AG (2006) Lateral acetabular growth stimulation following a labral support procedure in Legg-Calve-Perthes disease. *J Bone Joint Surg Am* **88**(7):1458–66.

16. Maxwell SL, Lappin KJ, Kealey WD, McDowell BC and Cosgrove AP (2004) Arthrodiastasis in Perthes' disease. Preliminary results. *J Bone Joint Surg Br* **86**(2):244–50.

17. Herring JA, Kim HT and Browne R (2004) Legg-Calvé-Perthes disease. Part II: prospective multicenter study of the effect of treatment on outcome. *J Bone Joint Surg Am* **86**-A(10):2121–34.

18. Wiig O, Terjesen T and Svenningsen S (2008) Prognostic factors and outcome of treatment in Perthes' disease: a prospective study of 368 patients with five-year follow-up. *J Bone Joint Surg Br* **90**(10):1364–71.

19. Kim HKW (2012) Pathophysiology and new strategies for the treatment of Legg-Calvé-Perthes disease. *J Bone Joint Surg Am* **94**(7):659–69.

20. Wright JG (2009) *Evidence-Based Orthopaedics. The Best Answers to Clinical Questions.* Philadelphia: Saunders.

21. Young ML, Little DG and Kim HK (2012) Evidence for using bisphosphonate to treat Legg-Calvé-Perthes disease. *Clin Orthop Relat Res* **470**(9):2462–75.

3.3 Developmental dysplasia of the hip

Background

Developmental dysplasia of the hip (DDH) is a spectrum of disorders of hip development that presents in different forms at different ages. This may range from:

1. Hip radiographic abnormalities, i.e. dysplasia found on ultrasound and radiographs with no clinical abnormalities. If untreated, these may present later as hip dysplasia or even frank dislocation.
2. Hip instability, such that the femoral head can be displaced partially (subluxated) or fully (dislocated) from the acetabulum by an examiner but relocated spontaneously (positive Barlow test).
3. A dislocated hip that is easily reducible on examination (positive Ortolani test).
4. Frank dislocation that cannot be reduced.

Teratologic dislocation of the hip is a distinct form of hip dislocation that is usually associated with disorders, such as arthrogryposis, myelodysplasia and neuromuscular diseases. These hips are dislocated before birth, have a limited range of motion and are not reducible on examination.

Klisic, in 1989, recommended the term 'developmental dysplasia of the hip' (DDH) instead of 'congenital dislocation of the hip' to indicate two facts:

1. The hip may be normal (or not dislocated) at birth.
2. The dynamic nature of the disorder: the hip may get better or worse as the child develops.

The incidence of DDH is difficult to determine because it is influenced by a number of factors, which include sex, race, age, type of examination and definition of the condition. The following are generally accepted:

- Ultrasound abnormality (8/100 births),
- Abnormal clinical finding (2.3/100 births),
- Dislocation (1.4/1000 births).

Aetiology

The cause of DDH is multifactorial, involving genetic, intra-uterine and environmental factors. The following are recognized risk factors (seven Fs):

1. **First baby** (the uterus is tighter and less elastic),
2. **Female** (lax ligament, by maternal hormones),

3. Family history (there may be a genetic predisposition),
4. Fetal malposition (extended knee, breech presentation),
5. Fetal packaging disorders (oligohydramnios, twins, feet metatarsus adductus and neck torticollis),
6. Left side (60% left hip, 20% right and 20% both; this may be related to the fetal position),
7. Other factors:
   a. Geographical and racial factors (more common in Europeans than Asians or Africans),
   b. Increased incidence in Native American and Lapp populations that use swaddling cloths and cradle boards. This limits hip mobility and positions the hip in adduction and extension.

Pathoanatomy

It is essential to understand normal growth and development of the hip joint, the pathoanatomy of DDH and its natural history.

The hip joint develops as a cleft in the primitive limb bud at about 7 weeks of gestation. The concave shape of the acetabulum is determined by the spherical femoral head within the acetabulum. The two bony ends are covered by fully formed cartilage by the 11th week of gestation. A failure in this stage of development leads to proximal femoral focal deficiency.

The entire upper femur (femoral head, neck, greater and lesser trochanters) is a cartilaginous structure. Its development occurs through a combination of appositional growth on the surfaces and physeal growth at the junction of the cartilaginous proximal femur and the femoral shaft.

The proximal femur has three ossification centres. An ossification centre appears in the centre of the femoral head between the 4th and 7th months of life. This centre grows until physeal closure between the ages of 14 and 17. The greater trochanter begins to ossify during the 4th year. It joins the shaft approximately 1 year after puberty. The lesser trochanter is the final centre to ossify and fuse; it does so at the onset of puberty (Figure 3.3.1).

At birth, the acetabulum is composed of hyaline cartilage, whose periphery is attached to the fibrocartilagenous labrum. The hyaline cartilage of the acetabulum is continuous with the triradiate cartilages, which interconnect the three bones of the pelvis (the ilium, ischium and pubis). Most acetabular development occurs by approximately 8 years of age (Figure 3.3.2) [1].

The final contour of the hip socket is further achieved by three acetabular epiphyseal centres, which appear around the age of 8 and fuse about the age of 18 [2]:

1. The anterior epiphyseal centre (os acetabulum) forms the anterior rim as part of the pubis.
2. The superior epiphyseal centre (acetabular epiphysis) forms along the superior edge of the acetabulum and the anterior inferior iliac spine (AIIS) as part of the ilium.
3. The posterior epiphyseal centre (os marginalis) forms the posterior rim.

In DDH, there are distinct pathological changes, which are initially reversible (Figure 3.3.3). At, or shortly after, birth, the affected hip spontaneously slides into and out of the acetabulum, leading to a flattening of the posterosuperior rim of the acetabulum. At this stage, the rim is made of hyaline cartilage and the attached fibrocartilagenous labrum. This rim usually becomes deformed and either everts or inverts, depending on the direction of the deforming forces (Ortolani called this deformed rim the neolimbus). Some hips spontaneously reduce and become normal, with complete resolution of the pathological changes. Other hips remain dislocated, leading to secondary pathological changes.

A fibrofatty tissue (known as the pulvinar) fills the shallow acetabulum and may impede reduction (this point is controversial). The ligamentum teres becomes hypertrophied and presses on the acetabular rim and the lower part of the femoral head. The transverse acetabular ligament is hypertrophic and tight, giving the socket a horseshoe shape. The growth of the acetabulum and the dislocated head causes the joint capsule to assume an hourglass shape with an isthmus that is narrower in diameter than the femoral head. The iliopsoas, which is pulled tight across this isthmus, contributes to this narrowing. The capsule also narrows through a 'Chinese finger-trap' mechanism. There is an associated increase in femoral anteversion and some flattening of the femoral head as it lies against the ilium or abductor muscles.

Clinical presentations

The clinical findings vary depending on age.

Neonates and infants

Most cases are asymptomatic with no discomfort or pain. There may be subtle clinical signs, such as asymmetrical skin folds (this is not very specific) or leg asymmetry (the Galezzi sign).

The Ortolani and Barlow tests are very important in the early weeks of life but their value is reduced as the child grows older. The **O**rtolani test identifies a dislocated hip (**O**ut) that can be reduced. After flexing the infant's hip and knee to 90°, the thigh is gently abducted with the middle finger over the greater trochanter to feel for the reduction of the dislocated head, as it comes from the dislocated position into the socket. With time, it becomes more difficult to reduce the femoral head into the acetabulum, and the Ortolani test becomes negative. The Barlow test is performed by attempting to subluxate or dislocate the femoral head from within the acetabulum. The hip is adducted and a gentle push is applied to slide the hip posteriorly. The Barlow test is rarely positive after 10 weeks.

Asymmetry may be identified as a leg length discrepancy (the Galeazzi test) and an external rotation deformity. Asymmetrical thigh creases have low specificity and many children with normal hips demonstrate this feature. Unilateral limited abduction in flexion has 70% sensitivity and 90% specificity for DDH in infants older than 3 months [3]. The Ortolani and Barlow tests have a 60% sensitivity and 100% specificity in

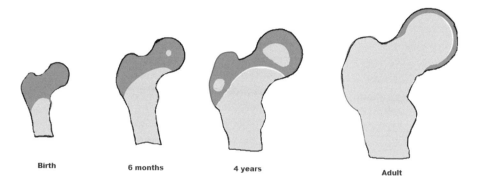

Figure 3.3.1 Proximal femur development.

Birth

6 months

4 years

Adult

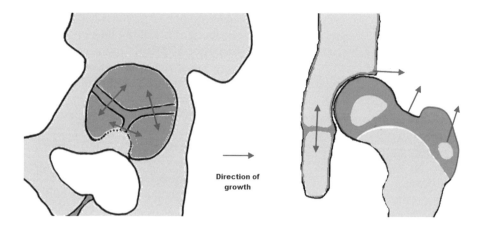

Figure 3.3.2 Acetabular development.

Direction of
growth

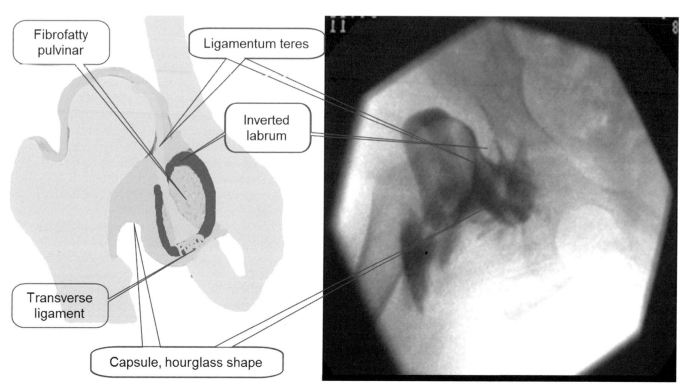

Fibrofatty
pulvinar

Ligamentum teres

Inverted
labrum

Transverse
ligament

Capsule, hourglass shape

Figure 3.3.3 Pathoanatomical changes in hip dislocation.

expert hands in comparison with ultrasound, which has 90% sensitivity and specificity [4].

The Klisic test can be used to detect dislocation, especially after 3 months. Place the index finger on the anterior superior iliac spine (ASIS) and the index finger on the greater trochanter. An imaginary line drawn between these two points should point toward or above the umbilicus. When the hip is dislocated, the more proximal greater trochanter causes the line to pass below the umbilicus.

In bilateral hip dislocation, there is no asymmetry of abduction and no leg length discrepancy, making detection more difficult.

Walking age

The presenting features are a limp, with the affected side appearing to be shorter. The child tends to toe-walk on the affected side to compensate for the shortening. In addition, there is a classical Trendelenburg gait (and a positive Trendelenburg's sign). Examination may demonstrate limited abduction on the affected side and a positive Galeazzi's sign – the knees are at different levels when the hips are flexed.

As with neonates and infants, bilateral dislocations in older children are more difficult to recognize than unilateral dislocation. There is a waddling bilateral Trendelenburg gait with a hyperlordosis secondary to a fixed flexion deformity. There is usually excessive internal and external rotation of the dislocated hips.

It is essential to examine the child for other congenital conditions in the neck, spine and feet.

Investigation
Ultrasound

The role of ultrasound is well established in diagnosing and grading DDH. There are two different techniques in use:

Graf   Static alpha and beta angles [5].

Harcke   Dynamic provocation test, in which the hip is moved to reproduce the Ortolani and Barlow tests, and the degree of subluxation is noted. A displacement of 4–6 mm is considered normal [6].

Dynamic assessment of hip stability is often considered to be of greater value in the management decision-making process than static images of morphology. Graf's angular measurements have weak inter-rater reliability, while Harcke's technique is subjective and requires significant experience to grade the laxity.

With experience and training, it is possible to identify the anatomical structures of an infant hip to decide whether they are normal or abnormal, and assess the severity of any dysplasia or dislocation.

The anatomical landmarks of normal infant hips revealed in an ultrasound scan include (Figures 3.3.4 and 3.3.5):

1. Chondro-osseous junction.
2. Femoral head.
3. Synovial fold.
4. Joint capsule.
5. Labrum.
6. Cartilaginous part of the roof. This is pliable and can be deformed with dislocation. The labrum and the cartilaginous part of the roof are sometimes collectively called the limbus.
7. Bony part of the roof.
8. Bony rim (or the turning point between concavity and convexity of the roof).
9. Ilium.

These landmarks should be identified in the same sequence every time, to enhance reproducibility.

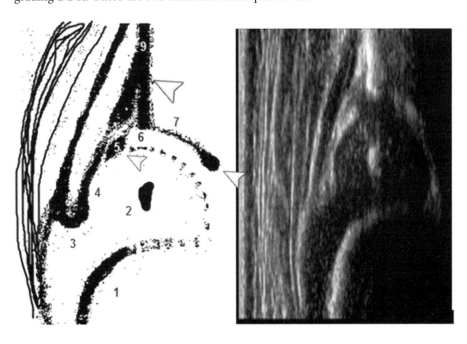

Figure 3.3.4 Infant hip ultrasound: anatomical landmarks (explanation in text).

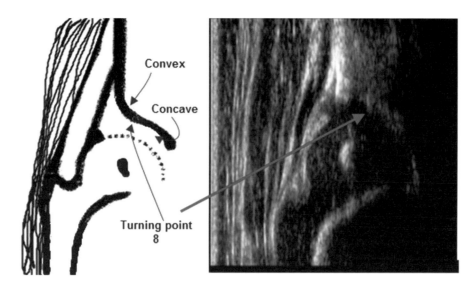

Figure 3.3.5 Infant hip ultrasound: turning point.

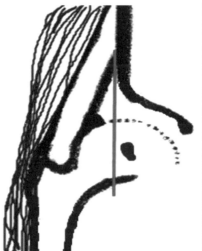 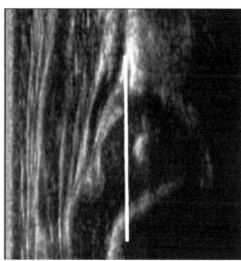

Figure 3.3.6 Infant hip ultrasound: the baseline.

Three landmarks (marked with arrowheads in Figure 3.3.4) are required, to establish the standard plane for an accurate infant hip ultrasonographic examination: the lower limb of the acetabular roof (usually it is the brightest and largest lower end of the bony roof); the midportion of the ilium and the labrum.

If any of these points is missing or not clearly shown, the sonogram is worthless and should not be used. The only exception is when the joint is decentred (dislocated) (Graf III and IV) [7].

Three important lines to be identified are:

1. The **baseline**, which runs tangentially to the outer surface of the ilium, where the cartilaginous roof meets the ilium. In a Graf Type I hip, this line bisects more than half of the head, as shown in Figure 3.3.6.
2. The **bony roof line**, which runs tangentially from the lower limb to the bony roof, as in Figure 3.3.7.
3. The **cartilaginous roof line** (or the inclination line); this is drawn from the turning point (the bony rim) to the centre of the labrum (Figure 3.3.8).

The angle between the bony roof line and the base line is the alpha angle (α). The angle between the cartilage roof line and the base line is the beta angle (β) (Figure 3.3.9). Note that the bigger the alpha angle and the smaller the beta angle, the better the hip, within limits.

Based on these angles, Graf classified infant hips into several types and subtypes (this has been updated on several occasions) (see Table 3.3.1). It is important to notice the following features.

In Graf Type I and II hips, the femoral head is centred within the acetabulum. The baseline bisects the head so that the acetabular coverage is more than 50% in Graf Type I hips and less than 50% in Graf Type II, III, and IV hips.

In Graf Type III and IV hips, the femoral head is decentred. In Graf Type III hips, the decentred femoral head pushes the cartilaginous acetabular roof upward; in Graf Type IV hips, the decentred femoral head pushes the cartilaginous acetabular roof downward.

The alpha (α) and beta (β) angles are not essential in distinguishing between Graf Types I, II, III and IV; however, they are confirmatory and guide subgrouping.

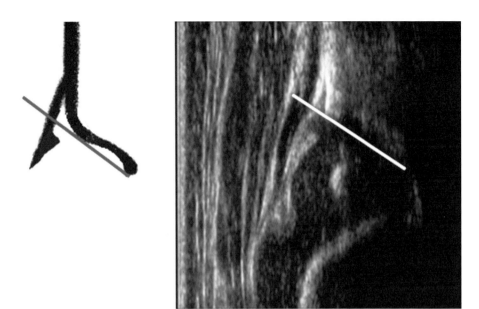

Figure 3.3.7 Infant hip ultrasound: the bony roof.

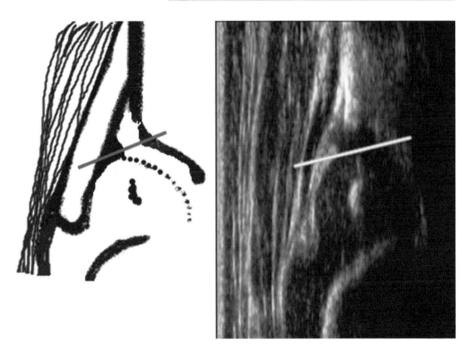

Figure 3.3.8 Infant hip ultrasound: the cartilaginous roof.

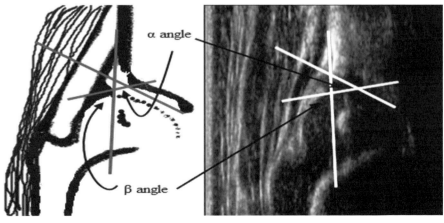

Figure 3.3.9 Infant hip ultrasound: the α and β angles.

α angle

β angle

Table 3.3.1 Graf sonographic grading for DDH

Type	Alpha angle (α)			Beta angle (β)		Description
I	>60°			<55° >55°	Ia Ib	Normal hip. This grade is further divided into Ia (β < 55°) and Ib (β > 55°). The significance of this subdivision is not yet established. Patients do not need follow-up.
II	50–59°	IIa		<77°		If the child is <3 months, this may be physiological and does not need treatment; however, follow-up is required.
		IIb		<77°		Child >3 months, delayed ossification
	43–49°	IIc	Stable Unstable	<77°		Critical zone, labrum not everted. This is further divided into stable and unstable, using the provocation test.
D	43–49°			>77°		This is the first grade where the hip becomes decentred (subluxed), so although it used to be called IId it is now identified as a distinct stage.
III	<43°	IIIa IIIb				Dislocated femoral head with the cartilaginous acetabular roof pushed **upward**. This is further divided into IIIa and IIIb, depending on the echogenicity of the hyaline cartilage of the acetabular roof (usually compared with the femoral head), which reflects degenerative changes (Figure 3.3.10).
IV	<43°					Dislocated femoral head with the cartilaginous acetabular roof pushed **downward** (Figure 3.3.11).

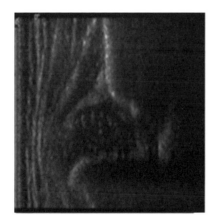
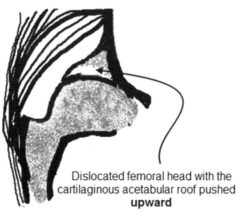

Dislocated femoral head with the cartilaginous acetabular roof pushed **upward**

Figure 3.3.10 Infant hip ultrasound: Graf III.

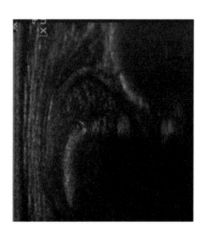
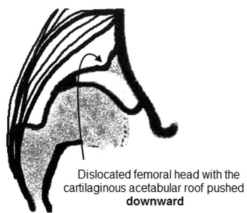

Dislocated femoral head with the cartilaginous acetabular roof pushed **downward**

Figure 3.3.11 Infant hip ultrasound: Graf IV.

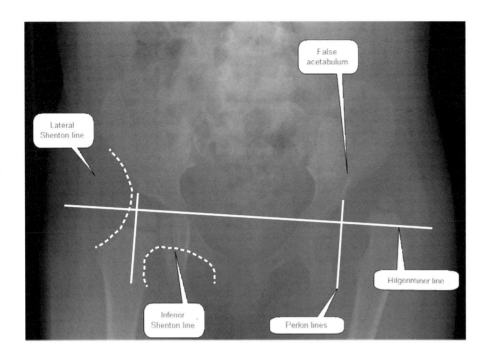

Figure 3.3.12 Plain X-ray of pelvis of 19-month-child with left dislocated hip.

Type I hips are normal and do not require treatment or follow-up. They only deteriorate if there is an abnormal pathological process, for example:

1. Wrong assessment (it was not Type I),
2. Neuromuscular disease,
3. Infection,
4. Trauma,
5. Previously decentred joints: hips that have been treated and have become Type I should be followed up radiologically until the end of growth. Disorders of growth may occur later; an initially 'healed' joint may later develop a secondary dysplasia.

Type IIa hips are physiologically immature; they do not need treatment but follow-up is required. Active treatment is recommended for all other hip types.

Universal hip ultrasound screening for DDH remains a complicated and controversial topic. Disparate findings in the literature and treatment-related problems have led to confusion about whether or not to screen for this disorder.

Universal screening is undertaken in Germany, Austria and Switzerland and has resulted in a reduction in the late presentation of hip dysplasia.

However, neonatal screening with ultrasonography will identify many infants with abnormal findings in the hip that may completely resolve if left untreated (i.e. a 'false-positive' ultrasound study). Hence, there remains a debate regarding the cost-effectiveness and efficacy of universal screening for hip dysplasia.

In the UK, hip ultrasound is used in high-risk groups (breech presentation, first-degree relatives, babies with risk factors) and neonates with abnormalities detected on clinical examination. There is concern over the large costs involved with universal screening and overtreatment of sonographically abnormal hips that would resolve without treatment.

The United States Preventive Services Task force concluded in 2006 [8] that 'evidence is insufficient to recommend routine screening' for hip dysplasia, because of the lack of clear scientific evidence favouring screening. The task force noted that they were 'unable to assess the balance of benefits and harms of screening' for DDH.

The major complication of treatment is avascular necrosis. Additional concerns would include examiner-induced hip pathology caused by vigorous provocative testing, an elevated risk of certain cancers from increased radiation exposure from follow-up radiographs, parental anxiety from the diagnosis and therapy, and false-positive results leading to unnecessary follow-up and potentially harmful interventions.

In an article in the *Journal of Bone and Joint Surgery* in 2009, Mahan *et al.* [9] recommended physical examination screening for all newborns and selective use of ultrasonography for those with a positive physical examination, breech delivery or positive family history of DDH. While Mahan *et al.* recognized the limitations inherent in the decision-analysis process, they thought it represented the best way to balance the risks and benefits of screening for hip dysplasia.

Radiography

Plain radiographs of the pelvis are useful when the capital femoral epiphysis begins to ossify, from 4 months of age. They can confirm a dislocated hip; however, an unstable hip may appear normal. On anteroposterior (AP) pelvic radiographs, several landmarks, reference lines and angles have been shown to be useful. These include:

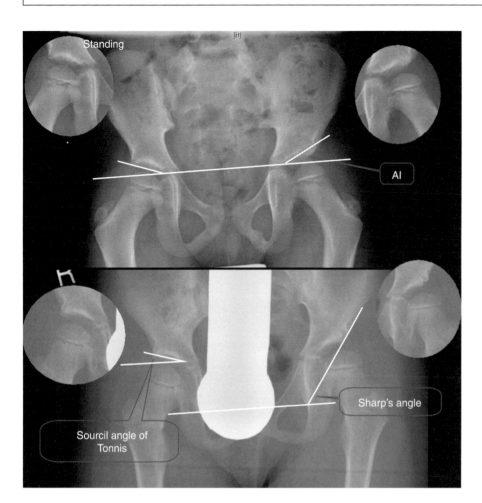

Figure 3.3.13 Plain X-ray of pelvis with residual dysplasia in left hip.

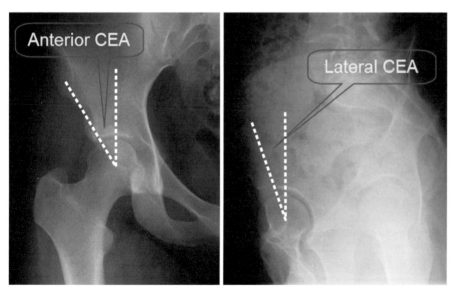

Figure 3.3.14 Centre edge angles (CEAs).

1. **H**ilgenreiner's line is a **h**orizontal line through the triradiate cartilages.
2. **P**erkin's line is a vertical line drawn at the lateral margin of the acetabulum **p**erpendicular to Hilgenreiner's line. These two lines create four quadrants. Most of the femoral head should normally lie in the inferomedial quadrant.

3. Shenton's line is a curved line that is drawn from the lesser trochanter, along the inferior femoral neck to the inferior border of the superior pubic ramus. It contrasts with the lateral Shenton's line, which is drawn from the greater trochanter, along the superior femoral neck and the ilium (Figure 3.3.12). Both lines should form a smooth curve without break.

4. The acetabular index is an angle formed by Hilgenreiner's line and a line drawn along the acetabular surface to the lateral edge of the acetabulum (Figures 3.3.13 and 10.6). The mean acetabular index (AI) is <30° at birth, 23° at 6 months and <20° by 2 years of age. After triradiate cartilage closure, a horizontal line can be drawn from the inferior tip of the teardrop to the lateral edge of the acetabulum; this is called Sharp's angle; it is less than 40°.

5. The acetabular index of the weight-bearing zone, or the sourcil angle (of Tonnis) is normally <15°.

6. The centre edge angle (CEA) of Wiberg (Figure 3.3.14) is useful after the age of 6 years.

   a. Anterior CEA (on the AP view): an angle between Perkin's line and a line to the centre of the femoral head. It is >20° by the age of 14 years and >25° in adult.

   b. Lateral CEA (on the false profile view): an angle between a perpendicular line of the acetabular edge on the false profile view and the line to the centre of the femoral head. Normally, it is >17°.

7. The teardrop is formed by the wall of the acetabulum laterally, the wall of the lesser pelvis medially, and the acetabular notch inferiorly. The teardrop appears between 6 and 24 months of age in a normal hip, later in a dislocated hip. A U-shaped teardrop is a good sign. Absent, widened or V-shaped teardrops are bad signs.

Treatment

The principles of treating DDH are:

1. Achieve a concentric reduction.
2. Maintain stability once concentric reduction is achieved.
3. Promote normal growth and development of the hip.
4. Minimize complications.

The management of DDH is based on the child age and reducibility of the dislocation:

1. Children from birth up to 6 months (Figure 3.3.15),
2. Children from 6 months to 18 months (Figure 3.3.16),
3. Children from 18 months to 30 months (Figure 3.3.17),
4. Children older than 30 months (Figure 3.3.18).

The age range is a rough guide and there is a significant overlap. The following sections represent accepted guidelines, which may be different from some local guidelines.

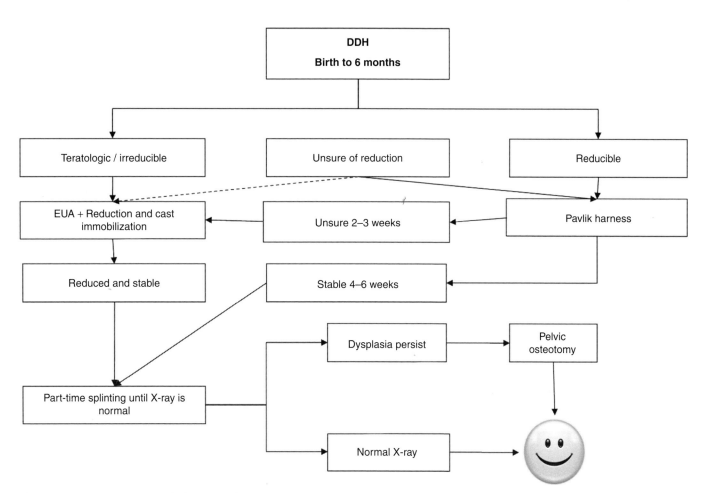

Figure 3.3.15 DDH management (birth to 6 months).

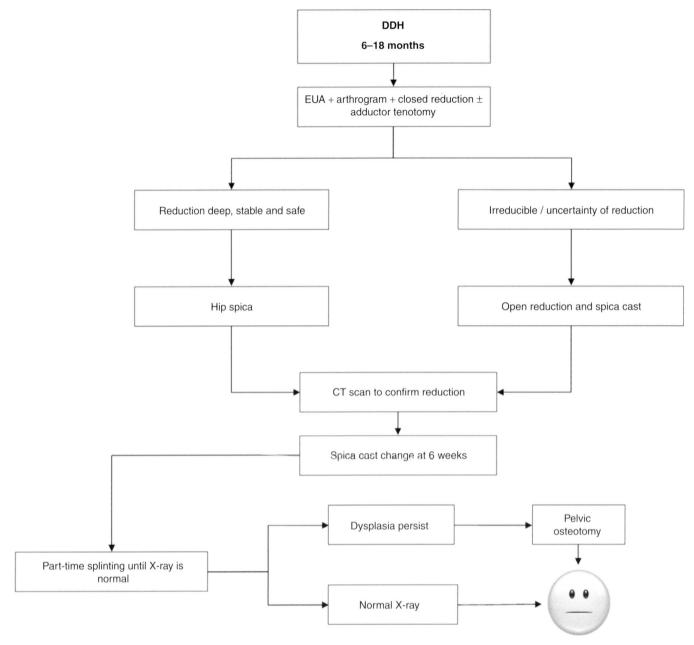

Figure 3.3.16 DDH management (6 to 18 months).

Children from birth to 6 months

The initial treatment of DDH in this age group involves the use of an abduction orthosis. Splinting the hip in a reduced position can be achieved by either:

1. Rigid splints, such as the Craig splint, the Von Rosen splint or hip spica. (Currently, these are out of favour. They may be useful in certain situations, such as respiratory compromise or shoulder anomalies.)

2. A dynamic splint, such as the Pavlik harness (PH) (Figure 3.3.19).

The Pavlik harness is designed to facilitate hip motion essential for joint cartilage nutrition, while maintaining hip flexion and limiting adduction. It has shoulder and leg straps. The anterior leg straps are to keep the hip flexion at around 100°, while the posterior leg straps are to keep hip abduction in the safe zone. The harness is sized by measuring the chest circumference. There are five sizes (premature, small, medium, large and extra-large). Excessive flexion may cause femoral nerve palsy or inferior dislocation, while too little flexion

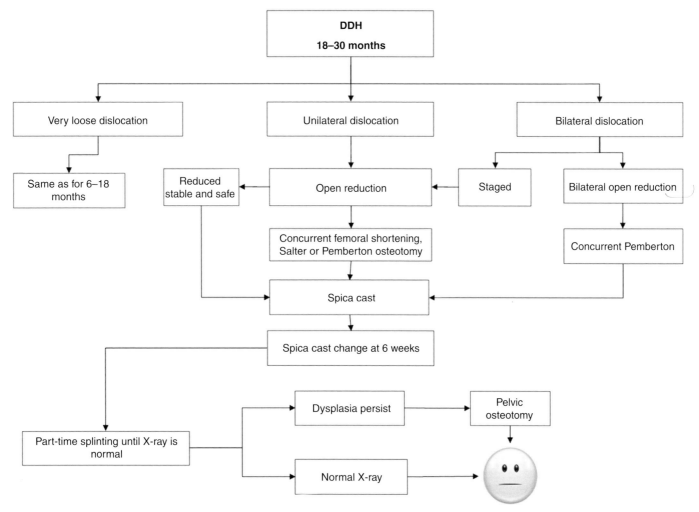

Figure 3.3.17 DDH management (18 to 30 months).

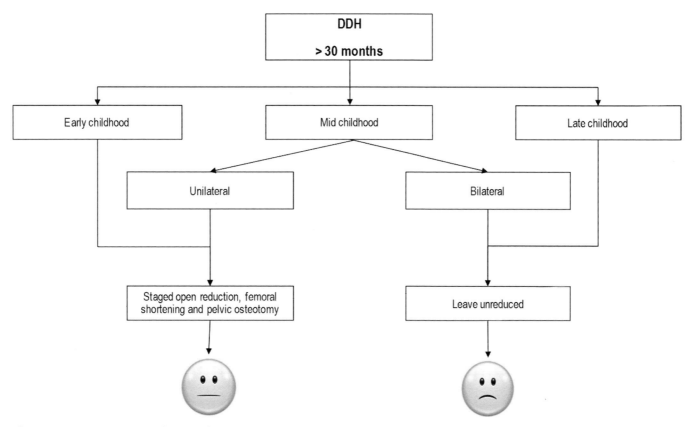

Figure 3.3.18 DDH management (>30 months).

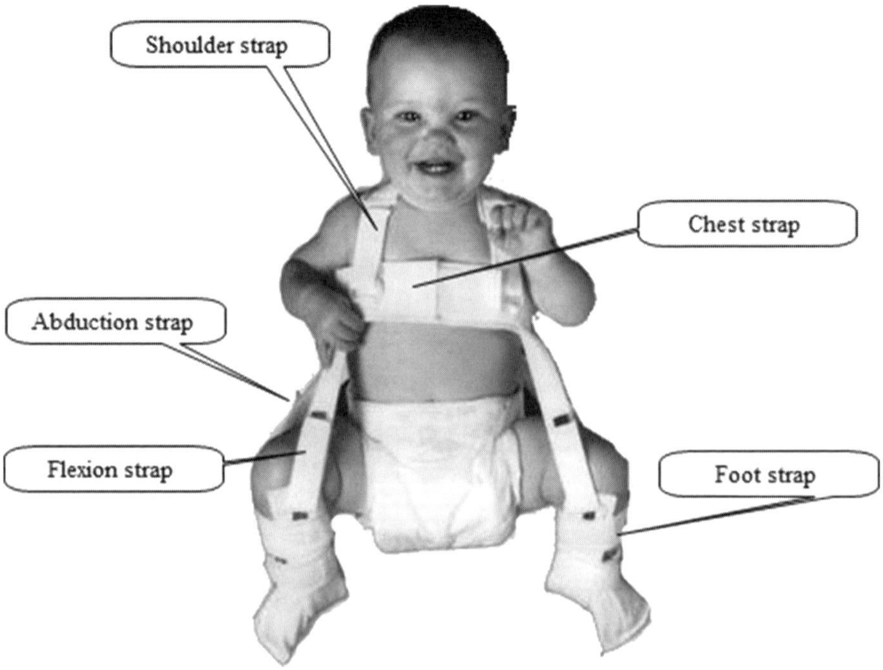

Figure 3.3.19 Pavlik harness (picture courtesy of Wheaton Brace Co.).

may cause the hip to re-dislocate. Forced abduction may lead to avascular necrosis of the femoral head.

It is essential to check a child with a Pavlik harness frequently (initially weekly then every 2 to 4 weeks) for reduction, ultrasound progression and fitness (as the child may outgrow the harness) and to document active knee extension (functioning femoral nerve). Pavlik harness treatment failure is predicted for children older than 7 weeks, bilateral hip dislocation and failure of reduction (negative Ortolani test).

Complications

1. Failure of reduction,
2. Damage to the posterior acetabular wall when there is a persistent posterior dislocation,
3. Avascular necrosis of the head of the femur (AVN) 2.4% (range, 0–15%),
4. Femoral nerve palsy,
5. Skin damage,
6. Brachial plexus injury,
7. Knee dislocation.

Murnaghan *et al.* [10] reported a femoral nerve palsy incidence of 2.5% (30 cases) in 1218 patients treated with a Pavlik harness, with 87% presenting within one week of harness application. Femoral nerve palsy was more likely in older, larger patients in whom the hip dysplasia was of greater severity. Patients whose femoral nerve palsy resolved within 3 days had a 70% chance of successful treatment using the Pavlik harness, whereas those who had not recovered by 10 days had a 70% chance of treatment failure. All patients had eventual complete return of full quadriceps function, with no clinically evident long-term motor or sensory deficit. The success rate associated with treatment with a Pavlik harness was 94% in the control group and 47% in the palsy group.

Contraindication of Pavlik harness

1. Major muscle imbalance, such as myelomeningocele,
2. Major stiffness as in arthrogryposis,
3. Ligamentous laxity, as in Ehlers–Danlos syndrome,
4. Severe respiratory compromise (a Craig splint may be useful),
5. Irreducible hip,
6. Age >6 months.

Children from 6 to 18 months

The goals of the treatment are to obtain and maintain reduction of the hip without damaging the femoral head. This can be achieved by either closed or open reduction. Closed reduction is the preferred treatment option.

Two controversial issues worth discussing are:

1. A preliminary period of traction before closed reduction,
2. The timing of reduction of the hip in relation to the appearance of the ossific nucleus of the femoral head.

Proponents of preliminary period of traction claim that it reduces the AVN rate and the need of open reduction. To reduce costs, they recommend a portable home traction device. Recent studies [11] have not supported this view and this practice is now less favoured.

In a retrospective study [11] of 49 children younger than 12 months old who had 57 hip dislocations, 18 hips developed partial or complete AVN and 39 hips did not. There was no significant difference in the occurrence of AVN with respect to such variables as preliminary traction, closed versus open reduction, Pavlik harness use or age at the time of operative intervention. However, the presence of the ossific nucleus before reduction, detected either by radiographs ($P < 0.001$) or ultrasonography ($P = 0.033$) was statistically significant in predicting AVN; one (4%) of 25 hips with an ossific nucleus developed AVN, whereas 17 (53%) of 32 hips without an ossific nucleus before reduction developed AVN.

Another study [12] of 48 patients who underwent successful closed reduction showed similar findings. At 2 years follow-up, AVN was noted post-reduction in 17 hips: 4 of 23 hips that had a nucleus at reduction, compared with 13 of 25 hips reduced before ossification of the nucleus.

Other studies disagreed with these findings, in a study [13] of 32 patients who underwent medial open reduction of 40 hips and follow-up of an average of 10.3 years, AVN developed in 11 hips (27.5%). Bilateral dislocations and age older than 1 year at surgery correlated with greater likelihood of AVN (<0.05), whereas absence of the ossific nucleus did not. Avascular necrosis developed in 4 of 13 hips (30.8%) that had a radiographic-apparent ossific nucleus at the time of reduction and in 7 of 27 hips (25.9%) that did not have an apparent ossific nucleus. The use of pre-operative traction was not protective against AVN, because 7 of the 11 hips with AVN had undergone pre-operative traction.

The authors believe that one should not wait to treat a hip until the nucleus appears. The growth potential of the acetabulum declines with age, and hips reduced later will not remodel as well as those reduced earlier.

Closed reduction

This is usually performed under anaesthesia. An arthrogram of the hip is obtained at the same time, to confirm reduction. An adductor or psoas tenotomy may also be needed, depending on the certainty of adequate joint reduction.

Once the hip is reduced, the range of motion in which the hip remains reduced must be determined. The hip is adducted to the point of re-dislocation and that position is noted. The hip is again reduced and then extended until it dislocates, and the point of dislocation is noted. These arcs represent the safe zone (of reduction). They can be improved by adductor tenotomy or psoas tenotomy, depending on the tightness of these structures. If the hip requires internal rotation to maintain reduction, this is also noted. The aim is to immobilize the hip within the safe zone without extremely abducting or flexing the hip. This usually occurs with hip abduction of about 45°, flexion greater than 90° and neutral hip rotation.

Hip arthrography

This can be done by either an anterolateral or a medial (or subadductor) approach (Figure 3.3.20). The medial approach is the preferred option for children of this age group because it is easier to perform and an extracapsular leak of the dye is less likely to obscure the important structures laterally (femoral head, labrum, cartilaginous part of acetabulum and amount of coverage).

The infant is placed in a supine position under general anaesthetic. The area is prepared and draped to allow easy access for the hip, in case an adductor tenotomy or open reduction is required. A needle attached to a 10 ml syringe containing saline is introduced underneath the adductor tendon, aiming for the ipsilateral shoulder. This is done under X-ray screening. Usually a 'give' is felt once the needle pierces the joint capsule. When the needle is in the joint, water is injected to fill the capsule. There should be a back-flow if the needle is in the right place. Next, 1–2 ml of contrast medium is injected slowly under X-ray control. Then the hip is screened for reduction and stability through the range of motion (ROM).

Open reduction

This is indicated when:

1. Closed reduction is not possible.
2. Closed reduction is not concentric.
3. The hip reduces but remains unstable or stability can only be achieved by holding the hip in extreme abduction or internal rotation. (This happens when the safe zone is narrow.) The former may cause re-dislocation while the latter may cause AVN.

Open reduction may be performed through a medial approach (<1 year) or an anterior approach (older children).

Medial approaches include:

Anteromedial (Iowa):	Interior to the pectineus and medial to the femoral sheath.
Medial (Ludloff):	Utilizes the interval between the pectineus muscle anteriorly and between the adductor longus and brevis muscles posteriorly.
Posteromedial (Ferguson):	Uses the interval between the adductor longus and brevis muscles anteriorly and the gracilis and adductor magnus muscles posteriorly.

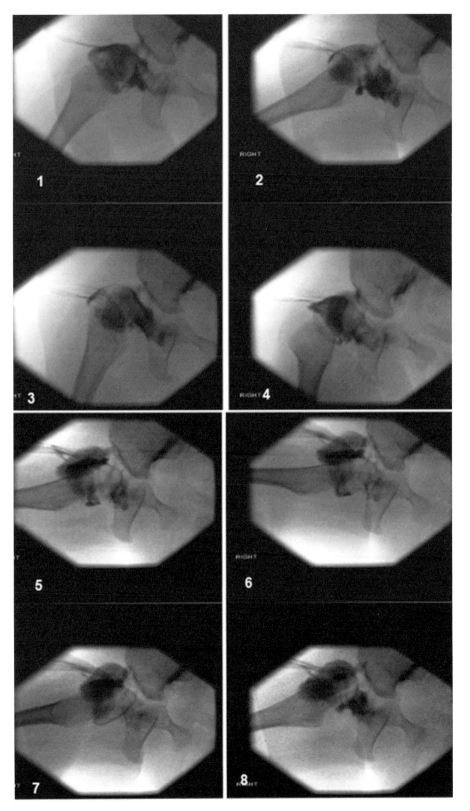

Figure 3.3.20 Hip arthrogram, showing the outline of the cartilaginous part of the femoral head. Panels 2 and 3 show the hourglass shape caused by the iliopsoas tendon (not visible) compressing the capsule in the middle. The top four pictures confirm hip dislocation; the head is not sitting in the acetabulum and there is significant medial dye pooling (>7 mm). The ligamentum teres is thickened and elongated (this is clearest in panel 3). Hip reduction is assessed in different positions; the hip is reduced in panels 5 to 7. Panels 7 and 8 show the effect of rotation on reduction, where external rotation led to dislocation anteriorly.

The disadvantages of the medial approach are a limited view of the hip, possible injury to the medial femoral circumflex artery (increased AVN rate), and inability or difficulty to perform a capsulorrhaphy.

The **anterior hip approach** (Smith-Petersen) utilizes the intervals between the tensor fascia lata and sartorius (superficial) and the rectus femoris and gluteus medius (deep). The reflected head of the rectus is detached

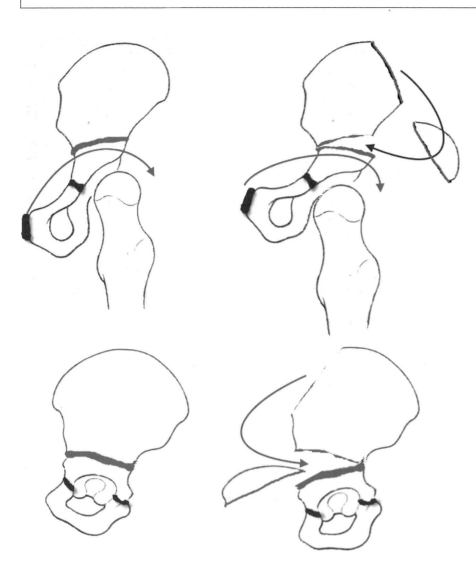

Figure 3.3.21 Salter's osteotomy. In Salter's osteotomy, a small arc of posterior column at the triradiate cartilage is left uncut and the acetabular roof is hinged on this arc to allow anterior or anterolateral coverage.

from the anterior lip of the acetabulum to reach the hip joint capsule.

The anatomical structures that can prevent reduction are:

1. Inverted limbus,
2. Thickened and elongated ligamentum teres,
3. Interposed iliopsoas tendon,
4. Pulvinar,
5. Contracted transverse ligament.

The large, redundant capsule should be tightened (T-V capsulorrhaphy) using non-absorbable sutures. The wound is closed in the routine manner. A hip spica is applied with the hip in 30° abduction, 30° flexion and 30° of internal rotation. The knee should be flexed to 30°, to relax the hamstrings and control rotation in the cast. This is different from the position of spica in closed reduction and there may be some variations between different centres.

A **femoral osteotomy** (shortening, varus, derotation or a combination) may be required. Shortening should be considered when excessive pressure is placed on the femoral head when it is reduced, particularly in a child older than 2. If the reduction is safe and not tight, the surgeon should be able to distract the joint a few millimetres without much force. If the joint remains stable only in wide abduction, a varus osteotomy is indicated. If there is excessive femoral anteversion and the reduction requires significant internal rotation to be stable, then a derotation osteotomy is needed.

Salter's innominate osteotomy [14] (Figure 3.3.21) may be indicated at the time of an open reduction, especially in children 18 months of age or older depending on the degree of acetabular coverage of the femoral head when the hip is placed in extension and neutral rotation and abduction. If more than one-third of the head is visible in this position, an innominate osteotomy will provide further hip coverage.

The **Pemberton pelvic osteotomy** is an alternative with several advantages. It is inherently stable, with no need for

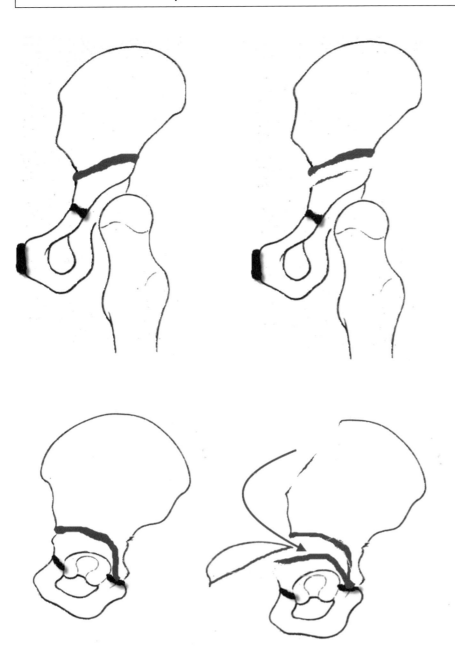

Figure 3.3.22 Pemberton osteotomy. In Salter's osteotomy, the ilium is completely divided, while in the Pemberton osteotomy it is not. Some obvious advantages of the Pemberton osteotomy are that it is more stable than Salter's osteotomy, does not require metal fixation, and rotation, rather than translation, is more likely.

metalware, is versatile in addressing femoral head coverage, and it reduces the size of the acetabulum (Figure 3.3.22).

Children from 18 to 30 months

The treatment of children of this age group is more challenging. They usually have a high dislocation and the muscles are more severely contracted. A femoral shortening is an essential part of management in the older child, who is more likely to need a primary pelvic osteotomy, such as Salter's osteotomy or the Pemberton osteotomy.

Children older than 30 months

There is some debate as to the upper age at which a successful reduction can be achieved. Reduction of bilateral dislocations is not recommended in children older than 8, while reduction of unilateral dislocations should be attempted for children up to 9 years of age. This is because gait asymmetry and function are more markedly affected in unilateral cases and the complication rate is considerably higher when both hips have to be reduced.

Residual dysplasia

It is important to follow-up children with dysplasia as persistent dysplasia is not uncommon (Figure 3.3.23). Surgery is generally indicated if:

1. The AI fails to improve over 18 months or normalize (AI $<$ 20°) by the age of 4 years,

2. Inadequate acetabular cover (CEA $<$15°, uncovering $>$30%),

Table 3.3.2 Residual dysplasia treatment [15]

	2–6 years		6 years to skeletal maturity		Skeletal maturity	
Concentric reduction	Achieved	Achieved	Achieved	Not possible	Achieved	Not possible
Size of acetabulum	Normal	Large	Normal	Small		Small
Required osteotomy	Salter's osteotomy	Pemberton or Dega osteotomy	Salter's osteotomy (<8 years) or Triple osteotomy	Shelf procedure or Chiari osteotomy	Triple osteotomy or Ganz osteotomy	Chiari osteotomy

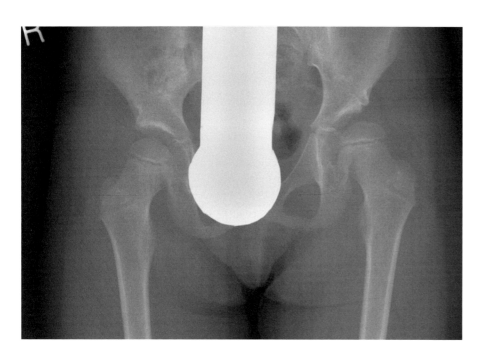

Figure 3.3.23 Persistent dysplasia. The radiograph shows a shallow acetabulum on the left side. Although, the femoral head is spherical and concentric in the acetabulum, it is not well covered. The AI (29° left; 21° right) and 50% of the head are uncovered.

3. Progressive subluxation and instability,
4. Pain with dysplasia.

The appropriate procedure should be selected based on the site of deformity, severity, joint congruity, age and available expertise. Table 3.3.2 summarizes the current recommended procedures for various persistent hip dysplasias. In severe dysplasia, pelvic osteotomy may be combined with femoral osteotomy to achieve the optimum result.

Each osteotomy provides anatomical advantages that may suit a particular clinical situation better than others. For example, Salter's osteotomy redirects the acetabulum forward, producing more anterior and lateral cover and improving the AI and CEA by about 15° at the expense of posterior cover. This is useful in mild and moderate dysplasia but it may be harmful in neuromuscular dysplasia, in which the posterior wall is usually deficient. Conversely, a Dega osteotomy provides lateral and posterior cover, which is useful in neuromuscular dysplasia.

Salter's osteotomy is hinged on the symphysis pubis, which makes it suboptimum in bilateral dysplasia. A Pemberton osteotomy overcomes this problem and is ideal for bilateral or severe dysplasia in children under 6 years. There are several types of triple osteotomy (Steele, Tönnis's), which provide the best choice for correcting dysplasia in young children when the triradiate cartilage is still open. A Ganz osteotomy achieves good correction without breaking the posterior column. Also, it does not affect the birth canal, which is an extra advantage in young women. However, the Ganz osteotomy is contraindicated if the triradiate cartilage is still open (as it interferes with the growth of the acetabulum).

The Chiari osteotomy and shelf procedures are salvage procedures, as they do not provide a hyaline cartilage-covered articulating surface. They are used in circumstances in which

Table 3.3.3 Avascular necrosis of the femoral head (Kalamachi and MacEwen classification)

Type I	Type II	AVN-III	AVN-IV
Small irregular epiphysis	Lateral physeal arrest leads to valgus neck and horizontal physis	Medial physeal arrest leads to varus neck and vertical physis	Central bridge cause total arrest and shortening of the neck
Usually resolves spontaneously	May require trochanteric epiphysiodesis (<8 years) or transfer ± varus femoral osteotomy	May require trochanteric epiphysiodesis (<8 years) or transfer ± valgus femoral osteotomy	May require trochanteric epiphysiodesis ± Wagner osteotomy ± contralateral distal femoral epiphysiodesis

there is irreducible subluxation or if other osteotomies cannot be performed due to previous surgery. A Chiari osteotomy is appropriate for a lateralized severely dysplastic hip. A shelf osteotomy is relatively safe and versatile, and can be used in a wide range of difficult situations (see Figures 10.7 and 19.6 for more details).

Avascular necrosis of the femoral head

Avascular necrosis is a major cause of long-term disability, which is directly related to the treatment. It does not occur in untreated DDH. Kalamchi and MacEwen [16] classified AVN following DDH treatment into four types. Table 3.3.3 summarizes these types, their features and treatments.

References

1. Herring JA (2008) *Tachdjian's Pediatric Orthopaedics*, 4th edition, volume 1. Philadelphia: Saunders Elsevier.

2. Scheuer L and Black SM (2000) *Developmental Juvenile Osteology*. Oxford: Elsevier.

3. Jari S, Paton RW and Srinivasan MS (2002) Unilateral limitation of abduction of the hip. A valuable clinical sign for DDH? *J Bone Joint Surg Br* **84**(1):104–7.

4. Jones D (1998) Neonatal detection of developmental dysplasia of the hip (DDH). *J Bone Joint Surg Br* **80**(6):943–5.

5. Graf R (1980) The diagnosis of congenital hip-joint dislocation by the ultrasonic Combound treatment. *Arch Orthop Trauma Surg* **97**(2):117–33.

6. Harcke HT, Clarke NM, Lee MS, Borns PF and MacEwen GD (1984) Examination of the infant hip with real-time ultrasonography. *J Ultrasound Med* **3**(3):131–7.

7. Graf R (2006) *Hip Sonography. Diagnosis and Management of Infant Hip Dysplasia*. Berlin: Springer.

8. US Preventive Services Task Force (2006) Screening for developmental dysplasia of the hip: recommendation statement. *Pediatrics* **117**:898–902.

9. Mahan ST, Katz JN and Kim YJ (2009) To screen or not to screen? A decision analysis of the utility of screening for developmental dysplasia of the hip. *J Bone Joint Surg Am* **91**(7):1705–19.

10. Murnaghan ML, Browne RH, Sucato DJ and Birch J (2011) Femoral nerve palsy in Pavlik harness treatment for developmental dysplasia of the hip. *J Bone Joint Surg Am* **93**(5):493–9.

11. Segal LS, Boal DK, Borthwick L, Clark MW, Localio AR and Schwentker EP (1999) Avascular necrosis after treatment of DDH: the protective influence of the ossific nucleus. *J Pediatr Orthop* **19**(2):177–84.

12. Carney BT, Clark D and Minter CL (2004) Is the absence of the ossific nucleus prognostic for avascular necrosis after closed reduction of developmental dysplasia of the hip? *J Surg Orthop Adv* **13**(1):24–9.

13. Konigsberg DE, Karol LA, Colby S and O'Brien S (2003) Results of medial open

reduction of the hip in infants with developmental dislocation of the hip. *J Pediatr Orthop* **23**(1):1–9.

14. Salter RB and Dubos JP (1974) The first fifteen years' personal experience with innominate osteotomy in the treatment of congenital dislocation and subluxation of the hip. *Clin Orthop Relat Res* **98**:72–103.

15. Joseph B, Nayagam S, Loder R and Torode I (2009) *Paediatric Orthopaedics: A System of Decision-Making.* Boca Raton, FL: CRC Press.

16. Kalamchi A and MacEwen GD (1980) Avascular necrosis following treatment of congenital dislocation of the hip. *J Bone Joint Surg Am* **62**(6):876–88.

3.4 Miscellaneous

Coxa vara

Coxa vara (CV) describes a proximal femoral varus deformity in which there is a reduction in the neck–shaft angle (NSA <110°) (Figure 3.4.1). It is not a single entity but rather a wide spectrum of different types, pathologies, aetiologies and natural history. These can be summarized as follows:

Congenital coxa vara (CCV)

This is more accurately described as congenital femoral deficiency with coxa vara: it is caused by a primary cartilaginous defect in the femoral neck. By definition, CCV presents at birth but it manifests clinically during early childhood and commonly follows a clinical course that is progressive with

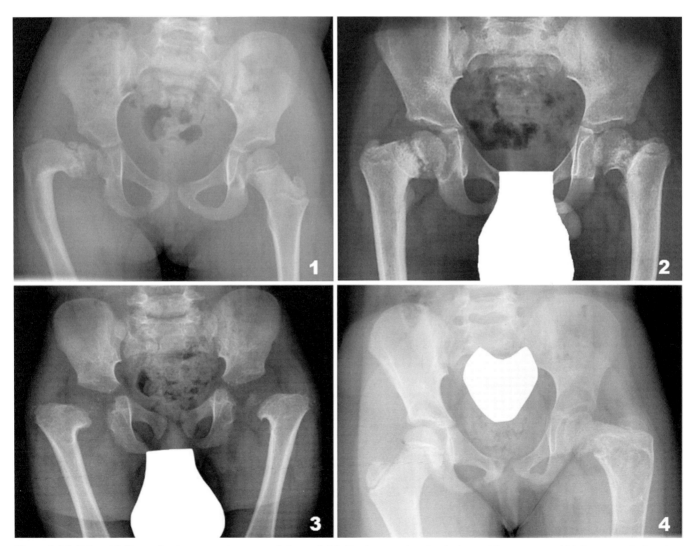

Figure 3.4.1 Plain pelvic X-rays of various types of coxa vara. 1: Congenital. 2: Developmental; notice the inverted Y appearance, which is more marked on the right hip. 3: Dysplastic; the underlying cause is chondrodysplasia punctata. 4: Acquired; the underlying cause is fibrous dysplasia.

Table 3.4.1 Summary of different types of coxa vara

	Congenital coxa vara	Developmental coxa vara	Acquired coxa vara[†]
Site	Subtrochanteric	Physis	Any (epiphysis, physis, metaphysis, subtrochanteric)
Pathology	Embryonic limb bud abnormality	Primary ossification defect in inferior femoral neck, predisposing the local dystrophic bone to fatigue and bend by shear stress of weight	Depends on cause; usually vascular insult (sepsis, AVN) or traumatic (fracture)
Age of onset	Birth	Walking age to 6 years	Usually older than CCV and DCV
Presenting feature	Unilateral short and deformed leg	Limping, Trendelenburg gait (unilateral) or waddling (bilateral) LLD rarely >3 cm	Presenting features of cause
Radiological features	Features of congenital femoral deficiency	Very typical: decreased NSA, vertical physis, a triangular metaphyseal fragment in the inferior femoral neck, inverted radiolucent Y pattern, decreased anteversion (may be retroversion)	Features of coxa vara and of the causative pathology
Natural history	Progression	Progression if HEA>60°	Progression if the physis or epiphysis is involved Fractures may remodel, resolving the varus deformity

[†] Features are closely related to the underlying pathology.

growth. It is usually associated with a significant limb length discrepancy, congenital short femur, proximal femoral focal deficiency (PFFD) and congenital bowed femur.

Developmental coxa vara (DCV)

This term is reserved for coxa vara of the proximal femur in early childhood with classical radiographic changes (inferior and posterior bony metaphyseal fragments) and no other skeletal manifestations. In the past it was also referred to as infantile or cervical coxa vara.

Acquired coxa vara

This is caused by several conditions, including:

1. Slipped upper femoral epiphysis,
2. Sequelae of avascular necrosis of the femoral epiphysis due to:
   a. Legg–Calvé–Perthes disease,
   b. Trauma,
   c. Femoral neck fracture,
   d. Traumatic hip dislocation,
   e. Post-reduction for developmental dysplasia of the hip,
   f. Septic necrosis,
   g. Other causes of avascular necrosis of the immature femoral head.
3. Coxa vara associated with pathologic bone disorders:
   a. Osteogenesis imperfecta,
   b. Fibrous dysplasia,
   c. Renal osteodystrophy,
   d. Osteopetrosis.

4. Association with a skeletal dysplasia (often referred to as dysplastic coxa vara; some authors classify this group under developmental CV):
   a. Cleidocranial dysostosis,
   b. Metaphyseal dysostosis,
   c. Other skeletal dysplasias.

Confusion and controversy exist in the literature as to terminology and classification of this disorder. Table 3.4.1 summarizes the differences among different types.

Presentation

Developmental coxa vara usually presents with a painless limp and progressive LLD. It may become painful toward the end of the day or after significant activity. There may be a family history and it can be bilateral (30–50%). Age of presentation is usually in the first 5 years of life, but older patients may be encountered. Patients may show prominent greater trochanters. There may be pelvic tilt secondary to LLD and there is usually a positive Trendelenburg or delayed positive Trendelenburg test.

Three important radiological measures quantify the coxa vara (Figure 3.4.2): the neck–shaft angle (NSA), the Hilgenreiner epiphyseal angle (HEA) and the articulotrochanteric distance (ATD). A decreased ATD indicates that the pathology is located in the physeal or intertrochanteric area, while a normal ATD indicates that it is in the subtrochanteric region.

Treatment

Treatment of CCV is discussed in the section on treating congenital femoral deficiency. The treatment for acquired

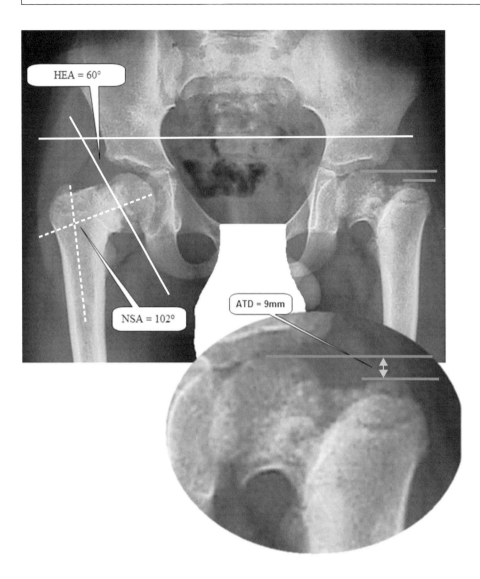

HEA = 60°

NSA = 102°

ATD = 9mm

Figure 3.4.2 Pelvic X-ray of a limping child with coxa vara.

CV is directed at the cause; however, anatomical correction may be necessary.

Weinstein [1] introduced the Hilgenreiner epiphyseal angle (HEA) to aid in surgical decision making. The average normal value is 20°.

- HEA < 45°; usually improves without intervention,
- HEA > 60°; usually worsens if left untreated and is an indication for surgery,
- HEA = 45–60°; require observation for either healing or progression. Surgical intervention is required if progressive.

Surgical treatment involves corrective osteotomy to achieve the following goals:

1. Neck-shaft angle (NSA) ≥140° and HEA to less than 35–40°,
2. Correction of femoral version to normal values (usually there is a retroversion),
3. Ossification and healing of the defective inferomedial femoral neck fragment,
4. Restoring ATD and abductor mechanism length-tension relationship,
5. Adductor tenotomy to remove deforming force.

Several osteotomies, such as Pauwels' Y-shaped osteotomy, Langenskiold intertrochanteric osteotomy and Borden's subtrochanteric osteotomy, have been described. Associated abnormalities, such as LLD, femoral retroversion or trochanteric overgrowth, can be corrected simultaneously or at a second stage, depending on severity.

Congenital femoral deficiency

Congenital femoral deficiency (Figure 3.4.3) is a spectrum of disorders, rather than a single disease entity. There are two distinct forms:

1. Proximal focal femoral deficiency (PFFD) describes a deformity in which the femur is shorter than normal and there is discontinuity (with loss of variable lengths of femur) between the femoral neck and shaft.

Table 3.4.2 Aitken's classification of congenital femoral deficiency

Type	Diagram	Description
A	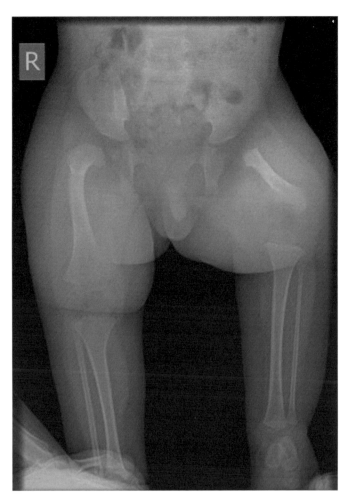	There is a normal acetabulum and femoral head. The femur is short. Bony connections exist between all components. The cartilaginous neck ossifies later on, although this is often associated with a pseudarthrosis. This may heal; however, X-rays show severe coxa vara with significant shortening of the femur.
B		The femoral head is more rudimentary and the deficiency of the proximal femoral shaft is more extensive. Pseudarthrosis between femoral shaft and head is always present.
C		The acetabulum is markedly dysplastic and the femoral head never ossifies. The femoral shaft is very short and its upper end tapers sharply to point. The hip is very unstable.
D		Both the femoral head and the acetabulum are absent and the deficiency of the femoral shaft is more significant.

Figure 3.4.3 X-ray of child with congenital femoral deficiency, showing short and dysplastic left femur. The proximal parts (head and trochanter) are not visible (may be absent or not ossified yet); features are consistent with proximal focal femoral deficiency (PFFD). There is coxa vara of the right side, indicating that the right side may be affected as well (bilateral involvement occurs in 15% of patients). The left fibula seems to be shorter than the right, raising the possibility of fibular hemimelia (2/3 of patients). It is difficult to comment on the hip and knee joints states from a single plain radiograph and further assessment is required.

2. Congenital short femur describes a short femur with no bony loss or discontinuity.

In most cases, the cause of the femoral deficiency is unknown; however, it may be part of genetically transmitted syndromes.

Presentation

The diagnosis may be made antenatally using ultrasonography or at birth. Patients with congenital femoral deficiency have a short thigh that is flexed, abducted and externally rotated. They may also have features of coxa vara and fibula hemimelia.

Several classifications have been developed to aid assessment and treatment:

Aitken's classification

This is shown in Table 3.4.2. If the femoral length is greater than 50%, the recommended treatment is reconstruction and lengthening (usually grade A and B, where there is a head). For a femoral length less than 50%, the treatment may be amputation, fusion or Van Ness rotational arthroplasty.

Gillespie and Torode classification

Group A: Congenital short femur by about 20% (the foot of the affected limb is at midtibia level or below compared with the normal side). The child can bear weight on the affected leg.

Group B: The LLD is around 40% (the foot of the affected limb is at a level between the knee and midtibia compared with the normal side). There is anterior projection of the thigh and flexed knee.

Group C: The thigh is short and bulbous and the leg is externally rotated with the foot at or near the level of the other knee.

Paley's classification

This is the most recent comprehensive classification; however, it is still not widely adopted.

Type I: Intact femur with mobile hip and knee:

a. Normal ossification of proximal femur,
b. Delayed ossification of proximal femur.

Type II: Mobile pseudarthrosis (hip not fully formed, a false joint) with mobile knee:

a. Femoral head mobile in acetabulum,
b. Femoral head absent or stiff in acetabulum.

Type III: Diaphyseal deficiency of femur (femur does not reach acetabulum):

a. Knee motion >45°,
b. Knee motion <45°.

Type I is further subclassified into:

0. Ready for surgery; no factors to correct before lengthening,
1. One factor to correct before lengthening,
2. Two factors to correct before lengthening,
3. Three factors to correct before lengthening,
4+. Etc.

Examples of factors requiring correction prior to lengthening of femur are NSA <90°, delayed ossification of the proximal femur, centre edge angle (CEA) <20°, a subluxing patella and a dislocating knee.

The management strategy is for staged corrections of the abnormalities to reach Stage I0, which is then amenable to lengthening. For example, Type Ia-3 is converted through Ia-2 and Ia-1 to Ia-0, before lengthening. Pre-existing knee stiffness is the most functionally limiting factor and should be considered a relative indication for amputation versus reconstruction. Hip dysplasia or deficiency is reconstructable and is not a limiting factor. Hip reconstruction should be performed prior to lengthening.

Treatment

Treatment is challenging and should be undertaken in specialized centres. The National Institute for Health and Clinical Excellence (NICE) has issued guidance to NHS hospitals on combined bony and soft-tissue reconstruction for PFFD [2]. Treatment must be tailored to individual patients and is based on leg length discrepancy, hip and knee-joint stability, proximal musculature, presence or absence of foot deformities,

availability of expertise, and patient and family motivation. The two broad options are reconstructive surgery or amputation and the use of a prosthesis.

First year of life

Usually no treatment is required. This is the period when the surgeon formulates a treatment plan and the family develop an understanding of the condition. The limb inequality at this stage will not prevent the child crawling or sitting.

Children from 1 to 3 years

Children with a deformed or functionless foot are best treated with a Syme's amputation followed by prosthetic fitting, while those with a satisfactory foot and ankle may only require a shoe raise initially.

Children from 3 to 15 years

In a child with a satisfactory foot and ankle, limb length equality must be achieved by skeletal maturity.

In general, prosthetic management is used when the femoral length is less than 50% of the opposite normal side and lengthening with or without contralateral epiphysiodesis is used if the femoral length is greater than 50%. Length discrepancy can be estimated by remembering that the relative proportions of the skeleton remain constant throughout life, i.e. a 20% discrepancy in infancy equates to a 20% discrepancy at maturity. Aitken's class A and B legs have a femoral head that allows for reconstruction including lengthening, while classes C and D present a more difficult situation.

Before undertaking any lengthening, hip dysplasia must be corrected by a pelvic osteotomy to prevent subluxation of the hip.

Coxa vara can be corrected by a subtrochanteric valgus osteotomy. Other options include Van Ness rotationplasty.

Traumatic disorders
Pelvis fractures
Background

Pelvic fractures in children are rare (<0.2% of all paediatric fractures) and are usually caused by road traffic accidents. It is vital to appreciate the high-energy mechanism of injury and the associated injuries to the neurovascular structures, abdominal viscera, genitourinary system, musculoskeletal zone and central nervous system (CNS). The mortality rate ranges between 2.4% and 14.8% with associated head injury cited as the most common cause of death [3]. Thorough primary and secondary Advanced Trauma Life Support surveys are essential in all pelvic injuries.

The pelvis of a child differs from that of an adult: the bone, ligament and joints are more elastic and provide a greater capacity for energy absorption than adults before they break. For the same reason, bones are less brittle and may break in only one area rather than two. (The 'Polo mint ring' analogue is not applicable.) Avulsion fractures through an apophysis occur more often in children and adolescents than in adults.

Table 3.4.3 Key and Cornwell's classification and treatment recommendation [**4**]

Type	Subtype	Treatment recommendation
I. Intact ring	a. Avulsion (ASIS, AIIS, ischial tuberosity)	Bed rest with hip flexed for 2 weeks, then protected weight-bearing for 4 weeks
	b. Pubis, ischium	Bed rest for 1 week, then partial weight-bearing
	c. Iliac wing (Duverney fracture)	Bed rest with abducted leg for 1 week then weight-bearing as tolerated
	d. Sacrum, coccyx	Severe sacral fractures may need 4–6 weeks bed rest
II. Single break in ring	a. Ipsilateral rami b. Symphysis pubis c. Sacroiliac joint (rare)	Bed rest for 2–4 weeks then progress to weight-bearing
III. Double break in ring	a. Bilateral pubic rami (straddle) b. Anterior and posterior ring with migration (Malgaigne)	Bed rest for 2–4 weeks then progress to weight-bearing Skeletal traction or external fixator for 3–6 weeks
IV. Acetabular fractures	a. Small fragment with dislocation b. Linear: non-displaced c. Linear: hip unstable d. Central	Reduce dislocation and ambulate as able Treat associated pelvic fracture Skeletal traction; open reduction and internal fixation if incongruous Lateral traction for reduction; open reduction and internal fixation if severe

Physeal injury in children can result in growth disturbances and may lead to significant deformity.

A single AP radiograph is usually sufficient to identify pelvic ring fractures in the acute situation. The inlet view is useful in determining posterior displacement of the pelvis. The outlet view is useful to demonstrate superior displacement of the posterior pelvis or superior or inferior displacement of the anterior portion of the pelvis. However, CT scanning has largely abolished the need for these views.

Classification

Several classifications have been proposed for pelvic fractures.

Torode and Zieg classified pelvic fractures in children into:

Type I: Avulsion fractures,

Type II: Iliac wing fractures,

Type III: Stable pelvic ring fractures,

Type IV: Any fracture pattern that creates a free bony fragment (unstable pelvic ring injuries).

Tile's classification is applicable in patients near skeletal maturity with more adult-type patterns of fracture:

A. Stable fractures:

  A1. Avulsion fractures,

  A2. Undisplaced pelvic ring or iliac wing fractures,

  A3. Transverse fractures of the sacrum and coccyx.

B. Rotationally unstable, vertically stable fractures:

  B1. Open-book fractures (anteroposterior compression fracture),

  B2. Lateral compression injuries (ipsilateral: the anterior and posterior fractures are on the same side),

  B3. Lateral compression injuries (contralateral: the anterior and posterior fractures are on opposite sides; contralateral bucket handle).

C. Rotationally and vertically unstable pelvic ring fractures:

  C1. Ipsilateral anterior and posterior pelvic injury,

  C2. Bilateral hemipelvic disruption,

  C3. Associated acetabular fracture.

The **Key and Cornwell's classification** is shown in Table 3.4.3.

Fractures of the head and neck of the femur

These fractures are exceedingly rare, accounting for less than 1% of all paediatric fractures. They are usually caused by high-energy trauma unless there is a pathology that has weakened the bone.

Delbet classified these fractures into four types (Figure 3.4.4). Type I is a transepiphyseal separation, with (Type IA) or without (Type IB) dislocation of the femoral head from the acetabulum. Type II is a transcervical fracture. Type III is a basocervical fracture. Type IV is an intertrochanteric fracture.

The aim of treatment is early anatomic reduction of these fractures with stable internal fixation and application of hip spica. There have been high rates of coxa vara, delayed union, and non-union in patients treated without internal fixation. Undisplaced fractures can be treated with percutaneous pinning using wires or cannulated screws, depending on the size of the bone. Displaced fractures must be reduced anatomically, either by closed methods or by open methods using a Watson–Jones type approach.

Avascular necrosis is the most serious complication (30% overall) and is highest after displaced Types IB, II and III

Table 3.4.4 Guidance on femoral-shaft treatment

Age	Treatment option
<6 months	Pavlik harness
	Immediate hip spica
6 months to 5 years	Immediate hip spica
	Traction
5 years to 11 years	Flexible nailing
	Early hip spica
	Delayed hip spica
>11 years	Flexible nailing
	Plating
	External fixator
	Locked nailing

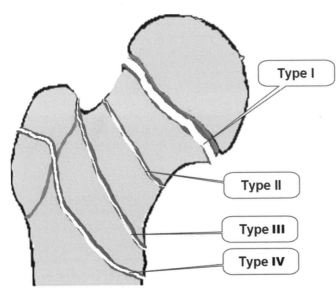

Figure 3.4.4 Delbet classification. Type I is a transepiphyseal separation, with (Type IA) or without (Type IB) dislocation of the femoral head from the acetabulum. Type II is a transcervical fracture. Type III is a basocervical fracture. Type IV is an intertrochanteric fracture.

fractures. Early treatment, anatomical reduction and evacuation of haematoma may reduce the risk of AVN. Signs and symptoms of AVN usually develop within the first year after injury, but sometimes develop as late as 2 years. Several joint-preserving procedures for AVN have been advocated, including core decompression, vascularized fibular grafting and the trapdoor procedure, but their therapeutic value remains uncertain in this age group.

Other complications include coxa vara (20–30%), premature growth arrest (28%) and non-union (8%) [3]. Coxa vara may be caused by malunion, AVN, premature physeal closure or a combination of these problems. The capital femoral physis contributes only 13% of the growth of the entire limb; hence, shortening due to premature growth arrest is not significant, except in very young children. Non-union is generally seen after Type II or III fractures and usually due to failure to obtain or maintain an anatomic reduction. A CT scan is

helpful to establish non-union, which should be treated operatively, either by using rigid internal fixation or by subtrochanteric valgus osteotomy, to allow compression across the fracture. Because the approach necessary for bone grafting is extensive, it should be reserved for persistent non-union [3].

Femoral fractures

Femoral-shaft fractures account for approximately 1.6% of all bony injuries in children. There is a bimodal distribution, with peak incidences at 2 and 12 years of age. Most femoral fractures unite rapidly without significant complications or sequelae. Although femoral fractures were traditionally treated with traction and casting, alternative treatment options, such as external fixation, compression or submuscular plating, and flexible or locked intramedullary nailing, have become available [3].

Classification of femoral fractures is based on the site (proximal, shaft or distal third), fracture configuration (transverse, oblique or spiral) or comminution (comminuted or non-comminuted).

Table 3.4.4 shows the treatment options. It is important to discuss these options with patients and parents, outlining the pros and cons of each option.

Children from 0 to 6 months

A femoral fracture in children of this age (or a small child up to 12 months of age) is best managed in a Pavlik harness, rather than a hip spica. A retrospective study of 40 patients by Podeszwa [5] compared application of the Pavlik harness and spica casting for the treatment of infant femoral-shaft fracture. No difference was found in radiographic outcomes, but approximately one-third of all spica patients experienced development of a skin complication. The authors conclude that all children younger than 1 year with a femoral-shaft fracture should be considered for treatment with a Pavlik harness, as it offers several advantages, including ease of application (no need for a general anaesthetic or sedation), short length of stay, the ability to adjust the harness when fracture manipulation is required, and ease of nursing.

Children from 6 months to 5 years

Immediate hip spica (single-leg spica) is preferred over double-leg spica [6]) and is the first-line treatment in this age group, unless there is an unacceptable deformity (shortening of >3 cm or angulation >30°), significant swelling or unsupportive social circumstances, in which case traction may be considered. In a multiply injured patient, traction may be used until associated injuries permit definitive treatment.

The spica should be placed with the thigh flexed approximately 60–90° (the more proximal the fracture, the more flexion is required) and abducted to 30°. In general, an acceptable reduction is no more than 30° sagittal plane angulation and 15° of coronal plane deformity with shortening not exceeding 3 cm.

Alternatives are Gallows traction or Bryant traction, where both legs are placed in traction with the thigh flexed to 45° and abduction of 30°. Traction is contraindicated in children younger than 2 or weighing less than 12 kg.

Children from 5 to 11 years

Flexible nailing is the preferred option in this age group, and offers excellent fracture union with few reported complications. Nails may be placed in an antegrade or retrograde fashion, depending on the location of the fracture site (insertion is preferable through the larger fragment) and the experience of the surgeon. The nail size is 1/3 of the bone diameter and the nails should be bent to three times the bone diameter with the apex of the bend at the fracture site.

A transverse fracture with minimal comminution is the ideal indication; however, flexible nailing can be used with caution for long oblique and spiral fractures. If there is any concern about the stability of the fracture, a hip spica can be used to supplement the fixation for a short period.

The nails should be left in place for a year before removal. There is some controversy about removing asymptomatic flexible intramedullary nails. The potential advantages of nail removal are: (1) elimination of stress risers at the insertion site and (2) the ease of nail removal at 1 year as opposed to years later, when the nail end is covered by bone [7].

In a retrospective series of 234 fractures of the femur in 229 children treated with flexible nailing between 1996 and 2003, Moroz *et al.* [8] reported excellent outcomes in 150 (64%), satisfactory outcomes in 57 (24%), and poor outcomes in 23 (10%) fractures. Poor outcomes were due to LLD in 5 fractures, unacceptable angulation in 17, and fixation failure in 1. There was a statistically significant relationship between age ($P = 0.003$), weight (54 kg vs 39 kg; $P = 0.003$) and outcome. Poor outcome was noted in children who were older than 11 years or heavier than 49 kg (odds ratio = 3.8 and 5, respectively).

In another comparative study [9], of 28 patients with femoral fractures (aged 8 to 13 years old): 14 patients (group I) were treated by conventional 90–90 balanced skeletal traction with late hip spica, while 14 (group II) with multiple associated injuries or hyperkinetic problems were treated with flexible nailing. Flexible nailing yielded results superior to the

hip spica with the advantage of early discharge from hospital and return to school.

In a randomized controlled trial [10], Bar-On and colleagues compared external fixation with flexible nailing in 20 femoral fractures, which were randomly assigned (10 fractures each) to have external fixation (EF) or flexible intramedullary nailing (FIN). The duration of the operation averaged 56 minutes for the EF group, with 1.4 minutes of fluoroscopy, compared with 74 minutes and 2.6 minutes, respectively, for the FIN group. The times to full weight-bearing, full range of movement and return to school were all shorter in the FIN group. Complications for the FIN group included one transitory foot drop and two cases of bursitis at an insertion site. In the EF group there were one refracture, one rotatory malunion requiring remanipulation and two pin-track infections. After an average follow-up time of 14 months, two patients in the EF group had mild pain, four had quadriceps wasting, one had leg length discrepancy of over 1 cm, four had malalignment of >5°, and one had limited hip rotation. In the FIN group, one patient had mild pain and one had quadriceps wasting; there were no length discrepancies, malalignment or limitation of movement. Parents of the FIN group were more satisfied. Bar-On and colleagues recommended the use of flexible intramedullary nailing for fractures of the femoral shaft that required surgery, and reserved external fixation for open or severely comminuted fractures.

Children 11 years and older

Despite poor results obtained from the Moroz series in older patients, most studies have reported good outcomes from flexible nailing in a selected group (stable fracture pattern) of patients. Submuscular plate fixation may be considered for unstable patterns. External fixators are an alternative, particularly with open fractures. A trochanteric entry rigid locked intramedullary nail has become more popular in older children, in spite of the risk of osteonecrosis.

In a study of 31 femoral-shaft fractures in 30 patients treated with interlocking intramedullary nails (average age 12 + 3 years) at the time of injury [11], all fractures united, and the average LLD was 0.51 cm. Two patients had an overgrowth of >2.5 cm; none had angular or rotational deformity. One patient (3%) developed asymptomatic osteonecrosis.

References

1. Weinstein JN, Kuo KN and Millar EA (1984) Congenital coxa vara. A retrospective review. *J Pediatr Orthop* **4**(1):70–7.

2. National Institute for Health and Clinical Excellence (2009) *Combined Bony and Soft Tissue Reconstruction for Hip Joint Stabilisation in Proximal Focal Femoral Deficiency (PFFD)*. London: NICE.

3. Beaty JH and Kasser JR (2006) *Rockwood and Wilkins' Fractures in Children*, 6th edition. Philadelphia: Lippincott Williams & Wilkins.

4. Brinker MR (2000) *Review of Orthopaedic Trauma*. London: WB Saunders.

5. Podeszwa DA, Mooney JF 3rd, Cramer KE and Mendelow MJ (2004) Comparison of Pavlik harness application and immediate spica casting

for femur fractures in infants. *J Pediatr Orthop* **24**(5):460–2.

6. Epps HR, Molenaar E and O'Connor DP (2006) Immediate single-leg spica cast for pediatric femoral diaphysis fractures. *J Pediatr Orthop* **26**(4):491–6.

7. Herring JA (2008) *Tachdjian's Pediatric Orthopaedics*, 4th edition, volume 1. Philadelphia: Saunders Elsevier.

8. Moroz LA, Launay F, Kocher MS *et al.* (2006) Titanium elastic nailing of

fractures of the femur in children. Predictors of complications and poor outcome. *J Bone Joint Surg Br* **88**(10):1361–6.

9. Kissel EU and Miller ME (1989) Closed Ender nailing of femur fractures in older children. *J Trauma* **29**(11):1585–8.

10. Bar-On E, Sagiv S and Porat S (1997) External fixation or flexible intramedullary nailing for femoral shaft fractures in children. A prospective, randomised study. *J Bone Joint Surg Br* **79**(6):975–8. Erratum in *J Bone Joint Surg Br* (1998) **80**(4):749.

11. Beaty JH, Austin SM, Warner WC, Canale ST and Nichols L (1994) Interlocking intramedullary nailing of femoral-shaft fractures in adolescents: preliminary results and complications. *J Pediatr Orthop* **14**(2):178–83.

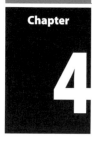

Chapter

The knee

4

Sattar Alshryda and Fazal Ali

Bow leg and knock knees

Bow leg (Figure 4.1) and knock knees are common referrals to children's orthopaedic clinics. Most are physiological; however, pathological causes must be excluded (Table 4.1).

The leg alignment in the coronal plane (varus and valgus) undergoes a unique pattern of changes from birth until adulthood, as described by Salenius and Vankka [1]. Most newborn babies have an average knee varus of 10°–15°. This begins to be corrected during the second year of life, reaching about 10° of valgus at around 4 years of age. The valgus alignment then gradually decreases, reaching the adult value (5° of valgus) around 8 years of age (see Figure 4.2). The standard deviation (SD) is 8° (more in the boys, 10°, and less in the girls, 7°).

Children with physiological genu varum and internal tibial torsion typically come to medical attention after the standing age (between 12 and 24 months), usually because of parental concern regarding the appearance of the legs, and these children have no other significant findings on clinical examination.

In most cases, a history and clinical examination is all that is required to differentiate between pathological and physiological bowing. A healthy child with normal developmental milestones, fairly symmetrical bowing and no other skeletal abnormalities is likely to have a physiological bowing. Radiographs are generally unnecessary, but may be required occasionally to help differentiate pathological from physiological bowing.

In physiological bowing, radiographs may show an apparent delay in ossification of the medial side of the distal femoral and proximal tibial epiphyses or flaring of the medial distal femoral metaphysis and a normal-looking physis. The following rules are helpful but not infallible.

Genu varum is more likely to be pathological if it is:

1. Present after 2 years,
2. Unilateral or there is asymmetry of more than 5°,
3. Associated with shortening of the limb (or stature),
4. Severe (beyond 2 standard deviations of the mean, as per Salenius chart; 1 SD = 8°),
5. Present in an obese child.

Genu valgus is more likely to be pathological if it is:

1. Severe (intermalleolar distance >10 cm at 10 years or >15 cm at 5 years),
2. Unilateral.

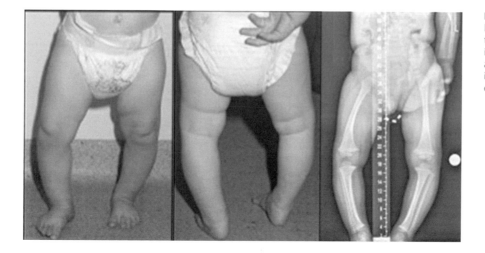

Figure 4.1 Standing child with symmetrical bow leg (bilateral genu varum). Both feet look normal, the right foot points forward and the left points inward. The appearance of the tibial tuberosities and the ankles give the impression that there is internal tibial torsion as well; however, this must be confirmed by further clinical evaluation.

Postgraduate Paediatric Orthopaedics, ed. Sattar Alshryda, Stan Jones and Paul A. Banaszkiewicz. Published by Cambridge University Press. © Cambridge University Press 2014.

The following radiological measurements (Figure 4.3) are useful (ensure that the patella is facing forward):

1. Tibiofemoral angle,
2. The mechanical and anatomical axes deviation,
3. Metaphyseal–diaphyseal angle (MDA) of Levine and Drennan (normal, <11°; abnormal, >16°),
4. Epiphyseal–metaphyseal angle (EMA) (normal, <20°).

The tibiofemoral angle is formed by the intersection of the two mid-diaphyseal lines of the femur and the tibia, respectively. The value should be within the normal range depicted by a Salenius curve.

The mechanical and anatomical axes deviation is the distance between the mechanical axes of the lower limb and the centre of the knee (the anatomic axes cross the knee almost at the centre). The normal mechanical axes pass 8 ± 7 mm medial to the centre of the knee.

The metaphyseal–diaphyseal angle (MDA) is the angle formed by a line connecting the most distal point on the medial and lateral beaks of the proximal tibial metaphysis

and a line perpendicular to the anatomic axis (or lateral cortex) of the tibia (see Figure 4.3).

Levine and Drennan [2] reported that a child was more likely to develop Blount's disease if the initial MDA were more than 11°.

The epiphyseal–metaphyseal angle (EMA) is determined by measuring the angle formed by a line through the proximal tibial physis parallel to the base of the epiphyseal ossification centre and a line connecting the midpoint of the base of the epiphyseal ossification centre to the most distal point on the medial beak of the proximal tibial metaphysis (see Figure 4.3).

Davids et al. [3] observed that children younger than 3 with a MDA >10° and an EMA >20° were at greater risk of developing Blount's disease and should be followed closely. In their study, none of the children with a MDA <10° and an EMA <20° developed Blount's disease.

Blount's disease

Blount's disease is a type of idiopathic tibia vara. It is uncommon, and is characterized by disordered ossification of the medial aspect of the proximal tibial physis, epiphysis and metaphysis.

Though the cause is unknown, it is thought to be a combination of excessive compressive forces on the proximal medial metaphysis of the tibia and altered enchondral bone formation. There are two recognized types of idiopathic tibia vara, infantile (<4 years) and adolescent (>10 years) (see Table 4.2).

A third type, juvenile tibia vara, has been described for Blount's disease in children aged 4 to 10 years.

Infantile tibia vara

This is bilateral in 80% of cases and more prevalent in girls, blacks and children with marked obesity (Figure 4.4). These children generally start walking early (before 10 months of age). Associated clinical findings include a lateral thrust of the knee when walking, internal tibial torsion and LLD.

Table 4.1 Causes of genu varus (bow leg) and genu valgus (knock knees)

Bow leg	Knock knees
1. Physiological	1. Physiological
2. Tumours such as osteochondroma	2. Tumours such as osteochondromas
3. Skeletal dysplasia	3. Skeletal dysplasia
4. Blount's disease	4. Primary tibia valga
5. Infection	5. Infection
6. Trauma	6. Trauma
7. Metabolic (vitamin D deficiency, fluoride poisoning, osteogenesis imperfecta)	7. Renal osteodystrophy
8. Focal fibrocartilaginous dysplasia	8. Neuromuscular disorders (polio) and tight iliotibial band

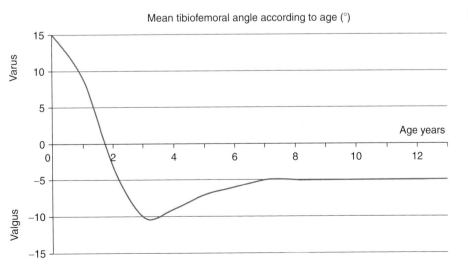

Mean tibiofemoral angle according to age (°)

Figure 4.2 Salenius curve.

Table 4.2 Summary of the differences between infantile and adolescent tibia vara [7]

	Infantile type	Adolescent type
Clinical	The typical patient is an obese female, <4 years with lateral knee thrust.	The typical patient is a male teenager, often black, whose body weight greatly exceeds 2 standard deviations (SD) above the mean.
Radiological	Medially sloped and irregularly ossified epiphysis, sometimes triangular. Prominent beaking of the medial metaphysis with lucent cartilage islands within the beak. Widened and irregular physeal line medially. Lateral subluxation of the proximal end of the tibia. Varus angulation at the epiphyseal–metaphyseal junction.	The shape of the epiphysis is relatively normal. Lack of beaking of the medial tibial metaphysis. Widening of the proximal medial physeal plate, sometimes extending across to the lateral side of the physis. Widening of the lateral distal femoral physis in comparison to either the medial femoral physis of the same knee or the distal femoral physis of the normal knee.
Treatment	Treatment is based on the stage of the disease. Orthosis is indicated in the early stages. The goal of surgical treatment is to overcorrect the mechanical axis. Hemiepiphysiodesis (alone) is not usually effective or adequate.	Treatment is usually surgical as orthosis is usually ineffective. The goal of surgical treatment is to correct the mechanical axis to normal (avoid overcorrection) so that physeal growth is restored and degenerative arthritis of the medial compartment of the knee can be avoided. Lateral hemiepiphysiodesis (alone) can be successful treatment in 50–70% of the cases.

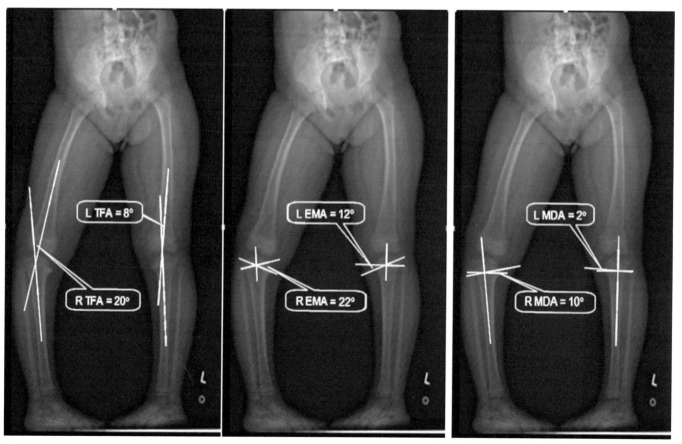

Figure 4.3 Radiological measurements in genu varum. EMA, epiphyseal–metaphyseal angle; MDA, metaphyseal–diaphyseal angle; TFA, tibiofemoral angle.

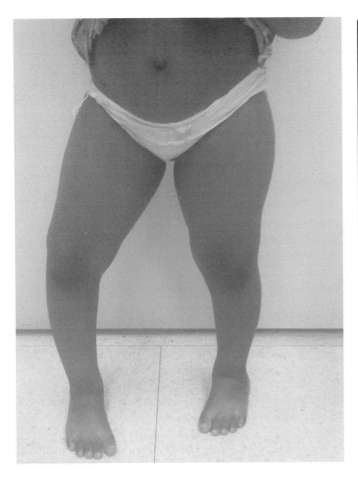

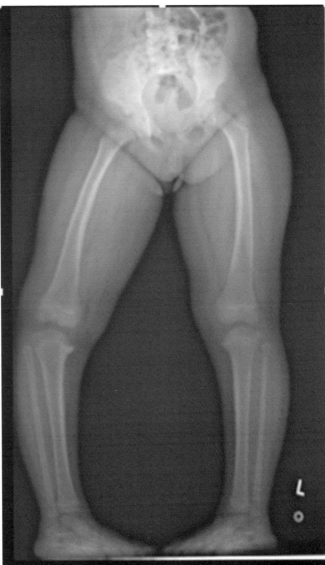

Figure 4.4 Photograph and X-ray of 5-year-old African child with Blount's disease. There is an obvious varus deformity of the right leg, specifically around the knee. The child is overweight. Both feet point inward (right > left), the patellae seem to be pointing outward, indicating bilateral tibial internal tibial torsion (right > left). The X-ray shows a varus angulation of the right knee and, to a much lesser extent, the left knee. There is a medially sloped and irregularly ossified epiphysis and prominent beaking of the medial metaphysis. It is difficult to visualize the physis.

Adolescent tibia vara

This is unilateral in 80% of cases. Patients are usually overweight and complain of pain at the medial aspect of the knee. A leg length discrepancy is generally observed and the femoral alignment is often abnormal.

Diagnosis

The diagnosis is made based on the characteristic clinical presentation and X-ray findings (Figures 4.3 and 4.5), which include:

1. Sharp varus angulation in the proximal tibial metaphysis,
2. Widened and irregular physeal line medially,
3. Medially sloped and irregularly ossified epiphysis,
4. Prominent beaking of the medial metaphysis with lucent cartilage islands within the beak.

Although rare, focal fibrocartilaginous dysplasia (FFD) has many similar features. Clinically, there is significant hyperextension of the knee in FFD. Radiologically there is an abrupt varus at the metaphyseal–diaphyseal junction of the tibia with surrounding cortical sclerosis; usually a radiolucent area just proximal to the area of cortical sclerosis and the physis appears normal.

It is important to assess the whole leg for any associated deformities. An increased mLDFA (mechanical lateral distal femoral angle) reveals a significant varus of both distal femurs (Figure 4.5). It is not unusual to have Blount's disease on a background of physiological varus.

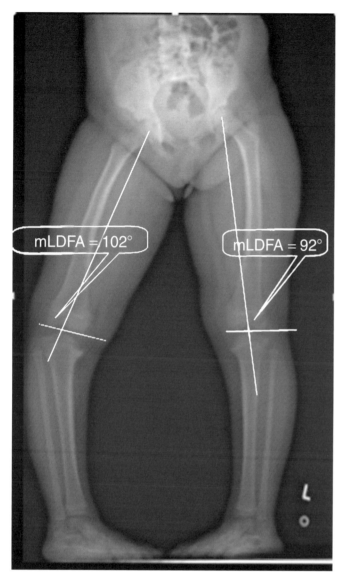

Figure 4.5 Femoral involvement in Blount's disease. There is bilateral increase in the mLDFA, indicating varus deformity of the distal femur and the proximal tibia.

Classification

Langenskiold [4] proposed a six-stage radiological classification (Figure 4.6). This classification was not intended for use in determining the prognosis or the most desirable type of treatment. However, it is generally accepted that surgical treatment is required for any child with Stage III–VI changes (Table 4.3).

Treatment in children younger than 3 years
Bracing

This is indicated in children younger than 3. Risk factors for failure are instability, obesity and delayed bracing. Raney *et al.* [5] reported their experience with 38 patients (60 tibia vara) with MDA of >16° or MDA between 9° and 16° with a clinical risk factor for progression, such as ligamentous instability, patient weight above the 90th percentile, bilateral involvement or late initiation of bracing. The success rate was 90% (54 tibias); 27 tibias were treated by full-time bracing, 23 by night-time bracing only and 4 by daytime use. Valgus correction should be increased every 2 months to promote correction; if no correction is achieved within a year, the brace has probably not been successful. Bracing is not recommended for children older than 3 years.

Treatment in children older than 3 years
Lateral tibial hemiepiphysiodesis (using 8-plate)

This may be the sole treatment or implemented as an adjunct to tibial osteotomy with variable success rates. Successful outcomes have been noted in adolescent tibia vara when the physis is sufficiently open, the varus deformity is mild to moderate and patients are younger than 10 [6].

Proximal tibial osteotomy

In the young child, an acute correction is undertaken and the osteotomy is stabilized with K-wires and a cast. In the older child, external fixators may be used to facilitate gradual correction.

Management of Langenskiold Stages V and VI needs special considerations. Patient age, future growth, magnitude of deformity and joint surface congruity all influence decision making. Additional surgical procedures required at the time of tibial osteotomy may include:

- Resection of the bony bridge and placement of interposition graft (fat). This is indicated in children <7 years of age, to enable physeal growth and reduce the risk of recurrence of the deformity.
- Epiphysiodesis: this is undertaken in the presence of large bony bridges that are not amenable to resection. If more than 2 years of growth are expected, a limb-lengthening procedure is required, to prevent a LLD developing. This can be done concomitantly.
- Significant incongruity and depression of the medial joint surface may require a curved osteotomy to facilitate elevation of the medial tibial plateau.

Table 4.2 summarizes the differences between infantile and adolescent tibia vara.

Bowing of the tibia

Three types of tibial bowing are described (Table 4.4), depending on the direction of the bow.

Posteromedial tibial bowing

This is seen shortly after birth and is often associated with a calcaneovalgus deformity of the foot (Figure 4.7). It is considered to be physiological and thought to be due to intra-uterine malposition. Spontaneous resolution is the rule, although

Table 4.3 Langenskiold classification of Blount's disease

Stage	Description	Treatment
I	Medial beaking, irregular medial ossification with protrusion of the metaphysis	Orthotic for <3 years old
II	Cartilage fills depression Progressive depression of medial epiphysis with the epiphysis sloping medially as disease progresses	Failure of full correction or progression to Type III → surgery
III	Ossification of the inferomedial corner of the epiphysis	Surgery around the age of 4
IV	Epiphyseal ossification filling the metaphyseal depression	
V	Double epiphyseal plate (cleft separating two epiphysis)	
VI	Medial physeal closure	

Table 4.4 Tibial bowing

Type	Cause	Treatment
Posteromedial	Physiological	Observation, rarely causes LLD
Anteromedial	Fibular hemimelia	Reconstruction vs amputation for severe deformities
Anterolateral	Congenital pseudarthrosis	Total contact brace, intramedullary fixation, external fixators or amputation

the child may develop a residual LLD. The foot deformity generally resolves by 9 months and the tibial bowing by the age of 2. The parents are encouraged to undertake stretching exercises to facilitate correction of the foot deformity and should be counselled about the probable need for limb lengthening if a LLD develops. In severe cases, it may be necessary to use serial casting into plantar flexion (Figure 4.8) followed by splints or bracing to maintain the position until weight-bearing is possible.

Anterolateral tibial bowing

This is commonly associated with tibial pseudarthrosis (see Figure 4.9), which is a rare, incompletely understood condition. Many cases have been linked to neurofibromatosis (50%, but only 10% of patients with neurofibromatosis have this disorder),

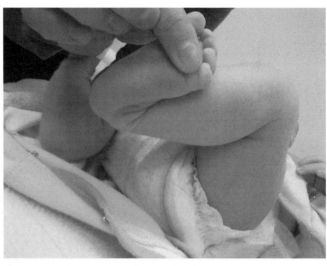

Figure 4.7 Calcaneovalgus deformity of the foot.

Figure 4.6 Langenskiold classification of Blount's disease.

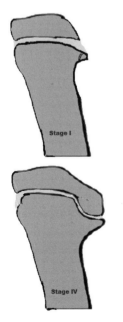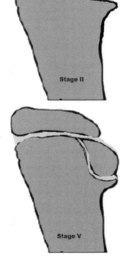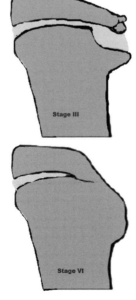

67

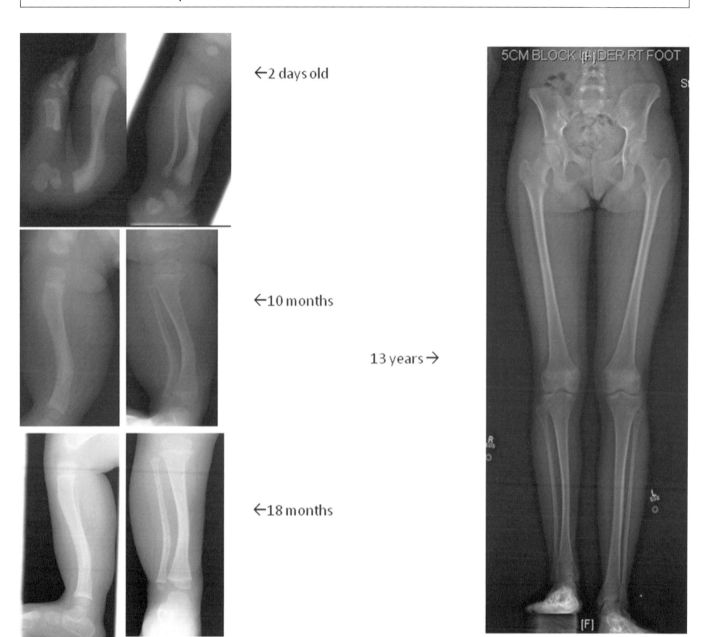

←2 days old

←10 months

13 years →

←18 months

5CM BLOCK [H]DER RT FOOT

Figure 4.8 Posteromedial bowing of the right tibia. These X-rays show a resolved posteromedial bowing of the right leg. The bowing was almost resolved at 18 months; however, the patient had a 5 cm LLD at 13 years of age.

fibrous dysplasia and amniotic band syndrome. A callus does not form at the fracture site, resulting in a pseudarthrosis. The site universally has fibrous tissue.

The diagnosis can be made at birth in severe deformities or in those with a fracture. Milder forms may present later in childhood with tibial bowing, a limp and an actual fracture.

Classifications, such as Boyd's and Crawford's, have been advocated. They are more descriptive and do not provide guidance on management or eventual outcome.

Crawford's four radiographic types are:

I. Anterolateral bowing. The medullary canal is preserved and dense. Cortical thickening might be observed. This type has the best prognosis and may never fracture.

II. Anterolateral bowing with thinned medullary canal, cortical thickening and trabeculation defect. This type should be protected with a brace and considered for surgery.

III. Anterolateral bowing with a cystic lesion. This type has a high risk of fracture and should be treated with fixation and bone graft.

IV. Anterolateral bowing with fracture or pseudarthrosis. This has the worst prognosis.

A simpler and probably more useful classification is based on age and the presence of a fracture:

I. With or without fracture,

II. Younger or older than 4 years of age.

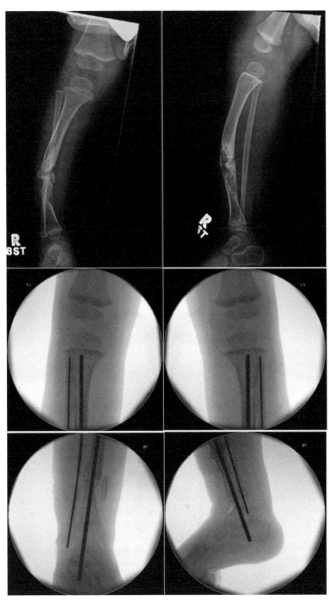

Figure 4.9 Anterolateral bowing with pseudarthrosis (common association). The X-ray shows tibial pseudarthrosis and anterolateral tibial bowing. There is bowing of the tibia anteriorly and laterally (hence, 'anterolateral' bowing) with narrowing of the tibial shaft and sclerosis encroaching on the medullary cavity at the apex. The apex of the curve is typically at the junction of the middle and distal thirds of the tibial shaft. The lower four intraoperative images show that the tibia and fibula were both nailed after excision of the pseudarthrosis and bone graft.

Treatment

Treating anterolateral bowing with pseudarthrosis and fracture is very challenging and the outcome may be unfavourable. Parental education is an essential part of the treatment.

- Braces, i.e. a clam shell, can be used to prevent fractures. If a fracture occurs, casting and bracing may achieve union in those younger than 4 years old or with first time fractures.
- For recurring or unhealed fractures, the alignment should be corrected and the fracture stabilized.

Several forms of surgical interventions have been tried with variable success rates. The current trend is excision of the pseudarthrosis, shortening of the tibia, stabilization with intramedullary telescopic nailing (through the foot or through the fracture site) and autologous bone graft. Bone morphogenic protein (BMP), particularly in Type II, has been shown to be a useful adjunct; however, the long-term safety and potential for neoplastic transformation is a concern.

Other treatment options include:

1. Excision of the pseudarthrosis and bone transport using a circular frame,
2. Ipsilateral or contralateral vascularized fibular graft,
3. Amputation may be considered if reconstructive surgery fails.

Anteromedial tibial bowing

This is usually caused by fibular hemimelia (Figure 4.10) and the treatment is directed toward the latter.

Fibular hemimelia is the most common long bone deficiency (1/600). The aetiology is unknown and the fibular deficiency may be intercalary or terminal.

Clinical features may include absence of the lateral foot rays, a hypoplastic foot, tarsal coalition, a ball-and-socket ankle joint, ankle instability, hindfoot valgus, a short tibial segment, the absence of knee ligaments (i.e. anterior cruciate ligament), a hypoplastic lateral femoral condyle with a valgus knee deformity, PFFD or significant LLD.

Various classifications have been advised to describe the condition and plan management.

Achterman and Kalamchi

Type I. Hypoplastic fibula:

    Ia. Proximal fibula is more distal and distal fibula is more proximal,

    Ib. At least 30–50% of the fibula is absent.

Type II. Complete absence.

Coventry and Johnson

Type I. Hypoplastic:

    Ia. Normal foot,

    Ib. Equinovalgus foot.

Type II. Complete absence,

Type III. Bilateral.

Birch's functional classification (Table 4.5)

The treatment options depend on the predicted LLD and foot function. Hip dysplasia must be treated before undertaking femoral lengthening, to prevent subluxation of the hip joint. In addition, the knee and ankle joints must be temporarily stabilized when undertaking femoral and tibial lengthening, thus preventing subluxation of these joints.

Table 4.5 Birch's functional classification and treatment guidelines

Classification			Treatment
Type I: functional foot	IA	0%–5% inequality	Orthosis, epiphysiodesis
	IB	6%–10% inequality	Epiphysiodesis with or without limb lengthening
	IC	11%–30% inequality	One or two limb-lengthening procedures or amputation
	ID	>30% inequality	More than two limb-lengthening procedures or amputation
Type II: non-functional foot	IIA	Functional upper limb	Early amputation
	IIB	Non-functional upper limb	Consider limb salvage procedure

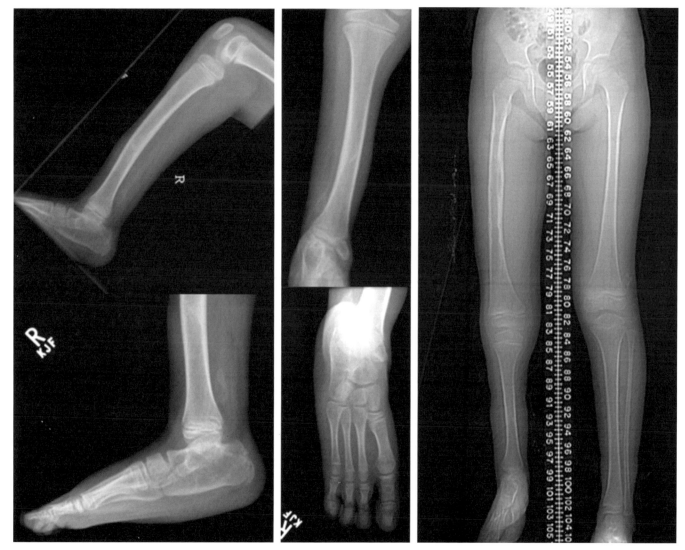

Figure 4.10 Anteromedial bowing associated with fibular hemimelia. There is an almost complete absence of the fibula (apart from high riding lateral malleolus) with slight anteromedial bowing and short right limb. There are four foot rays with absent lateral ray. There is some sclerosis and bony changes of the right femur; this may reflect an associated congenital short femur that had been lengthened.

Miscellaneous conditions

Tibial hemimelia

Tibial hemimelia has an autosomal dominant mode of inheritance and is less common than fibular hemimelia. However, it is more commonly associated with other bony anomalies (preaxial polydactyl, cleft hand) or syndromes (75% of patients) (Figure 4.11). Clinical features include a short tibia that is bowed anterolaterally with a prominent proximal fibula and equinovarus foot. There are two recognized classifications.

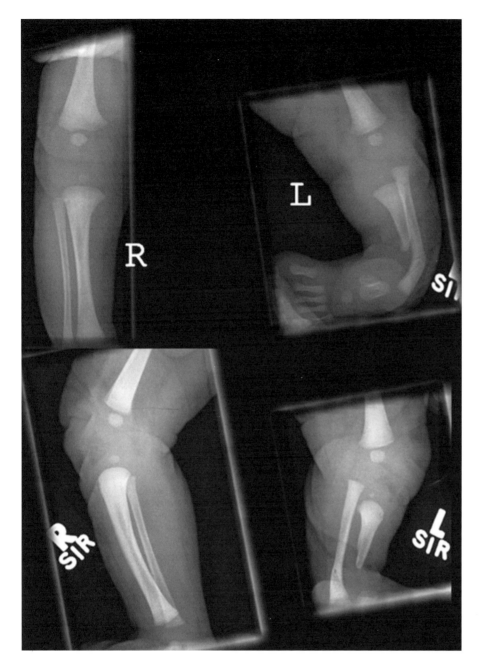

Figure 4.11 X-rays of a child with tibial hemimelia, showing left and right lower limb. There is a partial absence of the tibia (Type II) and a hypertrophied fibula, and the ankle is in severe varus. The foot has five rays and well-developed calcaneum, talus and cuboid. Before recommending any treatment, a thorough history should be obtained and thorough examination and investigation should be performed. Treatment should be provided by a multidisciplinary team. It is surgically possible to fuse the proximal tibia and fibula at this stage and perform lengthening in the future. The ankle should be stabilized in plantigrade or perform a Syme's amputation.

Kalamachi

Type I. Complete absence: the knee and ankle are grossly unstable.

Type II. Absence of distal half: the ankle is unstable.

Type III. Hypoplastic: the tibia is shortened, proximal migration of fibula and diastasis of distal tibia-fibular joint.

Jones' classification

See Table 4.6 [8].

Congenital dislocation of the patella

This is a rare condition with varying presentation. The patella is usually hypoplastic and laterally displaced with varying degrees of knee flexion (Figure 4.12).

Mild cases may not present until school age, with weak knee extension interfering with function. Severe cases are usually observed at birth and radiographic assessment is complicated by the fact that the patella may almost be confluent with the lateral femoral condyle. The severe form needs to be differentiated from other causes of congenital flexion contractures, such as:

1. Limb dysplasia, such as congenital femoral deficiency or tibial hemimelia,
2. Syndromes with soft-tissue contracture, such as arthrogryposis, pterygium syndromes and Beals syndrome (congenital contractural arachnodactyly),
3. Neurological syndromes, such as sacral agenesis and myelodysplasia,

Table 4.6 Jones' classification and treatment guidelines

Type	Radiological description	Clinical description
Ia	Tibia not seen with hypoplastic lower femoral epiphysis	Child has knee flexion contracture and hamstring function but not quadriceps function. The patella is typically absent and the foot, which is fixed in severe varus, has minimal functional movement. Treatment options are knee disarticulation or centralization of the fibula (Brown's procedure).
Ib	Tibia not seen but normal lower femoral epiphysis	Hamstring and quadriceps function is normal, and knee moves normally. The fibular head is displaced proximally and laterally, and the limb is in a varus position, with significant varus instability. The foot is displaced medially relative to the fibula and is in varus.
II	Distal tibia not seen	Good functional results can be obtained by fusing the proximal fibula to the upper part of the tibia (fusion cannot be obtained until there is sufficient ossification of the upper tibia to allow for successful synostosis with the fibula). A Syme's amputation with subsequent prosthetic management is the best treatment for the distal part of the limb because of the severe foot and ankle instability.
III	Proximal tibia not seen	Knee is unstable, and there are extra digits distally. The tibial shaft is palpable, and there is a severe varus deformity of the leg. Some of these patients may benefit from tibial lengthening with or without Syme's or Chopart amputation, depending on the anatomy of the ankle joint.
IV	Diastasis of tibia and fibula	There is a diastasis of the distal tibia and fibula, the limb is short, and the foot is in a severe rigid varus, positioned between the tibia and the fibula. This can be treated by Syme's ankle disarticulation performed at walking age. Tibial lengthening and foot repositioning may make it possible to retain a plantigrade foot. The functional outcome may not be better than amputation.

4. Skeletal dysplasia with bony flexion deformity, such as diastrophic dysplasia.

The treatment is surgical and involves a stepwise approach:

- Extensive lateral release and advancement of the vastus medialis obliquus (VMO) distally and medially,
- V-Y quadricepsplasty and Goldthwait transfer of the lateral half of the tendon,
- Immobilization of the knee at 20° for 6–8 weeks, followed by intensive physiotherapy.

Congenital dislocation of the knee

This is also referred to as congenital hyperextension of the knee (Figure 4.13). This is a relatively rare birth condition; babies with this condition have a hyperextended knee that may or may not be reducible. One or both knees may be involved and a calcaneovalgus deformity of the foot may also be observed.

Bilateral congenital dislocation is associated with such anomalies as Larsen, Beals or Ehlers–Danlos syndromes, arthrogryposis or spinal dysraphism. Unilateral dislocation may be an ipsilateral hip dislocation or congenital talipes equinovarus (CTEV) (70% and 50%, respectively). The dislocation is classified into three types, based on physical examination and radiographic assessment (Table 4.7).

Treatment should be started as early as possible and involves gentle manipulation and serial casting. Once a flexion of 90° is obtained, a removable splint can be used for a few months to maintain correction. Aggressive manipulation is to be avoided, as it causes fractures or epiphyseal injuries.

Surgery is indicated if serial manipulation fails and is usually done between 6 months to 1 year of age. It involves one or more of the following:

- V-Y quadricepsplasty,
- Posterior capsulorrhaphy,
- Femoral shortening,
- ACL reconstruction.

Osteochondritis dissecans

This condition commonly affects the knee, although it can occur in other joints, such as the ankle (talus) and elbow (trochlea). The cause is unknown. However, it is thought that articular trauma and subchondral ischaemia might be contributing factors.

In the knee, it occurs in the lateral aspect of the medial femoral condyle in 70% of cases (lateral condyle, 20%; patella, 10%). Boys are affected more commonly and the condition is bilateral in 25% of patients.

Patients may present with a limp, knee pain and clicking with or without swelling. There is often a history of an injury.

The diagnosis is confirmed by plain radiographs (Figure 4.14), including tunnel views, where it is best seen. MRI is useful for evaluating the status of the overlying cartilage and the amount of subchondral oedema. This helps in staging the lesion and, hence, predicting the outcome [9].

MRI classification (Guhl)

Type I. Signal change on MRI and the cartilage is intact.

Type II. High signal surrounding the bone portion, indicating detachment, but the cartilage is not breached.

Type III. Detachment of the bone and the cartilage is breached.

Type IV. There is displacement of the osteochondral fragment.

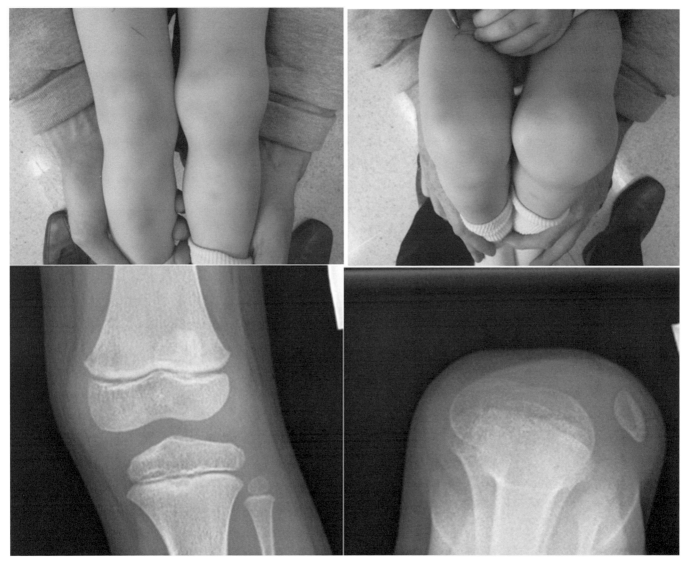

Figure 4.12 Congenital dislocation of the patella. The photographs show that the left patella is dislocated in flexion and partially reduced in extension. This is also shown on the X-radiograph. The patella does not normally ossify until about 3 years of age, and this may be delayed even further in the presence of congenital dislocation.

Good prognostic factors include early stage of the disease, small lesion (<20mm), location on the medial femoral condyle, younger age at presentation and open physis.

Treatment

Stable lesions are initially treated with activity modification, rest and sometimes area-specific offloading splintage. Surgical drilling may be considered if significant pain persists after 6 months of activity modification. This may be done arthroscopically using a transarticular approach or retro-articularly under image intensifier guidance. Although none of these approaches has been shown to be superior, the retro-articular approach is recommended if the lesion appears healed when viewed arthroscopically.

Unstable or loose lesions are treated by debridement of the bed followed by fixation with bio-absorbable pins or screws. Cancellous bone graft harvested from the tibia may be needed to restore the joint line. Non-viable fragments should be removed and the bed debrided and microfractured (Figure 4.15).

There is currently no evidence on the use of such techniques as osteochondral grafting, mosaicplasty or chondrocyte transplantation in the skeletally immature.

Traumatic injuries
Distal femur fractures

These injuries are classified by the Salter–Harris system. Type I and II injuries are usually treated conservatively. Other injuries may require closed or open reduction followed by

Table 4.7 Classification of congenital hyperextension of the knee

Grade	Descriptions
I: Congenital hyperextension	The knee can be flexed and reduced with gentle stretching of the quadriceps.
II: Congenital subluxation	The knee cannot be flexed beyond neutral. The femoral and tibial epiphyses are in contact and do not subluxate when flexion is attempted.
III: Congenital dislocation	Knee flexion is not possible and the tibia, which is anteriorly translated in the resting position, displaces laterally on the femur when more vigorous flexion is attempted. This is regarded as true irreducible congenital dislocation of the knee.

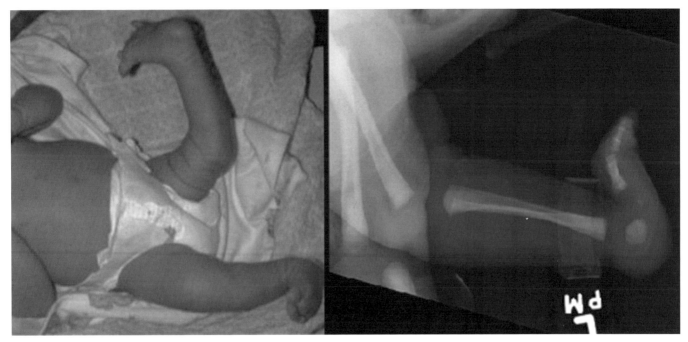

Figure 4.13 Photograph and X-ray showing marked left knee congenital hyperextension. There are abnormal skin creases. There are no obvious abnormalities in the feet.

internal fixation. With internal fixation, care should be taken to avoid the physis. If the physis does need to be crossed, smooth wires should be used and removed after 3–4 weeks (Figure 4.16).

Compartment syndrome and neurovascular injuries are rare but may be seen with displaced fractures, especially if the displacement is anterior.

Growth arrest is seen in 30%–50% of physeal injuries and may lead to angular deformities and LLD because of the rapid growth that takes place at the distal femur.

Patellar dislocation

Traumatic patella dislocation or subluxation is relatively common in children. It is probably the most common cause of a haemarthrosis in children. The incidence of recurrent dislocations is as high as 60% in patients aged 11–14 years and 30% in patients aged 15–18 years [10].

Risk factors include:

1. Female,
2. Q angle $> 20°$ (normal is 10° in boys and 15° in girls),
3. Genu valgus,
4. Rotational abnormalities, such as increased femoral anteversion or external tibial torsion,
5. Patella alta (Figure 4.17),
6. A shallow patella-femoral sulcus angle (ABC $> 144°$ is abnormal) (Figure 4.17),
7. Abnormal congruence angle of Merchant (OBX is normally $-6°$ to $-8°$). This angle is abnormal if it is more than $+16°$. Positive (+) means lateral while negative (−) means medial (Figure 4.17),
8. Vastus medialis obliquus hypoplasia,
9. Generalized ligamentous laxity,
10. Pes planus,
11. Lateral mobility greater than 3/4. (Medial mobility less than 1/4 indicates a tight lateral reticulum.)

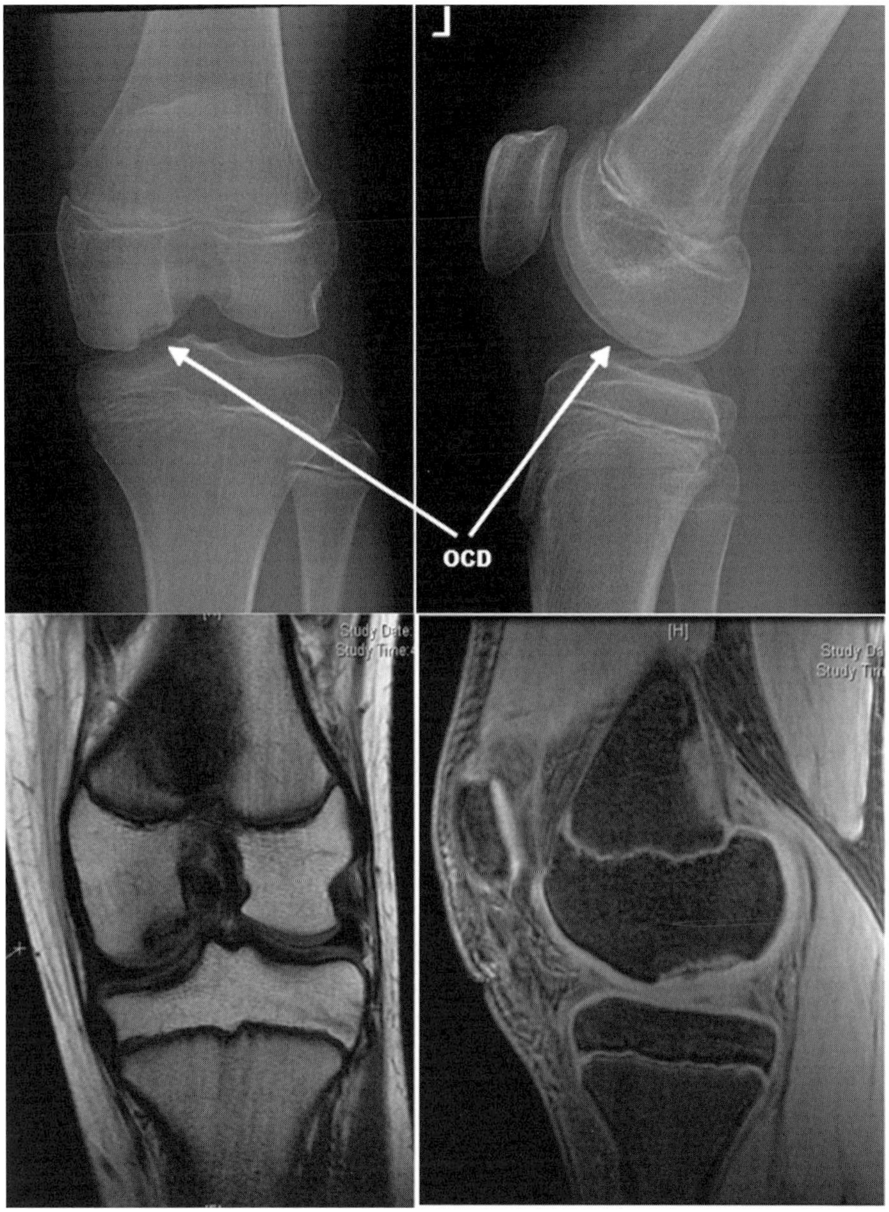

Figure 4.14 Osteochondritis dissecans (OCD).

Management

Most patellar dislocations are reduced spontaneously by simply extending the knee with or without gentle force directed anteromedially on the lateral patellar edge to lift the patella over the femoral condyle. Immobilization of the knee is in full extension for a maximum of 3 weeks to avoid muscle atrophy, knee-joint restrictions or retropatellar crepitation. This is followed by a period of physiotherapy [11].

Immediate surgery is recommended only in situations where there is an osteochondral fracture of the patella or femoral condyle (Figure 4.18). Small fragments are excised while large fragments are fixed.

Early medial patellofemoral ligament reconstruction has been suggested; however, a small randomized controlled trial (RCT) [12] of 62 patients that compared operative repair of the medial structures ($N = 36$) with non-operative treatment ($N = 28$) showed no difference in long-term outcome.

In patients with chronic patella instability that has failed to respond to physiotherapy, the consensus is to undertake surgery; this involves soft-tissue corrective procedures in the skeletally immature, with the addition of bony procedures in the mature individual.

The surgical interventions are summarized as:

- Proximal:
  - Lateral retinaculum release.
  - Medial (vastus medialis obliquus) advancement and reefing.

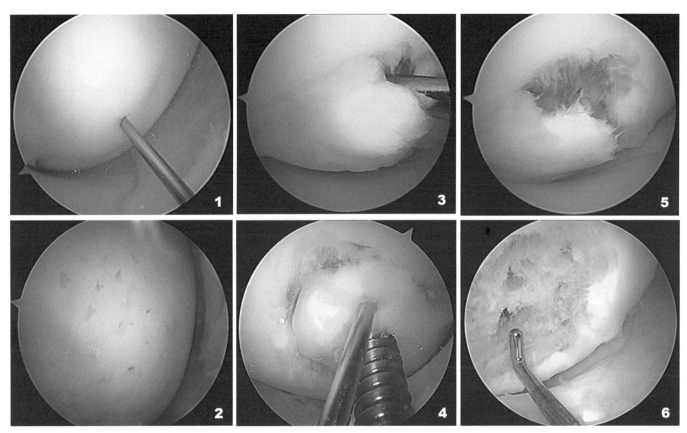

Figure 4.15 Arthroscopic pictures showing different interventions to treat osteochondritis dissecans of the knee. 1, 2: Transarticular drilling (notice the classical baseball on basketball appearance of the OCD). 3, 4: Fixation using headless screw. 5, 6: Debridement and microfractures.

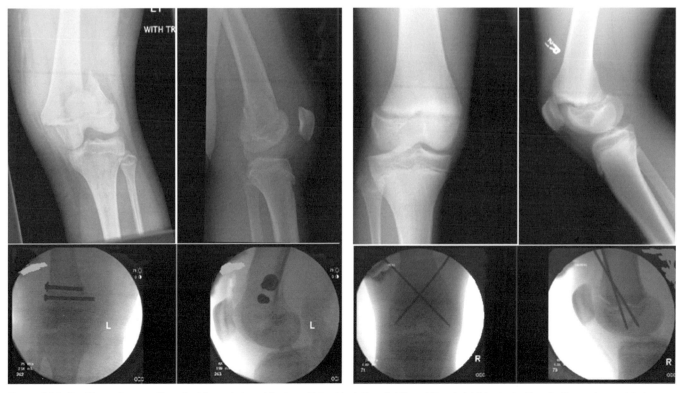

Figure 4.16 Distal femur fractures. Two distal femoral physeal fractures (Salter–Harris Type II, left, and Type I, right) treated with reduction and cannulated screws and fine K-wires, respectively.

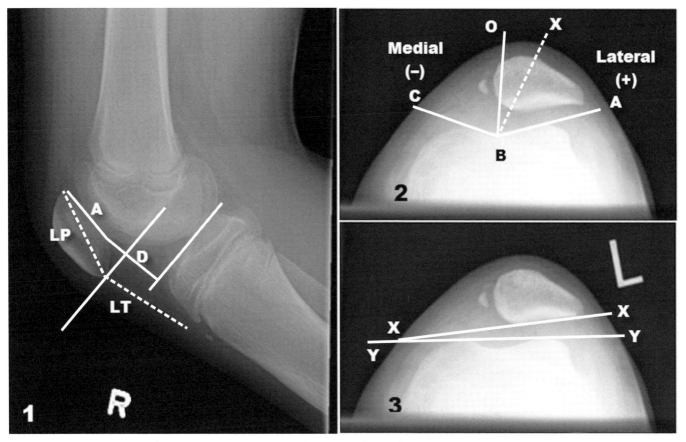

Figure 4.17 Radiological markers for patellar instability. Image 1 (knee lateral): With the knee flexed 30°, Blumensaat's line touches the lower border of the patella. Insall–Salvati index: the ratio, or index, of patella tendon length (LT) to patella length (LP) should be 1.0. An index of 1.2 is alta and of 0.8 is baja. Blackburne–Peel index: the ratio of the distance from the tibial plateau to the inferior articular surface of the patella (D) to the length of the articular surface of the patella (A) should be 0.8. An index of 1.0 is alta. Image 2: Sulcus angle ABC of 150°. Line BO is the bisector of the sulcus angle ABC. Line BX passes through the lowest point of the patella. Angle OXB is the congruence angle of Merchant, which is abnormally high (+20°) in this image. Also, notice the avulsion fracture of the MPFL. Image 3: The lateral patellofemoral angle should open laterally, as in this example.

Distal (not recommended in the presence of a normal Q angle):

- Roux–Goldthwait: half of the patellar tendon is transferred to the sartorius insertion.
- Elmslie–Trillat procedure: osteotomy of tibial tuberosity, preserving the distal attachment of the patellar tendon; the tuberosity is then moved medially and fixed with a single screw.
- Fulkerson technique: similar to Elmslie–Trillat, but a longer osteotomy; the direction of the cut should allow anteromedialization of the tibial tuberosity. It is then usually fixed with two or three screws.
- Galeazzi (for immature skeleton): semitendinosus is released proximally and passed through the patella and resutured on itself.
- Combined.
- Others:
  - MPFL (medial patella-femoral ligament) reconstruction.
  - Medial hemiepiphysiodesis in patients with bilateral genu valgum.

- Derotation osteotomy if there are significant torsional abnormalities (see Chapter 16).

Patellar fractures

These usually result from a direct blow or a forced flexion injury to the knee. If the fracture is through the bony part of the patella, the diagnosis is usually obvious from the radiographs. This must be differentiated from a bipartite patella. In a bipartite patella, the edges are typically rounded and are characteristically located in the superolateral part of the patella.

A patella sleeve fracture is a variation seen in children (Figure 4.19). The bony component is usually small but there is a large chondral segment that is attached to the bone. This chondral part is not seen on the radiographs and the only clue on the images may be a small bony fragment or a patella alta (or baja with proximal pole injuries). Hence, these injuries are frequently missed in the initial assessment.

Fractures through the bone may be treated as in adults with plaster immobilization for undisplaced fractures and tension band or cerclage wires for displaced fractures.

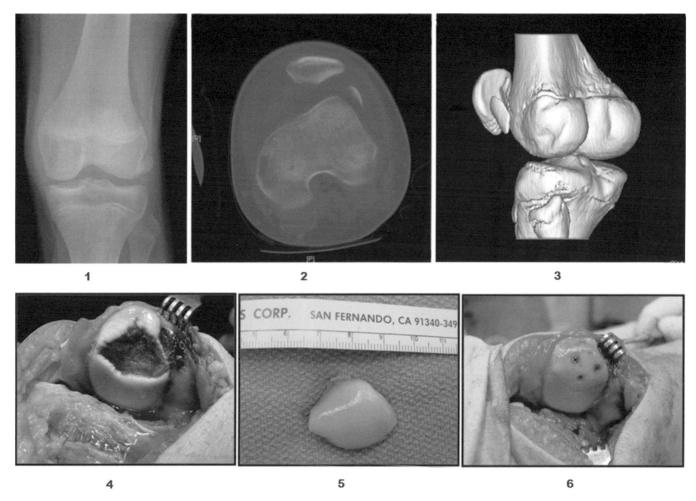

Figure 4.18 Patellar dislocation with osteochondral fragment.

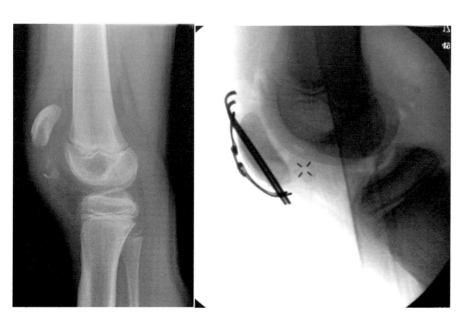

Figure 4.19 Sleeve fracture of the patella treated with tension band.

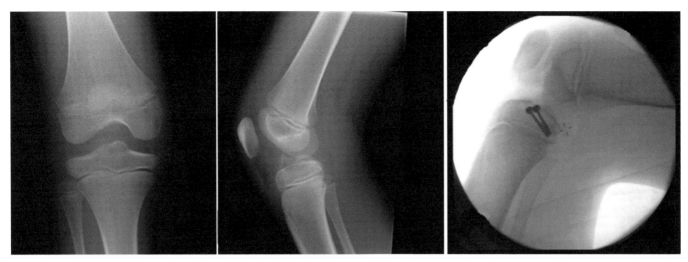

Figure 4.20 Type III tibial spine fracture treated with arthroscopic-assisted fixation.

Sleeve fractures are treated by repairing the associated retinacular tears as well as inserting strong sutures through the cartilaginous and bony parts of the fracture.

Tibial spine fractures

These fractures typically occur in children 8–14 years of age. They are the result of forced hyperextension of the knee or a direct blow to the distal femur with the knee flexed. These mechanisms create excessive tension on the bone and, because of the decreased resistance to tensile stress, the bone fractures while the anterior cruciate ligament is spared.

Meyers and McKeever classified these injuries into Types I–III:

I. The fracture is undisplaced.

II. The fracture is hinged posteriorly but lifted anteriorly.

III. The spine is completely displaced (Figure 4.20).

IV. This is a displaced and comminuted fracture (later addition).

Treatment

Type I and some Type II injuries can be treated non-operatively in a plaster cylinder. The knee should be immobilized in 20°–30° of flexion, avoiding hyperextension.

Surgery is required for Type III and IV fractures and for Type II fractures that cannot be reduced closed. It is not uncommon for the anterior horn of the meniscus to block the reduction. Reduction and fixation can be achieved by open or arthroscopic techniques.

Fixation may be by sutures, wires or screws. Care must be taken not to cross the proximal tibial physis when using screws.

Complications of this injury include ACL laxity and sometimes loss of full extension if there is malunion of the tibial spine fragment resulting in notch impingement on extension of the knee.

Proximal tibial physeal fractures

These are classified by the Salter–Harris method. Treatment is dictated by the degree of displacement.

- Undisplaced fractures can be treated by cast immobilization.
- Displaced Type I and II fractures require reduction and fixation using smooth wires, which need to be removed after 3–4 weeks.
- Displaced Type III and IV fractures and Type II fractures with a large metaphyseal fragment are treated by reduction and screw fixation. These screws are placed parallel to the physis.

Neurovascular complications occur in 10%–15% of injuries and include compartment syndrome, peroneal nerve injury and popliteal artery damage. Popliteal artery damage is most common after hyperextension injuries where the distal fragment is displaced posteriorly. Growth arrest occurs in 25% of patients with physeal injuries.

Tibial tubercle fractures

Tibial tubercle fractures occur in adolescents; the mechanism of injury is passive flexion of the knee with active quadriceps contraction, usually while jumping. There is a spectrum of injuries, ranging from an undisplaced fracture involving the tibial tubercle to injuries where the fracture line extends into the knee joint. Tibial tubercle fractures were classified by Ogden after modifying the Watson–Jones classification (Figures 4.21 and 4.22). An avulsion of the patella tendon with a periosteal sleeve can also be seen.

These injuries are usually treated surgically. An exception is the undisplaced fracture with no extensor lag, which can be treated in a plaster cast.

Though complications from this injury are uncommon, genu recurvatum may develop if there is damage to the anterior part of the physis.

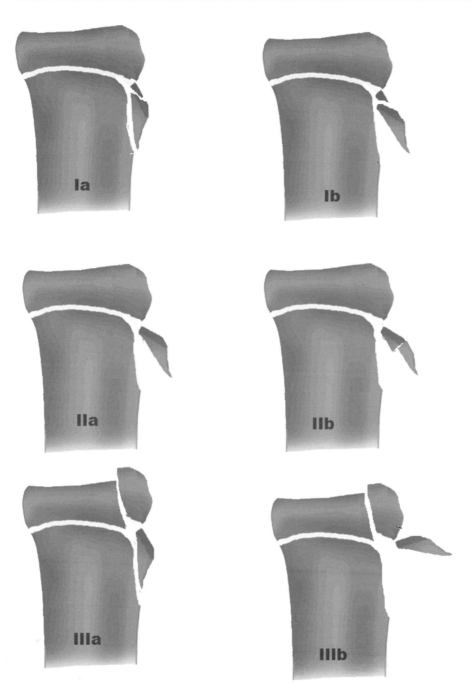

Figure 4.21 Ogden classification of the tibial tuberosity. Type I tuberosity fracture is distal to the physis: Ia, undisplaced; Ib, displaced. Type II fracture is through the physis: IIa, not comminuted; IIb, comminuted. Type III fracture crosses the physis: IIIa, not comminuted; IIIb, comminuted.

Proximal tibia metaphyseal fracture (Cozen fracture)

A characteristic pattern of injury occurs with some metaphyseal fractures (Cozen fracture) (Figure 4.23). Here, the proximal tibial fracture results in a valgus deformity, possibly due to medial overgrowth. The child's parents need to be warned that this may happen and that usually no treatment is needed as the tibia will remodel with time, although this may take up to 3 years. The deformity progresses rapidly in the first year and may continue to progress over 20 months after injury.

Surgery in the form of corrective osteotomies within the first 2–3 years after the injury has not yielded better results than non-operative treatment. The valgus deformity is thought to recur because the corrective surgery recreates the conditions of the initial fracture [13]. Persistence of the deformity after 3 years may warrant surgery, e.g. medial hemiepiphysiodesis or osteotomy.

Knee ligament injuries

Knee ligament injuries are rare in the skeletally immature patient. This is because the mechanisms that cause these injuries in the adult will result in a physeal or an avulsion-type fracture in children.

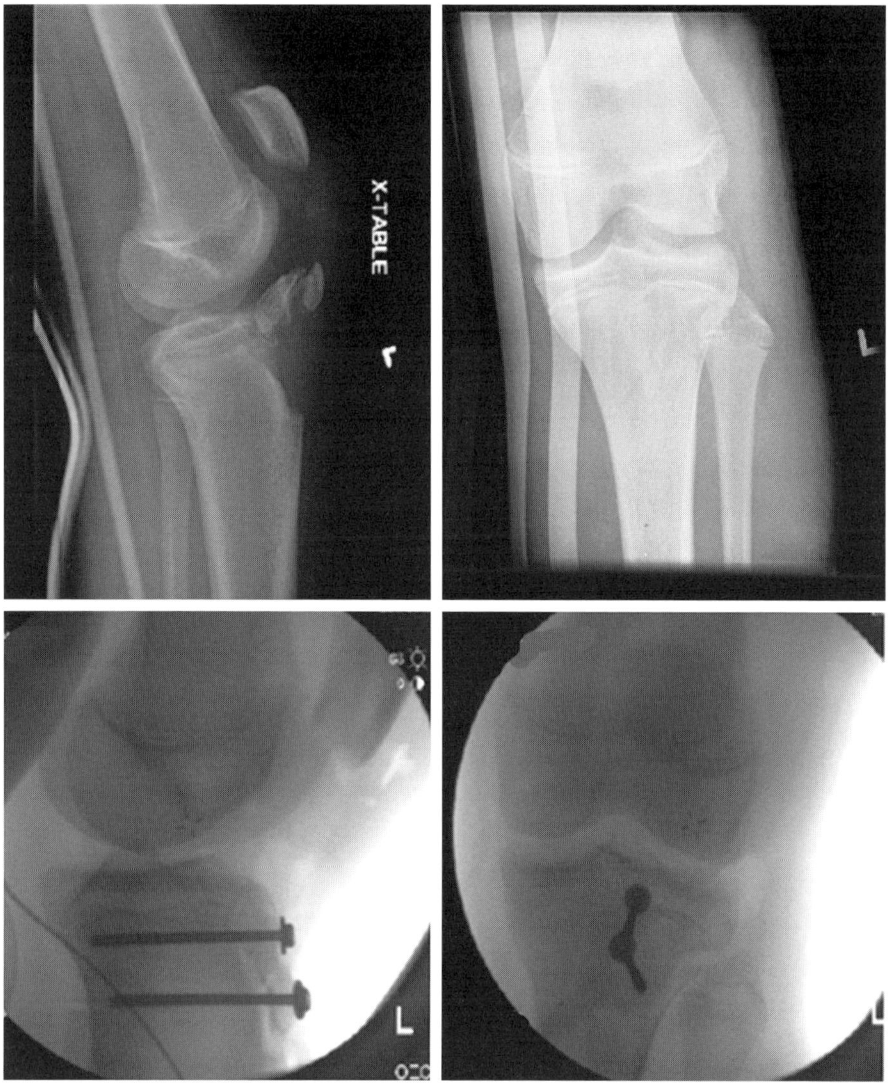

Figure 4.22 Type IIIb tibial tuberosity fracture.

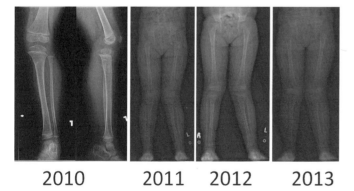

| 2010 | 2011 | 2012 | 2013 |

Figure 4.23 Cozen fracture.

A medial collateral ligament (MCL) rupture is the most common knee ligament injury, followed by an anterior cruciate ligament (ACL) rupture. Injuries to the posterior cruciate ligament (PCL) and the lateral collateral ligament (LCL) are very uncommon. Most controversies surround the management of ACL injuries, as these injuries are more likely to require surgical treatment.

Collateral ligament injuries

- Isolated MCL and LCL tears are usually treated non-operatively in a locked brace for 2 weeks, followed by a hinged brace for 2 weeks.
- MCL and LCL tears combined with other injuries, such as ACL injuries and some isolated Grade III injuries, may need direct repair.

Posterior cruciate ligament injuries

These are rare. When they occur, they are frequently combined with other ligament injuries and require surgery. Isolated PCL injuries can be effectively treated by non-operative means. Quadriceps strengthening exercises are the mainstay of treatment.

Anterior cruciate ligament injuries

The mechanism of injury is the same as in the adult. The younger patient is more likely to sustain a tibial spine fracture, while the older child will suffer an ACL rupture. A haemarthrosis is usually present and the diagnosis is confirmed by a positive Lachman test and with MRI. Plain radiographs may show a lateral capsule avulsion fracture (Segond fracture) (Figure 4.24).

Because of the potential damage to the physis associated with reconstructive surgery and the resulting growth disturbance, the following factors must be considered before undertaking reconstructive surgery:

- The age of the patient,
- Time to skeletal maturity,
- Level of planned activity,
- Parental influence.

Non-operative treatment is a viable option and involves hamstring rehabilitation, ACL brace and activity modification. If instability is a significant symptom, surgery should be undertaken, to prevent subsequent damage to the knee [14].

The following points should be considered when undertaking an ACL reconstruction in a skeletally immature patient:

- The skeletal age should be assessed using clinical and radiological methods.
- It is relatively safe to proceed to an ACL reconstruction within 2 years of skeletal maturity using transphyseal techniques (Figure 4.25) with low risk of growth disturbance (girls over 13 years and boys over 14 years).
- If surgery is to be performed in the younger patient, consider using physeal-sparing techniques such as all-epiphyseal or extra-articular reconstructions.
- With transphyseal techniques, a central tibial tunnel of minimal size and an over-the-top femoral tunnel technique are advised, to avoid the femoral physis.
- A hamstring graft is preferred over bone-patella tendon-bone, as it avoids spanning the physis with bone.
- Bioabsorbable screws are preferred. Avoid using metal screws near to the physis.
- Use an image intensifier for tunnel positioning and fixation.
- The results of most studies shows that the incidence of growth disturbance following ACL reconstruction is low [15].

Meniscal injuries

Meniscal tears are much less common in children than in adults. The mechanism of injury is usually a twisting force on a planted knee. The diagnosis can usually be made with a history of pain, giving way and locking, and joint line tenderness on clinical examination. MRI is not as accurate in diagnosing a tear as in adults because of the increased vascularity of the meniscus, resulting in false-positive findings (Figure 4.26).

Treatment

The aim in treating symptomatic cases should be to preserve the meniscus by repairing it where possible. If the meniscus is irreparable, a partial meniscectomy should be performed. Total meniscectomy should be avoided, as it leads to early degenerative changes in the knee. The success of meniscal repair is largely based on the blood supply, with the outer third (red zone) being better than the inner third (white zone).

Meniscal repair methods include:

- Inside-out repair (gold standard),
- Outside-in (especially for anterior horn repair),
- All-inside technique: at present this is the most popular method using modern suture equipment.

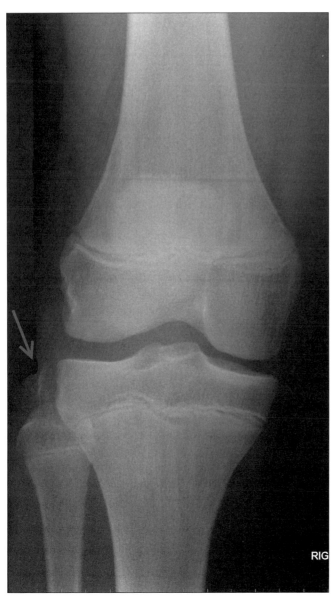

Figure 4.24 Knee X-ray showing a Segond fracture.

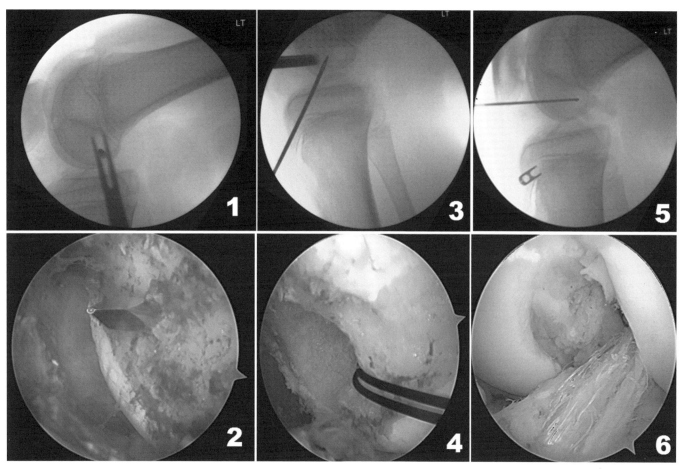

Figure 4.25 All-epiphyseal technique of ACL. All-epiphyseal ACL reconstruction involves creating tunnels in the distal femoral (images 1, 2) and proximal tibial (image 3) epiphyses using image intensifier and arthroscope. A direct endobutton (image 5) was used to secure the graft distally first, and was then pulled through the femoral tunnel (images 4, 6) and secured using a bioabsorbable interference screw.

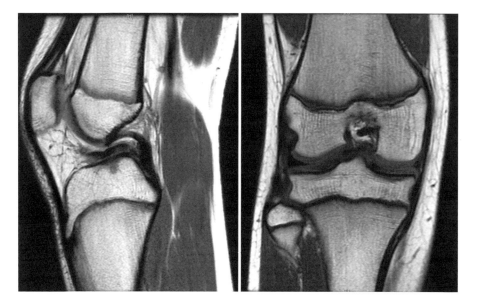

Figure 4.26 This MRI scan of the knee shows a large bucket handle tear of the medial meniscus, evident by a double PCL sign on the sagittal section. Compare the shape of the normal wedge-like lateral meniscus with that of the torn medial meniscus and note its presence in the notch on the coronal section.

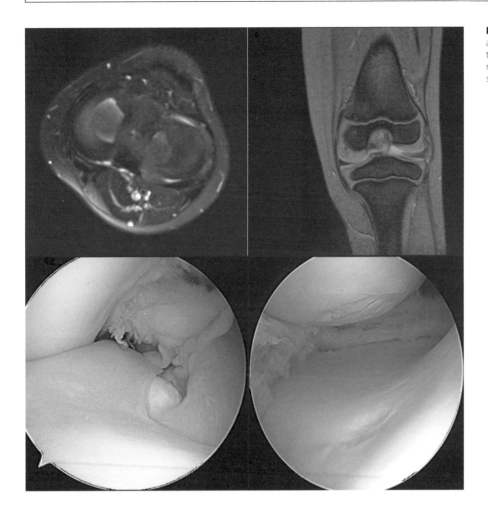

Figure 4.27 This MRI scan of the knee shows an almost complete discoid meniscus. The bottom two arthroscopic pictures show the discoid meniscus before (left) and after (right) saucerization.

The use of a fibrin clot may improve the healing potential of the meniscus.

Discoid meniscus

This is an abnormally thick meniscus that covers a large proportion of the tibial surface and is thought to be congenital in origin. It is almost always located in the lateral side. The incidence varies from 1.5% to 15% and occurs mostly in girls.

Discoidal meniscus presents in various ways, from an incidental finding on MRI or arthroscopy to a frank tear. Children frequently describe a 'popping', 'locking' or 'snapping'.

The diagnosis can be confirmed by MRI. The most accurate criterion for a diagnosis of discoid meniscus on MRI is a ratio of the minimal meniscal width to maximal tibial width on the coronal slice of more than 20% (Figure 4.27).

A less precise criterion is continuity between the anterior and posterior meniscal horns on three consecutive sagittal images. Radiographs characteristically show a widened lateral joint space and squaring of the lateral femoral condyle.

Watanabe classified the discoid meniscus into three types:

- Complete,
- Incomplete,
- Wrisberg type.

The complete and incomplete types have a stable posterior attachment via the meniscotibial ligaments. The difference is that the complete type covers the whole of the tibial surface whereas the incomplete type does not. The Wrisberg type is the most mobile, as it is bounded posteriorly only by the meniscofemoral ligament of Wrisberg.

Treatment

- If asymptomatic, discoid menisci are left alone.
- Tears are excised to a stable margin (saucerization), if the meniscus has adequate peripheral attachment.
- A hypermobile meniscus (Wrisberg type) may be repaired onto the capsule. In some cases a complete meniscectomy may be necessary.

References

1. Salenius P and Vankka E (1975) The development of the tibiofemoral angle in children. *J Bone Joint Surg Am* **57**(2):259–61.

2. Levine AM and Drennan JC (1982) Physiological bowing and tibia vara. The metaphyseal–diaphyseal angle in the measurement of bowleg deformities. *J Bone Joint Surg Am* **64**(8):1158–63.

3. Davids JR, Blackhurst DW and Allen BL Jr (2001) Radiographic evaluation of bowed legs in children. *J Pediatr Orthop* **21**(2):257–63.

4. Langenskiold A (1952) Tibia vara (osteochondrosis deformans tibiae); a survey of 23 cases. *Acta Chir Scand* **103**(1):1–22.

5. Raney EM, Topoleski TA, Yaghoubian R, Guidera KJ and Marshall JG (1998) Orthotic treatment of infantile tibia vara. *J Pediatr Orthop* **18**(5):670–4.

6. Park SS, Gordon JE, Luhmann SJ, Dobbs MB and Schoenecker PL (2005) Outcome of hemiepiphyseal stapling for late-onset tibia vara. *J Bone Joint Surg Am* **87**(10):2259–66.

7. Herring JA (2008) *Tachdjian's Pediatric Orthopaedics*, 4th edition, volume 1. Philadelphia: Saunders Elsevier.

8. Jones D, Barnes J and Lloyd-Roberts GC (1978) Congenital aplasia and dysplasia of the tibia with intact fibula. Classification and management. *J Bone Joint Surg Br* **60**(1):31–9.

9. Pill SG, Ganley TJ, Milam RA *et al.* (2003) Role of magnetic resonance imaging and clinical criteria in predicting successful nonoperative treatment of osteochondritis dissecans in children. *J Pediatr Orthop* **23**(1):102–8.

10. Cash JD and Hughston JC (1988) Treatment of acute patellar dislocation. *Am J Sports Med* **16**(3):244–9.

11. Maenpaa H and Lehto MU (1997) Patellar dislocation. The long-term results of nonoperative management in 100 patients. *Am J Sports Med* **25**(2):213–17.

12. Palmu S, Kallio PE, Donell ST, Helenius I and Nietosvaara Y (2008) Acute patellar dislocation in children and adolescents: a randomized clinical trial. *J Bone Joint Surg Am* **90**(3):463–70.

13. Dormans JP (2005) *Pediatric Orthopaedics: Core Knowledge in Orthopaedics*. Philadelphia: Elsevier Mosby.

14. Larsen MW, Garrett WE Jr, Delee JC and Moorman CT 3rd (2006) Surgical management of anterior cruciate ligament injuries in patients with open physes. *J Am Acad Orthop Surg* **14**(13):736–44.

15. Kocher MS, Saxon HS, Hovis WD and Hawkins RJ (2002) Management and complications of anterior cruciate ligament injuries in skeletally immature patients: survey of the Herodicus Society and The ACL Study Group. *J Pediatr Orthop* **22**(4):452–7.

16. Bowen JR, Torres RR and Forlin E (1992) Partial epiphysiodesis to address genu varum or genu valgum. *J Pediatr Orthop* **12**(3):359–64.

The foot and ankle

Anthony Cooper and Stan Jones

Congenital talipes equinovarus (club foot)

Overview

Club foot is a congenital foot deformity consisting of hindfoot equinus and varus as well as forefoot adduction and cavus (Figure 5.1).

Incidence varies with race. In Europe, the incidence is 1 in 1000 live births, with boys twice as commonly affected as girls. In 50% of cases, both feet are affected. In affected families, the likelihood of club foot occurring in the offspring is 30 times greater than in the general population.

Pathoanatomy

The exact cause is unknown but is thought to be multifactorial. Various aetiologies have been proposed, including primary muscle, bone, nerve or vascular pathology, developmental arrest and retracting fibrosis.

Anomalies are present in the bones, muscles, tendons and ligaments. Key components of the deformities are medial and plantar subluxation of the navicular on the talar head, and a medially rotated calcaneum, such that the talus and calcaneum are parallel in all three planes (sagittal, coronal and axial).

Diagnosis and evaluation

The diagnosis is often made prenatally by ultrasonography. In the absence of a prenatal diagnosis, diagnosis is made at birth by clinical examination.

Club foot may be positional, idiopathic or syndromic. Syndromic club foot is associated with such conditions as arthrogryposis, myelodysplasia, amniotic band syndrome and diastrophic dysplasia.

Common clinical findings are a small foot, thin calf and prominent medial and posterior skin creases. A full clinical examination is required to determine whether a child presenting with club feet has an associated syndrome.

Minimal ossification of the bones in the foot limits the usefulness of radiographs in the newborn. In addition, radiological appearances correlate poorly with clinical outcome.

Classification

The most commonly used classifications are those described by Pirani (Table 5.1) and Diméglio.

Both classifications assign points based on the severity of the clinical findings and the correctability of the deformity.

Treatment

The aim of treatment is to achieve a mobile, pain-free and functional foot that will fit in a shoe.

The initial treatment is non-operative and the Ponseti [1] method of manipulation and serial casting followed by bracing is the technique most commonly favoured. (An 80–90% success rate is achieved with the Ponseti method.) The French method is another non-operative treatment but it is not popular in the UK. It involves daily manipulations of the newborn's club foot by a specialized physical therapist, stimulation of the muscles around

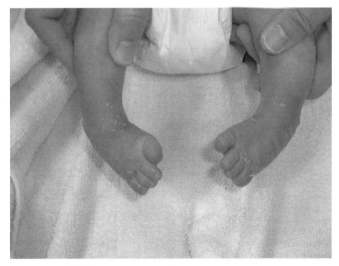

Figure 5.1 Club feet.

Postgraduate Paediatric Orthopaedics, ed. Sattar Alshryda, Stan Jones and Paul A. Banaszkiewicz. Published by Cambridge University Press.
© Cambridge University Press 2014.

Table 5.1 Pirani score for club feet (pictures courtesy of Dr Lynn Staheli and Global Help Publication): total Pirani score, 0–6

	Clinical sign	0	0.5	1.0
Hindfoot contracture score (0–3)	Equinus	Dorsiflexion	Comes to neutral	Cannot reach neutral
	Deep posterior crease	Multiple fine creases (normal)	Superficial single crease, which is obliterated on dorsiflexion	Deep persistent crease
	Empty heel	Easily palpable calcaneum	Deep calcaneum	Not palpable
Midfoot contracture score (0–3)	Curved lateral border	Straight	Mildly curved	Severely curved
	Medial crease	Multiple fine creases (normal)	Superficial single crease, which is obliterated on dorsiflexion	Deep persistent crease
	Lateral head of talus	Fully covered with the navicular bone	Partially covered	Not covered at all

87

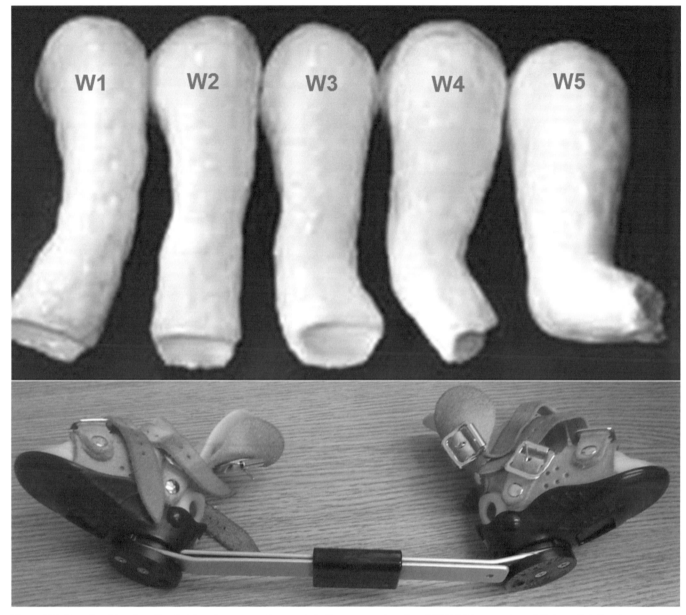

Figure 5.2 Ponseti serial casting. Top: Serial casting to correct cavus, abduction, varus and equinus (CAVE) (picture courtesy of Dr Lynn Staheli and Global Help Publication). Bottom: Denis Browne brace; the bar should be of sufficient length that the heels of the shoes are at shoulder width. This can be adjusted using the sliding clamp in the middle. The bar should be bent 5°–10° to hold the feet in dorsiflexion. For unilateral cases, the brace is set at 60°–70° of external rotation on the club foot side and 30°–40° of external rotation on the normal side. In bilateral cases, it is set at 70° of external rotation on each side.

the foot and temporary immobilization of the foot with elastic and inelastic adhesive taping. A comparative study [2] of 176 patients treated with the Ponseti method and 80 patients treated by the French functional method showed improved results with use of the Ponseti method, although the difference was not statistically significant.

Ponseti method

Treatment starts soon after birth but may be delayed for a few weeks in a premature baby.

The sequence of deformity correction is cavus, abduction, varus and finally equinus (CAVE) (Figure 5.2).

The forefoot is held supinated and not pronated. Lateral pressure with the thumb is over the neck of the talus and not the calcaneocuboid joint.

Long leg POP (plaster-of-Paris) casts are applied with the knee in flexion. (This prevents the cast falling off and controls tibial rotation.)

Casts are changed on a weekly basis, although this may be done at 5-day intervals.

Equinus should be corrected without causing a midfoot break and correction should start after achieving forefoot abduction of about 60° with the heel moved into the valgus position.

Residual equinus is corrected by a percutaneous Achilles tenotomy using a single incision. (Required in up to 90% of feet); this is followed by a last cast for 2–3 weeks.

After removing the last cast, a foot abduction orthosis (Denis Browne boots and bar, Figure 5.2) is applied and worn 23 hours a day, initially for 3 months then only at nap- and night-time for 2–4 years. This is required to facilitate remodelling of the foot and prevent relapse of the deformity.

The most common cause of relapse of the deformity is poor compliance with the Denis– Browne boot and bar. Relapse is treated by further serial casting with or without an Achilles tenotomy.

Table 5.2 Indications for surgery in club foot

Persistent supination	Whole or split tibialis anterior tendon transfer
Relapse despite repeat serial casting	Limited posteromedial release or soft-tissue distraction using a circular external fixator
Severe multiplanar residual deformity in the older child	Osteotomies of the mid ± hindfoot with or without external fixators

Surgery

The indications for surgery are shown in Table 5.2.

Metatarsus adductus

Overview

This deformity is characterized by medial deviation of the forefoot relative to a naturally aligned hindfoot. The incidence is 1 in 1000 live births.

Pathoanatomy

The cause is unknown though *in-utero* positioning may contribute to this deformity.

Diagnosis and evaluation

The diagnosis is clinical and the deformity is usually noted at birth, although it may be recognized at any age.

The foot has concave medial and convex lateral borders and when viewed from the sole assumes the shape of a bean. In addition the space between the great and second toe is wider than normal and internal tibial torsion may be present.

Classification

Bleck classified metatarsus adductus into mild, moderate and severe using the heel bisector line (Figure 5.3). Normally, this line passes between the second and third toes [3].

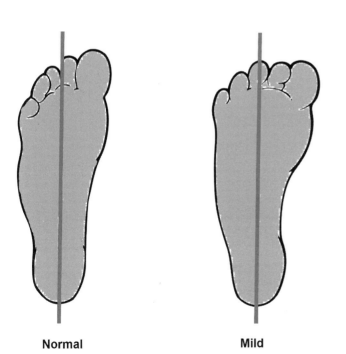
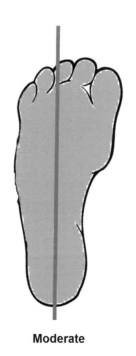
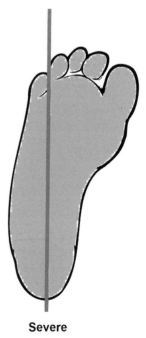

Normal   Mild   Moderate   Severe

Figure 5.3 Bleck's classification of metatarsus adductus.

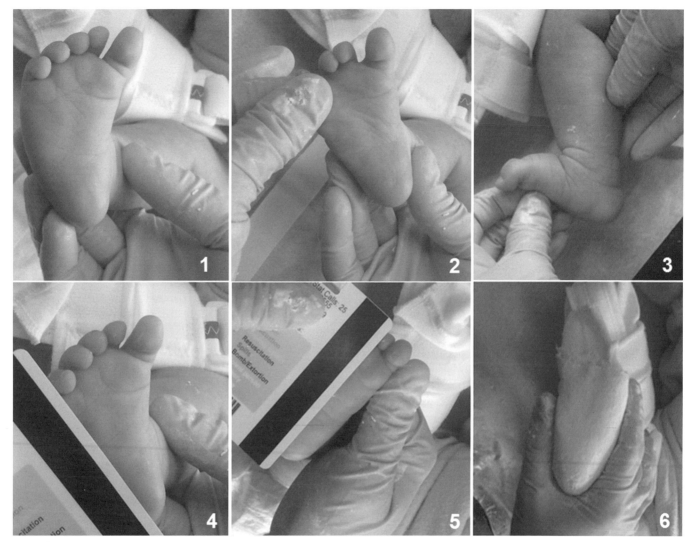

Figure 5.4 Severe metatarsus adductus (images 1, 4), which was fully correctable (images 2, 5) and treated by serial casting (image 6). Image 3 shows a normal hind foot with no equinus of the heel; an important differentiation from a club foot.

Treatment

Most cases (86%) resolve without active treatment and only parental reassurance is required.

Non-surgical

For mild deformities, the parents should be taught passive stretching exercises. Serial casting is recommended for moderate or severe deformities (Figure 5.4).

Surgery

Surgery is rarely required and only if the deformity does not resolve after serial casting.

In the younger child, the abductor hallucis may be released; in the older child (>7 years), a medial column lengthening (opening wedge osteotomy of the medial cuneiform) and lateral column shortening (closing wedge osteotomy of the cuboid) produces good results.

Flexible flatfoot (pes planovalgus)
Overview (epidemiology)

A flat foot is a foot with a large plantar contact area and an abnormal or absent longitudinal arch.

Though flexible flatfeet are present in nearly all infants and many children, the exact incidence is unknown. It is present in 20–25% of adults and runs in families.

Pathoanatomy

The cause is unknown, though it is more common in children with generalized ligamentous laxity.

In the infant's foot, the longitudinal arch is usually obscured by subcutaneous fat. As the child grows older, the fat atrophies and the longitudinal arch develops.

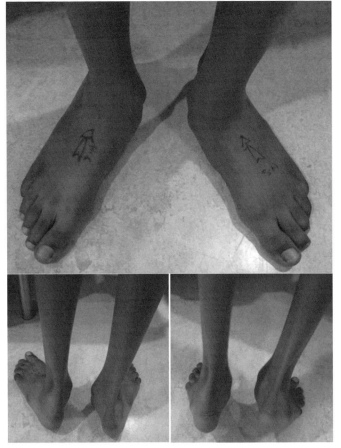

Figure 5.5 Bilateral severe flexible flat feet. Also shows bilateral forefeet abduction (too-many-toes sign) and valgus heels that move to varus on tiptoeing (see Figure 5.9 for comparison).

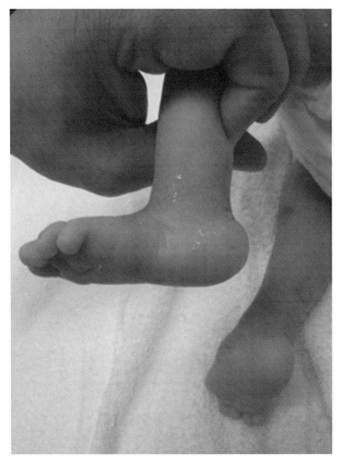

Figure 5.6 Rocker bottom foot in congenital vertical talus.

Evaluation

Clinical examination of the child while standing will reveal an absent or low longitudinal arch and the hindfoot may be in valgus. The medial arch reappears on tiptoeing or on passive dorsiflexion of the great toe with the child seated (Jack's test).

Subtalar motion should be full. The gastrocnemius or Achilles tendon may be tight; passive dorsiflexion of the foot with the heel inverted will demonstrate this. Features of generalized ligamentous laxity may be present and documented using the Beighton score.

Plain radiographs are not required to make a diagnosis; however, a standing lateral radiograph allows measurement of Meary's angle (lateral talus-first metatarsal angle) which is normally 0° but in a flexible flatfoot will be greater than 0° (Figure 5.5).

Classification

Flexible flatfeet may be divided into those with or without a tight gastrocnemius or Achilles tendon complex.

Treatment

In a young child with a flexible flatfoot deformity, treatment is not required and the parents should be reassured.

Non-surgical

Orthoses (medial arch supports) have not been shown to promote the development of the longitudinal arch and should not be routinely prescribed. They may, however, relieve pain if present.

Calf-stretching exercises may be helpful if the Achilles tendon or gastrocnemius is tight.

Surgery

Surgery is reserved for the older child with intractable symptoms unresponsive to non-surgical options.

A joint-sparing osteotomy, such as a lateral column lengthening procedure with or without release of the gastrocnemius or Achilles tendon is the procedure of choice.

Arthroereisis of the subtalar joint (using an implant) is an option but is not without complication and parents should be advised appropriately. Arthrodesis is not recommended.

Congenital vertical talus

Overview [4]

Congenital vertical talus (convex pes valgus) is an irreducible dorsal dislocation of the navicular on the talus. The foot assumes a rocker bottom shape (Figure 5.6).

The incidence is 1 in 150 000 births with no sex predilection and is bilateral in 50% of cases. It may occur as an isolated foot anomaly or in association with other neuromuscular conditions, such as myelomeningocele, arthrogryposis or chromosomal abnormalities.

Pathoanatomy

The cause is unknown but muscle imbalance, intra-uterine compression and growth arrest during fetal development have been suggested.

The navicular articulates with the dorsal aspect of the neck of the talus. The calcaneum is displaced posterolaterally with respect to the talus and is in equinus.

Diagnosis and evaluation

The diagnosis is made by clinical and radiological examination (lateral radiograph of the foot in maximum plantarflexion).

On clinical examination, the foot has a convex plantar surface, the talar head is prominent medially, the midfoot is dorsiflexed and abducted on the hindfoot and the hindfoot is in equinovalgus, giving the appearance of a Persian slipper. In addition, the Achilles, tibialis anterior and peroneal tendons are contracted. Passive correction of this deformity is not possible.

On a lateral radiograph taken with the foot in maximum plantarflexion, the hallmark of vertical talus is that a line drawn along the long axis of the talus appears vertical (almost parallel to the tibia) and also passes plantarward to a line drawn along the first metatarsal cuneiform axes (Figure 5.7).

Differential diagnosis

Oblique talus is a benign condition with a good prognosis and must be distinguished from vertical talus.

In oblique talus, the valgus deformity of the hindfoot is passively correctible and this restores the medial arch. Moreover, on a lateral radiograph, the navicular is reduced on the talus with the foot maximally plantarflexed.

Treatment

Non-surgical

Initial treatment involves manipulation and serial casting with the corrective forces applied opposite to that required during Ponseti casting for CTEV (often termed a reversed Ponseti method).

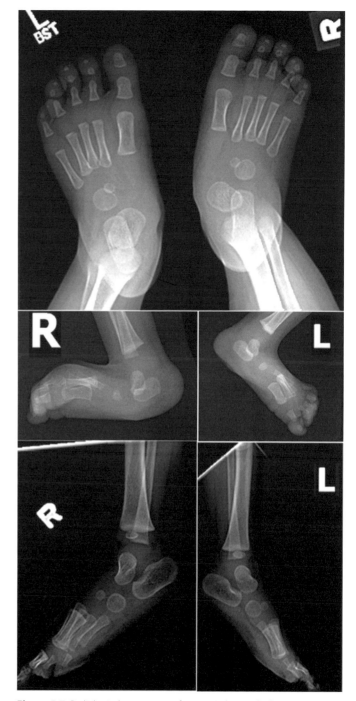

Figure 5.7 Radiological assessment of congenital vertical talus.

Manipulation and serial casting is usually not sufficient to correct the deformity fully and surgery is often required (Figure 5.8).

Surgical

Surgery is usually undertaken around 12 months of age and involves soft-tissue releases including Achilles tendon lengthening, reduction of the talonavicular joint and K-wire stabilization. Additional surgery may be required, such as transfer of the tibialis anterior tendon to the dorsum of the talus. In the older child (>3 years), it may be necessary to excise the navicular and carry out more extensive surgery. The outcome is less predictable.

Tarsal coalition

Overview

Tarsal coalition is an abnormal connection between two or more bones in the foot. The connection may be fibrous, cartilaginous or bony. The reported incidence varies between 1% and 6%; in 50% of affected individuals it is bilateral.

Coalitions may be solitary or multiple. The most common site is calcaneonavicular, followed by talocalcaneal. Talocalcaneal coalitions usually involve the middle facet. Coalitions are associated with limb abnormalities, such as fibular hemimelia and proximal femoral focal deficiency.

Pathoanatomy

Tarsal coalitions are thought to be the result of failure of segmentation of mesenchymal tissue in the developing foot.

Although coalitions may be present at birth, symptoms such as pain appear later in life, usually between 10 and 12 years of age for calcaneonavicular and 12 and 15 years, for talocalcaneal [5].

Evaluation

The presenting history and physical examination are suggestive but radiographs, CT or MRI are required to confirm the diagnosis. (MRI is more accurate than CT in demonstrating fibrous coalitions.)

Pain is usually the initial complaint and is typically localized over the sinus tarsi, although it may be present in other parts of the foot. It is aggravated by sporting activities.

Clinical evaluation reveals a planovalgus foot. On tiptoeing, the hindfoot valgus does not correct and the medial arch does not reconstitute (Figure 5.9). In addition, the range of movement to the subtalar joint is decreased.

A standing oblique radiograph provides the best view for diagnosing a calcaneonavicular coalition. A CT scan may be required to diagnose a talocalcaneal coalition and in addition to determine the size of the coalition, as this provides useful information regarding surgical options.

Lateral standing radiographs will show features, such as an anteater sign and a C sign, that are suggestive of calcaneonavicular and talocalcaneal coalitions, respectively (Figure 5.10).

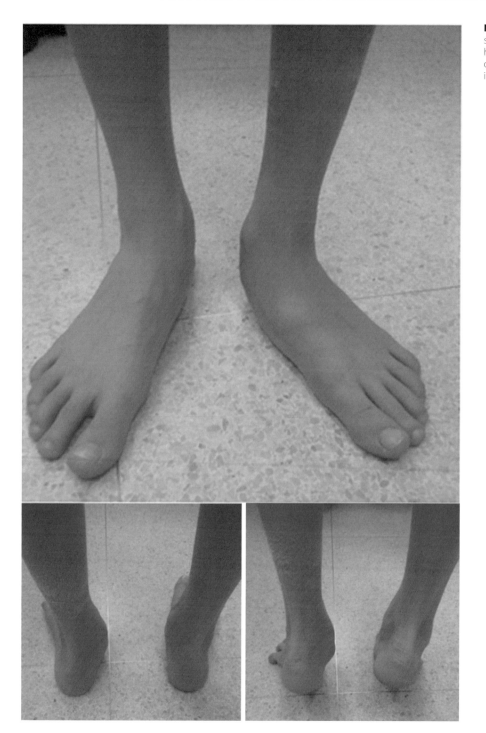

Figure 5.9 Tarsal coalition. The photograph shows a left flat foot, abducted forefoot and valgus heel that does not correct to varus on tiptoeing in comparison to the right foot. Underlying diagnosis is tarsal coalition.

Treatment

The goal of treatment is pain relief and to improve joint motion.

Non-surgical

An initial trial of non-operative management is recommended; this involves the use of non-steroidal anti-inflammatory drugs (NSAIDs), activity modification, orthoses or insoles and a period of immobilization in a below-knee weight-bearing cast for 4–6 weeks.

Surgery should be considered in patients who continue to have symptoms despite a period of non-operative management.

Surgery

Calcaneonavicular coalitions are excised, utilizing a modified Ollier incision. It is advisable to interpose extensor digitorum brevis or fat in the gap left, to reduce the risk of recurrence.

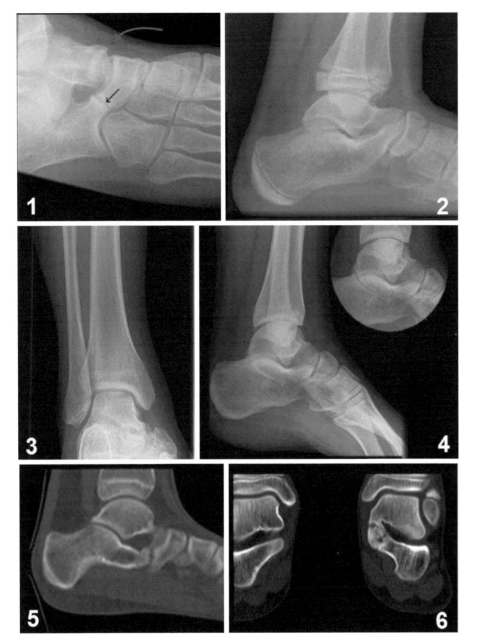

Figure 5.10 Tarsal coalition radiology. These X-rays show various recognized radiological signs of tarsal coalitions seen in different patients. 1: Calcaneonavicular coalition marked by a straight black arrow. The anterior process of the calcaneum can be elongated, mimicking an anteater nose (image 2). Talar peaking is another sign of tarsal coalition and is marked by a curved grey arrow. 3: Ball-and-socket ankle joint secondary to remodelling of the joint to compensate for the lost subtalar motion. 4: C sign. 5: Sagittal CT scan shows a calcaneonavicular fibrous tarsal coalition. 6: Coronal CT scan shows a talocalcaneal tarsal coalition on the right in comparison with the normal left side.

Talocalcaneal coalitions may be excised if less than 50% of the middle facet is involved. A medial hindfoot approach is recommended.

A triple or subtalar arthrodesis may be required in the presence of degenerative changes, multiple coalitions or if symptoms persist despite previous surgery to excise a coalition.

Accessory navicular

Overview

An accessory navicular is an accessory ossification centre at the medial side of the navicular; it is considered a normal anatomical variant. It is observed in 12% of the population.

Evaluation

Most accessory naviculars are asymptomatic and are diagnosed incidentally following radiographic examination after an injury of the foot (Figure 5.11).

A child with a symptomatic accessory navicular will present with pain over the medial aspect of the midfoot that is usually aggravated by tight-fitting shoes. A tender prominence will be observed to this area of the foot and resisted inversion may be painful.

Treatment

If asymptomatic, reassurance is usually all that is required.

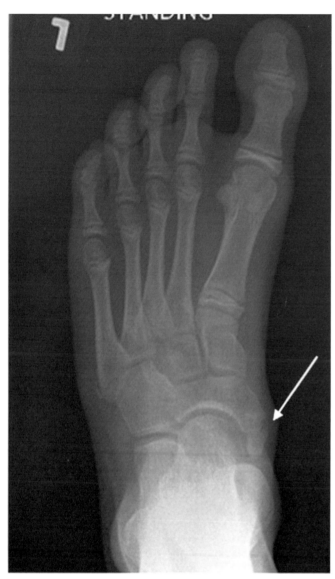

Figure 5.11 Accessory navicular.

It is a self-limiting condition and resolves over a period of 18 months to 3 years.

Pathoanatomy

Like other osteochondritidies, it is thought to be due to avascular necrosis.

The navicular is the last tarsal bone to ossify (after 2 years) and it is thought that it is therefore more susceptible to mechanical compression injury causing avascular necrosis.

Evaluation

Patients present with midfoot pain. Tenderness and swelling may be observed over the dorsum of the midfoot; in addition, the child may have a limp.

Radiographs confirm the diagnosis. Flattening, sclerosis or fragmentation of the navicular is observed (Figure 5.12). These radiographic changes disappear over time.

Treatment

The mainstay of treatment is activity modification. Immobilization of the affected limb in a below-knee weight-bearing cast for 4–6 weeks may be required and has been shown to reduce the duration of symptoms. Surgery is never indicated.

Freiberg's disease

Overview

Freiberg's disease is osteochondritis of the metatarsal head. The second metatarsal is most commonly affected, though occasionally the third may be involved. It is commonly seen in girls over the age of 13 years.

The cause is unknown but it is thought to be due to avascular necrosis of the metatarsal head due to microfracture secondary to repetitive stresses.

Evaluation

Patients may present with pain with or without a prominence to the dorsum of the foot overlying the second metatarsal head, although occasionally the diagnosis is made incidentally after radiographic examination of the foot following an injury.

Clinically localized tenderness with or without a swelling may be observed. There may also be an associated deformity of the respective toe, and the patient may have a limp.

An MRI scan may help make the diagnosis before radiographic changes occur. Radiographs show irregularity of the articular surface, sclerosis and fragmentation of the metatarsal head (Figure 5.13).

If symptomatic, the initial management is non-operative and involves the use of orthosis or a below-knee weight-bearing cast for a short period, to relieve pressure.

If pain persists despite a trial of non-operative treatment, surgery may be required to excise the accessory navicular through a tibialis posterior tendon splitting approach.

Kohler's disease

Overview

Kohler's disease is osteochondritis of the tarsal navicular. It is frequently bilateral, and is seen more commonly in boys (4:1), usually between the ages of 2 and 8 years.

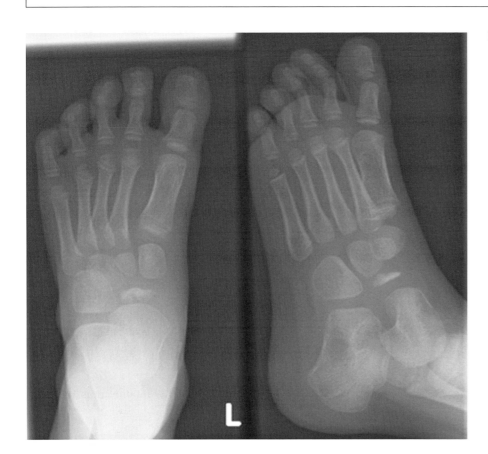

Figure 5.12 Kohler's disease.

Treatment

A trial of conservative management is usually advised in symptomatic cases. The options include rest, activity modification, the use of hard-soled shoes and a below-knee weight-bearing cast.

Surgery may be required if the patient is symptomatic despite a trial of non-operative treatment. The surgical options include joint debridement or cheilectomy, or a dorsiflexion osteotomy of the metatarsal neck.

Hallux valgus

Overview

Hallux valgus or juvenile bunions are often familial but may be seen in children with neuromuscular disorders (cerebral palsy or connective tissue diseases, such as Ehlers–Danlos syndrome).

It is often bilateral.

Evaluation

The diagnosis is clinical but radiographs are required to assess the severity of the deformity. In addition to examination of the foot, a full examination is required, to check for signs of generalized ligamentous laxity or other underlying causes, such as cerebral palsy.

Standing anteroposterior and lateral radiographs of the foot help define the severity of the deformity. The intermetatarsal angle (≤10°), hallux valgus angle (≤15°) and distal metatarsal articular angle (≤15°) and the length of the first metatarsal relative to the second are important parameters to be measured (Figure 5.14).

Hallux valgus may be classified into mild, moderate or severe, based on radiographic measurements (Table 5.3).

Treatment

Some conservative treatment options may help relieve pain but do not correct the deformity.

Toe spacers and splints worn around the great toe have been shown to be ineffective, though a medial arch support may be of benefit in a patient with associated flat foot.

Patients should be encouraged to wear comfortable shoes.

Surgery may be considered if the symptoms are unacceptable and non-surgical measures fail. Patients and their parents must be warned of the high rate of recurrence after surgery and complications such as overcorrection, hallux varus and joint stiffness.

The surgery options are distal soft-tissue release, distal first metatarsal osteotomies, such as the Scarf, often combined with an Akin osteotomy of the proximal phalanx (Akin), or a Lapidus procedure, which is a corrective fusion of the first tarsometatarsal joint with distal soft-tissue corrective procedures [6].

Table 5.3 Hallux valgus treatment recommendation

	Hallux valgus angle	Intermetatarsal angle	Distal metatarsal articular angle	Treatment
Normal	<15°	<10°	<15°	
Mild	<30°	<12°		Distal osteotomy, e.g. Chevron, Scarf
Moderate	30°–40°	13°–15°		Distal osteotomy, e.g. Chevron or Scarf + Akin
Severe	>40°	16°–20°		Double osteotomy Scarf + Akin, Lapidus

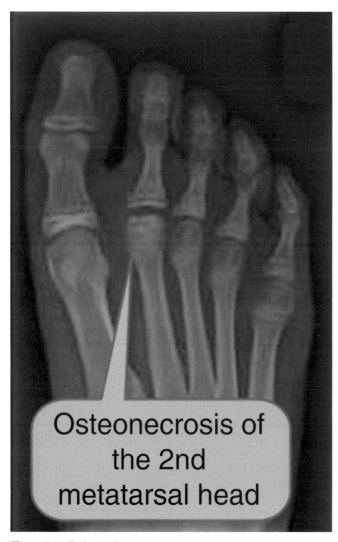

Figure 5.13 Freiberg's disease.

Overlapping fifth toes

Overview

An overlying fifth toe (Varus fifth toe) is a dorsal adduction deformity of the fifth toe. It is usually present at birth and is typically familial and bilateral. The extensor digitorum longus tendon is contracted.

Evaluation

The diagnosis is clinical (Figure 5.15). Pain may develop over time due to footwear irritation.

Treatment

Conservative measures, such as buddy strapping, are ineffective and surgery is usually advised.

Surgery involves a double-racquet skin incision around the toe, tenotomy of the extensor digitorum longus and dorsal capsulotomy of the metatarsophalangeal joint, with or without temporary stabilization of the toe with a K-wire in a corrected position for 2–4 weeks.

The risk of vascular injury with surgery is real and parents must be warned accordingly.

Curly toes

This deformity is characterized by flexion and medial deviation of the proximal interphalangeal joint of the affected toe and results in the affected toe underlying an adjacent one (Figure 5.15). Contracture of the flexor digitorum longus and brevis tendon is the most common cause.

Curly toes are usually bilateral; the third and fourth toes are commonly affected. There is often a positive family history.

In 76% of affected children, the deformity persists and surgery may be required, as toe strapping only improves the deformity temporarily. The recommended surgical option is an open tenotomy of the flexor digitorum longus and brevis tendons. A randomized controlled trial did not show a superior result with flexor-to-extensor tendon transfer. Rarely when there are bony changes, osteotomy may be required.

Pes cavus

Overview

Pes cavus is a foot with a high longitudinal arch (Figure 5.16). It is often associated with clawing of the toes and a varus

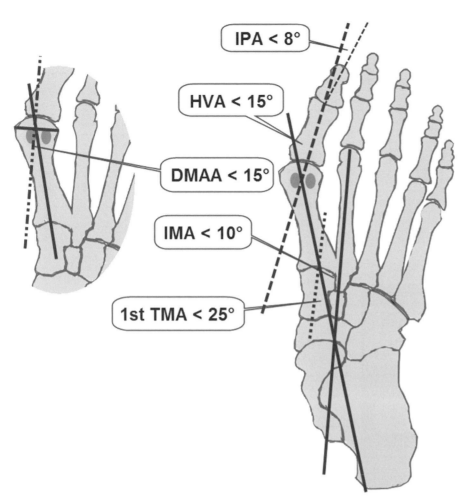

IPA < 8°

HVA < 15°

DMAA < 15°

IMA < 10°

1st TMA < 25°

Figure 5.14 Hallux valgus radiology measurements. Excessive IPA (interphalangeal angle) can be corrected with Akin osteotomy. The HVA (hallux valgus angle) indicates the severity of the valgus deformity. The distal metatarsal articular angle (DMAA) is the angle between the first metatarsal longitudinal axis and the line perpendicular to the articular line. Some books use the angle between the articular line and the main axis, quoting 85° as a normal value.

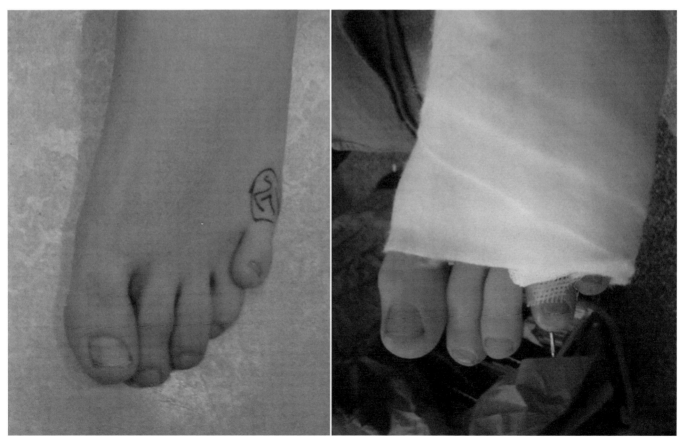

Figure 5.15 Overlapping and curly toes. This teenager had bilateral overlapping fifth toes and curly (underlapping) fourth toes. He underwent bilateral Butler's procedure for the fifth toes and lateral closing wedge of the middle phalanx of the fourth toes.

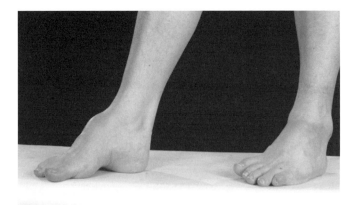

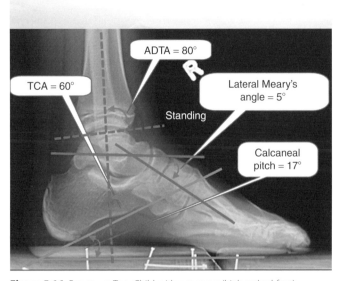

Figure 5.16 Pes cavus. Top: Child with pes cavus (high-arched foot). Bottom: Common radiological measures around the foot and ankle in the context of pes cavus. ADTA (anterior distal tibial angle) = 80° (78°–82°); lateral Meary's angle (talus longitudinal axis and first metatarsal axis) = 5° (1°–9°); calcaneal pitch = 17° (11°–23°); TCA (talocalcaneal angle: longitudinal axis of the tibia and the calcaneum; more useful than calcaneal pitch if there is associated equinus deformity) = 60° (60°–80°); the Hibbs angle (not shown) is the angle between the longitudinal axis of the calcaneum and the first metatarsal axis and is 150°. Some references quote slightly different values of these angles or use the complementary angles instead, which can create some confusion.

hindfoot. Two-thirds of patients with pes cavus have an underlying neurological condition, such as hereditary sensorimotor neuropathy, e.g. Charcot–Marie–Tooth disease (CMT), cerebral palsy, spinal dysraphism, poliomyelitis or Friedreich's ataxia. It may also be secondary to compartment syndrome following an injury of the leg.

Cavus deformities can be divided into pes cavus with hind foot varus (cavovarus) and pes cavus with hindfoot calcaneus (calcaneocavus). Calcaneocavus is observed in poliomyelitis or myelomeningocele; the deformity is due to weakness of the gastrocnemius muscle.

Pathoanatomy

In cavus with a neurological cause, imbalance is a common finding. In CMT, the tibialis posterior and peroneus longus tendons are strong, causing the hindfoot to invert and the first metatarsal to be depressed, while the tibialis anterior and peroneus brevis tendons are weak, leading to weakness of ankle dorsiflexion and eversion of the foot. The long toe extensors compensate for tibialis anterior weakness, thus leading to clawing of the lesser toes.

Evaluation and diagnosis

The diagnosis of the cavus deformity is usually made after a thorough examination of the foot and ankle.

A family history and a full neurological examination, including examination of the spine, are paramount. A hairy patch on the back is suggestive of spinal dysraphism.

Unilateral limb involvement suggests a focal diagnosis, i.e. spinal cord or nerve injury, while bilateral involvement suggests CMT. In CMT, examination of the dorsum of the hand may reveal guttering due to intrinsic muscle wasting.

In a cavovarus foot, it is essential to carry out a Coleman block test to determine whether the hindfoot varus is flexible or fixed. This has important implications when planning surgical treatment.

In unilateral cavus feet, calf muscle atrophy may be observed and the affected foot often appears shorter.

Standing radiographs of the foot and ankle help to quantify the severity of the deformity. Meary's angle (normal = 1°–9°) is increased in cavus feet while the Hibbs angle (normal >150°) is usually decreased (Figure 5.16).

Consultation with a neurologist is useful. Nerve conduction studies, MRI of the brain and or spine, muscle biopsy and DNA assay may be required to help establish the underlying cause.

Treatment

The aim of treatment is to relieve symptoms (pain, ankle instability), correct deformity and minimize the risk of recurrence of the deformity.

Asymptomatic patients do not usually require treatment. Conservative treatment options, such as orthosis, muscle stretching and strengthening exercises, play a limited role.

The mainstay of treatment is surgical: the options include plantar fascia releases, tendon transfers, calcaneal and other osteotomies, and triple arthrodesis. The type of surgery undertaken depends on the age of the patient, symptoms, muscle strength or weakness and rigidity of the deformity.

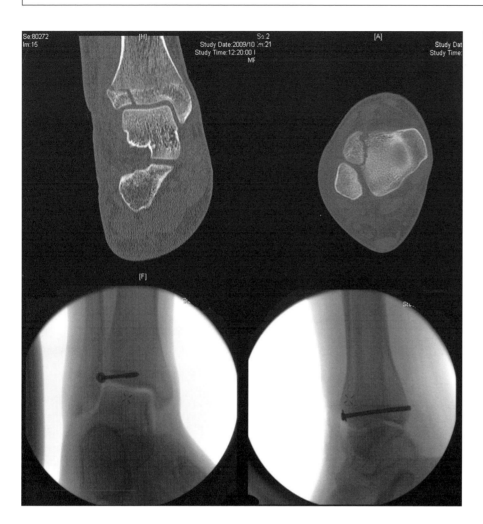

Figure 5.17 Tillaux fracture.

Transitional fractures

The distal tibial physis closes in an asymmetric fashion over a period of 18 months between the ages of 13 and 15 years. Thus, injuries sustained during this period can produce unusual fracture patterns not usually seen in younger children.

These fractures are called transitional fractures, as they occur during a transition toward skeletal maturity, and include Tillaux fractures and triplane fractures. They are commonly intra-articular. The treatment priority is to restore joint congruity.

Juvenile Tillaux fractures

These are Salter–Harris Type II fractures involving the antero-lateral distal tibia (Figure 5.17). The part of the physis not involved in the fracture is closed. These fractures are caused by external rotation forces.

Treatment usually involves open reduction and internal fixation with a screw to restore joint congruency and retension ligaments.

Triplane fractures

As the name implies, these fractures occur in three different planes (x, y, z). On anteroposterior radiographs, the fracture appears as a Salter–Harris Type III while on lateral views, it appears as a Type II (Figure 5.18). They are usually caused by external rotation forces, which are believed to be greater than that required to produce a Tillaux fracture.

Radiographs centred on the ankle are usually diagnostic but CT scans are usually required to define the fracture better and help in pre-operative planning.

Open reduction and internal fixation using screws is advised if there is >2 cm joint incongruency. The screws may be inserted percutaneously but a short skin incision is usually required to visualize restoration of joint congruency.

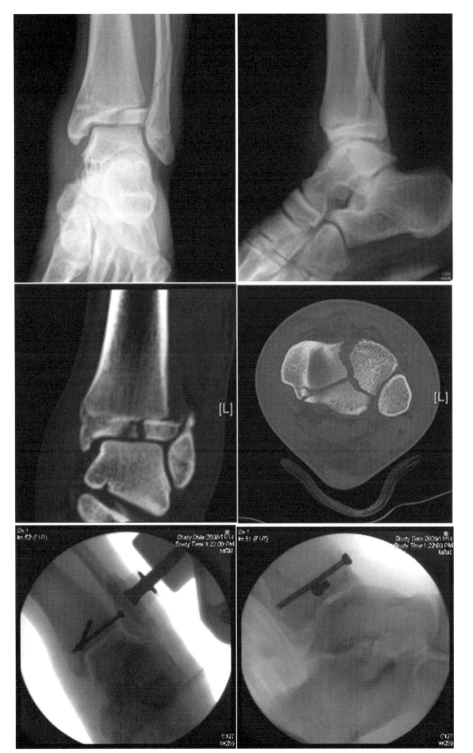

Figure 5.18 Triplane fracture. AP radiograph shows a Salter–Harris Type III fracture, while on the lateral view it appears as a Type II. This is often called two-part triplane (the number of the distal fragments: a small anterolateral and large posteromedial). In a three-part triplane fracture, the lateral view shows a Salter–Harris Type IV, where the posteromedial fragment is split into two parts (epiphyseal and metaphyseal).

References

1. Laaveg SJ and Ponseti IV (1980) Long-term results of treatment of congenital club foot. *J Bone Joint Surg Am* **62**(1):23–31.

2. Steinman S, Richards BS, Faulks S and Kaipus K (2009) A comparison of two nonoperative methods of idiopathic clubfoot correction: the Ponseti method and the French functional (physiotherapy) method. Surgical technique. *J Bone Joint Surg Am* **91**(Suppl 2):299–312.

3. Bleck EE (1983) Metatarsus adductus: classification and relationship to

outcomes of treatment. *J Pediatr Orthop* **3**(1):2–9.

4. Drennan JC (1996) Congenital vertical talus. *Instr Course Lect* **45**:315–22.

5. Mubarak SJ, Patel PN, Upasani VV, Moor MA and Wenger DR (2009) Calcaneonavicular coalition: treatment by excision and fat graft. *J Pediatr Orthop* **29**(5):418–26.

6. Robinson AH and Limbers JP (2005) Modern concepts in the treatment of hallux valgus. *J Bone Joint Surg Br* **87**(8):1038–45.

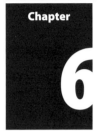

Chapter

6

The spine

Ashley A. Cole and Lee M. Breakwell

Spinal deformity

Spinal deformities can be divided into scoliosis and kyphosis, which affect either the whole spine or a region thereof, or spondylolisthesis, which usually affects a localized section of the spinal column.

Scoliosis

Scoliosis is defined as a frontal or coronal plane curvature with a Cobb angle of greater than 10°. The Cobb angle is defined as the maximal angle subtended by the endplates of the vertebrae within the curve.

Classification

1. Congenital,
2. Idiopathic,
3. Syndromic,
4. Neuromuscular,
5. Degenerative,
6. Paralytic.

Congenital

Congenital scoliosis is due to a developmental defect in the formation of the mesenchymal anlage. The resulting abnormal vertebra conveys uneven growth, creating angulation of the endplates and leading to unbalanced growth in adjacent vertebrae (Figure 6.1).

The defects are due to:

- Failure of formation: the commonest abnormality in this group is a hemivertebra, which may be fully, partially or unsegmented.
- Failure of segmentation: this results in block vertebrae, and unsegmented bars.
- A combination of these.

Associations

Once a diagnosis of congenital scoliosis has been made, the following associated anomalies must be sought and excluded:

- Spinal abnormalities (21–37%, MRI):
  - Hairy patch,
  - Dysraphism,
  - Myelomeningocele,
  - Diastematomyelia.
- Cardiac anomalies (12–26%, echo),
- Renal anomalies (20%, renal ultrasound),
- VACTERL association.

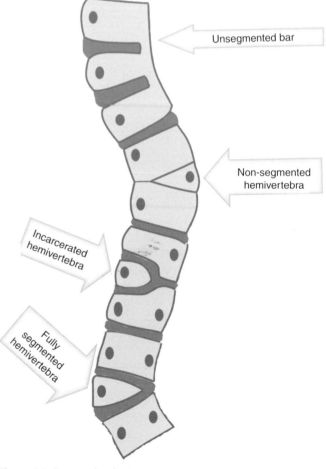

Figure 6.1 Congenital scoliosis.

Postgraduate Paediatric Orthopaedics, ed. Sattar Alshryda, Stan Jones and Paul A. Banaszkiewicz. Published by Cambridge University Press. © Cambridge University Press 2014.

Risk of progression

Several factors will help to indicate the risk of progression and hence the indications for treatment:

1. Age of patient (remaining growth),
2. Site of the anomaly (worse at junctional regions, such as thoracolumbar and lumbosacral),
3. Type of anomaly (from worst to best):
   i. Unilateral unsegmented bar with contralateral fully segmented hemivertebra,
   ii. Unilateral unsegmented bar,
   iii. Fully segmented hemivertebra,
   iv. Partially segmented hemivertebra,
   v. Incarcerated hemivertebra,
   vi. Non-segmented hemivertebra.
4. Size of curve at presentation.

Idiopathic

Idiopathic scoliosis is by far the commonest form of scoliosis and affects approximately 3% of girls. Although the aetiology is unknown, there is growing evidence of a genetic causation.

Right thoracic curves are the commonest, followed by double major (right thoracic and left lumbar) then left lumbar.

Idiopathic scoliosis is subdivided into three forms based on the age of onset:

1. Infantile (0–3 years),
2. Juvenile (4–10 years),
3. Adolescent (>10 years).

Infantile

This represents less than 1% of all idiopathic curves, is commonly seen in boys and is usually a left thoracic curve.

It is the only true scoliosis that can resolve spontaneously: this can be predicted by measuring the rib–vertebra angle difference (RVAD) of Mehta on an AP radiograph.

This is derived by taking the angle of the concave and convex ribs to the apical vertebra bisector, and subtracting the concave from the convex angles (Figure 6.2).

An angle difference of greater or less than 20° implies a significant chance of progression or resolution respectively; 83% of the curves that resolved had an initial RVAD measuring less than 20°, whereas 84% of the curves that progressively worsened had an RVAD exceeding 20° [1].

Juvenile

Juvenile curves have a relatively high risk of progression due to the remaining growth potential. Approximately 70% will progress and many will require treatment. As many as 1 in 10 juvenile scoliosis patients are revealed to have a neural axis abnormality by MRI.

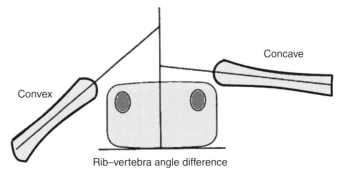

Figure 6.2 Congenital scoliosis, showing rib–vertebra angle difference.

Adolescent

This is the most common form of idiopathic scoliosis; it is commonly seen in girls.

Factors that aid in identifying risk of progression:

1. Curve size (>20°),
2. Remaining growth (curves worsen with growth). This is usually assessed:
   i. Clinically (menarche and peak height velocity (PHV)),
   ii. Radiological triradiate cartilage closure and Risser's stages (Figure 6.3).
3. Curve type (double curve and thoracic curve, thoracolumbar then lumbar).

In clinical practice, the PHV (i.e. growth spurt) is documented by serial measurement of the patient's height over time. The average age of the PHV is approximately 11.5 years in girls. Triradiate cartilage closure, a radiographic index of maturity, occurs after PHV and before Risser grade 1 and menarche.

Factors of no predictive value for curve progression before skeletal maturity include:

1. A family history of scoliosis,
2. Patient height-to-weight ratio,
3. Lumbosacral transitional anomalies,
4. Thoracic kyphosis,
5. Lumbar lordosis,
6. Spinal balance.

Syndromic

Scoliosis is a common feature of many well-known syndromes. In addition, it is present in many rare syndromes that are regularly seen in spinal clinics. Common syndromes with scoliosis include:

- Neurofibromatosis,
- Marfan syndrome,
- Ehlers–Danlos syndrome.

Rarer syndromes with scoliosis include:

- Rett,
- Sotos,
- Prader–Willi.

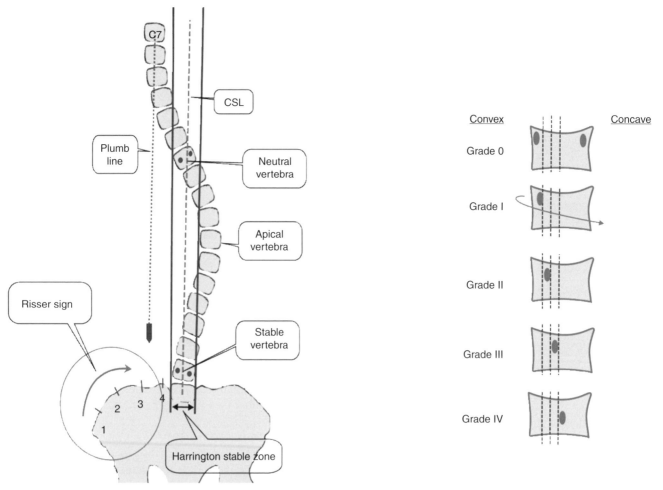

Figure 6.3 Scoliosis radiology. Left: Diagram showing various radiological terms of scoliosis. Right: Nash–Moe method for assessing vertebral rotation. Grade 0: Both pedicles are symmetric, Grade I: the convex pedicle has moved away from the side of the vertebral body. Grade III: the convex pedicle is in the centre of the vertebral body. Grade II: the rotation is between Grades I and III and Grade IV when the convex pedicle has moved past the midline. The curved arrow denotes the direction of the rotation. CSL, central sacral line.

The majority of these patients already have a diagnosis prior to identification of the scoliosis; however, in some patients, the spinal deformity is the index problem.

Neurofibromatosis scoliosis is the most common skeletal manifestation of neurofibromatosis.

The cause is unknown but various theories have been proposed, such as primary mesodermal dysplasia, erosion or infiltration of the bone by localized neurofibromatosis tumours, and endocrine disturbances.

Neurofibromatosis scoliosis can be either:

- Non-dystrophic,
- Dystrophic.

Differentiation between the two types is important because the prognosis and management differ significantly.

Dystrophic scoliosis is more common (Figure 6.4), usually located in the thoracic region, and has a short (4–6 vertebrae), sharply angled curve. It has a greater tendency to progress, and is at risk of developing neurologic deficits. Non-dystrophic

scoliosis more closely resembles idiopathic scoliosis in both curve patterns and behaviour.

Neuromuscular

These curves are usually long, less likely to have compensatory curves and may progress after maturity. Pulmonary problems, such as decreased lung function, are observed.

This form of scoliosis is divided into two subgroups:

- Cerebral palsy,
- True neuromuscular diseases, in which there is primary nerve or muscle disorder, e.g. Duchenne muscular dystrophy.

Cerebral palsy

The incidence of spinal deformity increases with the severity of cerebral palsy. It is around 20%; however, in the quadriplegic group, the incidence is in excess of 70%.

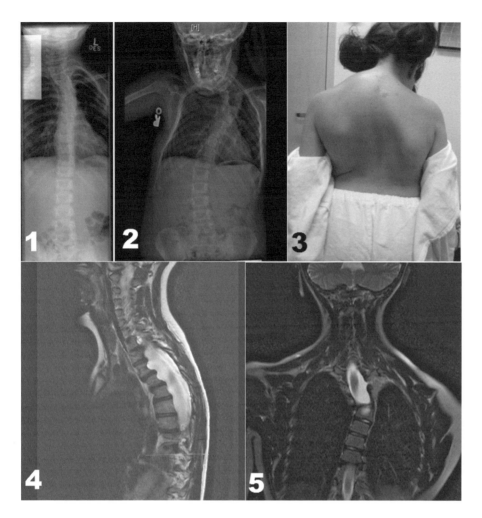

Figure 6.4. Dystrophic scoliosis in a child with neurofibromatosis scoliosis. 1, 2: There was a rapid progression in the severity over 2 years. 3: Café au lait spots and a sharply angled kyphoscoliosis. The kyphosis is more pronounced than the scoliosis. 4, 5: MRI scan shows large dural ectasia and scalloping of the posterior vertebrae. 5: There is a large plexiform neurofibroma in continuity with a nerve root.

The ability to walk is relatively protective, and therefore wheelchair dependence is a risk factor for development and progression of a spinal curvature.

Duchenne muscular dystrophy

This X-linked recessive condition, affecting the production of dystrophin, almost exclusively affects boys, with their mothers as the carrier. Historically, wheelchair dependence happened at about 10 to 11 years of age, following which the patient developed a scoliosis. Curves beyond 20° were seen to progress inexorably and surgery was advised at an early stage, to prevent further respiratory embarrassment.

Since the advent of steroid treatment, the progression of weakness has significantly slowed, and many subjects continue with some form of ambulation into their teens. This, coupled with the fact that treated curves do not always progress, means that the indication for surgery has changed, and not all patients require surgery.

The decision to undertake corrective surgery can now often be left until the curve has progressed to 40° or more, as the child is often older, and the lung function better than the historical cohort.

Spinal muscular atrophy

This autosomal recessive muscular wasting disease commonly causes scoliosis, which is often progressive. A defect in the *SMN1* gene leads to loss of the SMN protein, which is vital for muscle function. There are three types of spinal muscular atrophy in children, with function and life expectancy increasing from Type I through to Type III. Respiratory function can be severely restricted; hence, scoliosis is a major concern. The median survival in Type I spinal muscular atrophy is 7 months, with a mortality rate of 95% by the age of 18 months. In Type II spinal muscular atrophy, the age of onset is between 6 and 18 months and the age of death varies. The decision to undertake surgery for spinal deformity must be made in close collaboration with respiratory physicians, ideally considering life expectancy and function, as well as risk of curve progression.

Degenerative

This form of curve typically develops in the fifth or later decade of life, often in a previously normal spine; hence, it is beyond the scope of this book.

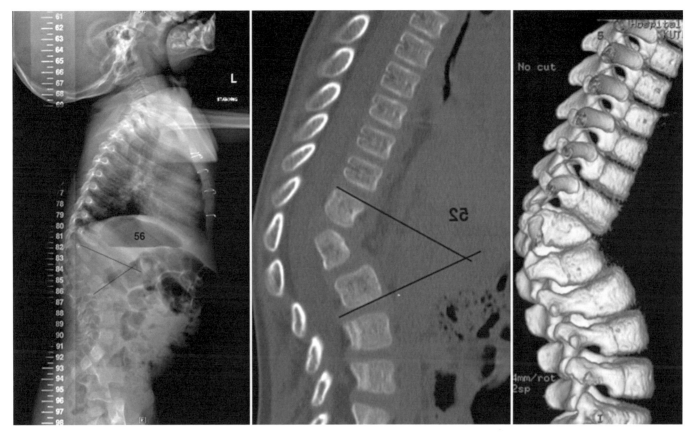

Figure 6.5 Congenital kyphosis.

Paralytic

Spinal cord injury with resultant paralysis before the onset of the adolescent growth spurt leads to the development of scoliosis in 97% of patients [2].

Kyphosis

Kyphosis is a forward curvature of the spine in the sagittal plane. A certain degree of thoracic kyphosis (20°–50°) is normal and desirable for spinal balance. Thoracic kyphosis does not strictly have a normal value, as it exhibits a range throughout different body shapes.

Classification

1. Congenital,
2. Idiopathic,
3. Neuromuscular,
4. Syndromic,
5. Traumatic,
6. Degenerative.

Congenital

As in scoliosis, this deformity develops due to an underlying structural disorder. The same basic types exist as in the coronal plane scenario.

A hemivertebra positioned posteriorly (Figure 6.5) will gradually deform the spine in a kyphotic direction. This causes a localized angular, deformity called a gibbus.

As the angulation progresses with growth, the centre of gravity of the body moves forward, increasing the load on the anterior aspect of the vertebral ring apophysis. This impedes anterior growth, in compliance with the Hueter–Volkmann law, unbalancing in favour of posterior height increase and leading to worsening of the kyphosis. By this process, kyphosis progresses throughout growth, and, if beyond 90°, continues into adulthood.

Whereas scoliotic deformity causes neurological deficit extremely rarely, congenital kyphosis has a relatively high risk of curve progression and neurological deficit when the angle is localized and beyond 90°.

Idiopathic

Scheuermann's kyphosis is seen in children older than 10 years and is more common in boys. The incidence ranges from 1–8%.

The accepted pathoaetiology is that slight kyphosis in the growing spine causes an anterior shift in the body weight centre, unevenly loading the anterior apophysis. This then leads to fragmentation and poor growth, as seen in the anterior vertebral body. It is characterized by vertebral wedging, disc space narrowing, endplate irregularities, including Schmorl's nodes, and kyphosis (Figure 6.6).

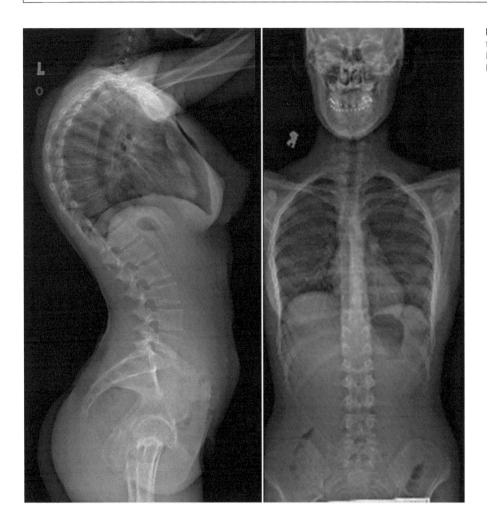

Figure 6.6 Scheuermann's kyphosis is traditionally defined by anterior wedging by at least 5° of three or more adjacent thoracic vertebral bodies.

Long-term natural history studies have shown that pain and function levels are not affected until the kyphosis progresses beyond 75° [3].

Neuromuscular

This is often noted in the wheelchair-dependant patient, as it is related to seating position and a preference to leaning forward when sitting. It is typically passively correctable.

Syndromic

Kyphosis is a common feature of some syndromes, in particular the mucopolysaccharidoses with Hurler (Type I), Hunter (Type II) and Morquio (Type IV) being the commonest.

Severe localized kyphosis can occur in the presence of abnormal bone, making surgical treatment very complex.

Natural history

Scoliosis is not always progressive and, in the infantile group, can resolve spontaneously in a large proportion of patients. Many curves, however, do progress, and it is important to understand the natural history in order to plan management.

In normal healthy subjects, lung alveolar budding is completed by 4 years and full lung structure at 8 years of age. After this, the lungs expand significantly due to thoracic spine and ribcage growth.

Any effect on thoracic spine growth before 8 years of age can be catastrophic, and beyond this age can affect long-term cardiorespiratory function.

Spinal deformities are often associated with complex rib and cardiac anomalies. These anomalies infer a risk to the long-term health of a patient, and quantification of this risk will aid the decision whether to correct a spinal deformity surgically.

Early-onset idiopathic scoliosis (onset before 10 years) carries a significant mortality risk.

Adolescent scoliosis rarely causes major health concerns, and only affects respiratory function when the curve progresses beyond 90°.

The major problem in the more severe syndromic and neuromuscular cases is the ability to sit, as many patients are non-ambulant. Respiratory embarrassment may be a feature, particularly in those with muscular weakness or thoracic cage restriction.

Kyphosis beyond 90° will progress beyond maturity, and carries a significant neurological risk in adult life. The cord becomes progressively draped and stretched over the apex, leading to myelopathic change. In general, angular kyphosis is more problematic than global kyphosis for neural structures.

Assessment

The main areas of concern for the doctor and the patient are:

- Risk to long-term health,
- Risk to neurological structures,
- Cosmesis,
- Pain,
- Function.

Clinical examination aims to assess first the likely type of scoliosis, and then the nature of the curve itself.

Observation of the child for skin markers, such as hairy patches, café au lait spots, axillary freckling and sacral dimples, may indicate underlying disorders (see Figures 2.2 and 2.3).

Assessment of the overall standing or sitting balance is next, with a plumb line from the vertebra prominens, which should pass through the natal cleft. Leg length discrepancy, real or apparent, must be calculated.

Curve geometry gives the most basic form of classification, such as right thoracic, when the apex of the curve is in the thoracic spine convex aspect to the patient's right.

The flexibility of the curve can be estimated by bending the spine left and right or, if the child is small enough, by suspension.

Rotation of the spine, a fundamental aspect of the deformity in scoliosis, can be estimated by Adam's forward bend test. On flexing forward such that the spine is horizontal in the sagittal plane, the true rotation of the curve apex can be measured with a scoliometer (Figure 6.7).

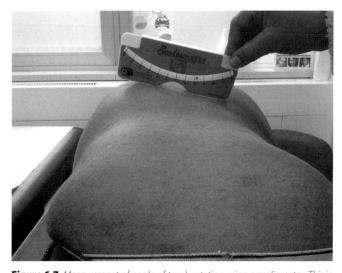

Figure 6.7 Measurement of angle of trunk rotation using a scoliometer. This is the paraspinal rib hump that is accentuated by forward bending in structural scoliosis (it is not seen in non-structural scoliosis curves). An angle of trunk rotation of 5°–7° is associated with a Cobb angle of 15°–20°.

Neurological examination, including abdominal reflexes, will help identify a neural axis abnormality, while inspection of the feet may show cavus deformities due to hereditary motor and sensory neuropathy.

Investigations

A full PA and lateral spine film, standing where possible, will allow diagnosis of a congenital anomaly and estimation of the Cobb angle. Plain X-radiographs are the most commonly used modality for assessing progression over time. Most studies suggest an increase in the Cobb angle greater than 5°–6° as indicative of definite progression. Bending views may be requested to confirm flexibility and aid classification. The majority of classification systems are based upon this imaging modality (King [4] and Lenke [5]) (see Chapter 19 for more details).

The following radiological terms are useful to assess radiographs:

Cobb angle:	The maximal angle subtended by the endplates of the vertebrae within the curve.
Harrington's stable zone:	This is defined by two vertical lines drawn up from the lumbosacral facets.
Plumb line:	A line drawn vertically from the midbody of C7 toward the floor.
Central sacral line (CSL):	This is drawn as a vertical line extended cephalad from the spinous process of S1.
Apical vertebra:	This is the name given to the vertebra at the apex of a curve.
Apical vertebra translation:	The distance of the apical vertebra of the thoracic curve from the plumb line and the lumbar curve from the CSL.
Apical vertebral rotation:	This indicates the magnitude of the apical vertebral rotation. There are two methods to measure the vertebral rotation, the Perdriolle and the Nash–Moe methods. The former uses a transparent torsionometer that is overlaid on the radiograph. In the Nash–Moe method, the relationship of the pedicle to the centre of the vertebral body is observed on AP radiographs (Figure 6.3).
Stable vertebra:	The most caudal vertebra that is bisected by the CSL.
Neutral vertebra:	The most cephalic vertebra that has neutrally rotated pedicles.

Major curve:	The largest curve and the one with the greatest degree of rotation. The direction of the curve is determined by its convex side.
Rib–vertebra angle difference (RVAD):	This is derived by taking the angle of the concave and convex ribs to the apical vertebra bisector, and subtracting the concave from the convex angles (Figure 6.2).

The following signs of skeletal maturity are used to assess the remaining growth:

i. Risser's sign: the iliac crest is divided into four quarters (Risser 1 = no ossification through Risser 4 = complete ossification and Risser 5, when the apophysis is fused with the iliac wing).
ii. Triradiate closure.
iii. Vertebral apophysis fusion on the lateral X-ray is a good indicator of skeletal maturity of the vertebra.

MRI is excellent at identifying cord (tethered cord and Chiari malformations) and hindbrain anomalies present in congenital deformities and can also be used to demonstrate the stretched or compressed cord sometimes seen in severe kyphosis.

As noted, early-onset scoliosis has a relatively high incidence of neural axis abnormality; hence, routine MRI scans are performed as part of the assessment of these subjects. Adolescent scoliosis patients very rarely exhibit MRI positive findings (1:1000), so in our practice the scan is reserved only for those undergoing surgery. All ambulant patients undergoing corrective spinal surgery require an MRI scan as part of the preoperative work-up.

In deformity, MRI is used for:

1. All ambulant patients undergoing surgery,
2. Severe kyphosis,
3. Early-onset scoliosis,
4. Congenital deformity,
5. Significant pain,
6. Neurological deficit.

Computed tomography (CT), in particular 3D reconstruction imaging, is helpful in understanding and planning treatment of complex deformities, such as congenital scoliosis and dystrophic curves. This is especially the case for identifying the posterior element anatomy.

Treatment

The aim of treatment is to maintain as many motion segments at maturity, while giving as normal a spine as possible.

Congenital

The mainstay of treatment is observation, as the large majority of congenital curves result in minor deformity. Bracing is of little value in this type of abnormality. Surgical management has three broad principles:

- Convex growth arrest, to allow corrective growth,
- Correction and fusion of an abnormal section, to arrest abnormal growth and correct malalignment,
- Excision of abnormal bone and correction of surrounding vertebrae.

Idiopathic

Infantile

Early treatment can, in this group, reverse the deformity, leading to normal growth of the spine. EDF (elongation, derotation and flexion) casting has been shown to treat infantile scoliosis successfully, if applied in the first year of life. Casting in even severe curves can significantly delay progression and prevent serious cardiorespiratory harm developing [6].

Surgery may be required if repeated casts fail to control the curve. This involves the use of growing rods (Luque trolley, single or dual growing rods) without spinal fusion. The concept is for the rods to maintain an applied correction while the spine grows.

Juvenile

This group attracts the most interest in terms of varied treatments. Various forms of braces exist, the evidence for which is weak. The aim of bracing is to prevent progression, or at least delay surgery long enough to allow for lung development.

It is advisable to delay surgery until the adolescent growth period, as spinal fusion before the age of 10 years reduces the final lung volume and chest expansion, thus compromising respiratory function. Apparent trunk shortening can also be a cosmetic issue in some patients, as can the crankshaft phenomenon [7], which occurs in posterior-only fusions in immature spines with significant remaining anterior growth.

Various 'growing' constructs exist for the surgical treatment of the immature spine (Figure 6.8). The basic concept is for an implant to hold an applied correction while the spine continues to grow, allowing lung volume increase and trunk: lower limb ratio maintenance.

Types of growth implants include:

- Luque trolley [8],
- Single or dual growing rod,
- Magnetically driven expandable rods,
- Shilla technique.

Adolescent

Reassurance is the most commonly required treatment in this group as the vast majority of curves will not progress, and if they do, will not exceed cosmetic or health-challenging proportions. Long-term studies have shown very little impact on the health of patients with curves below 80°.

Curves less than 40° at skeletal maturity, do not progress during adult life while curves above 50° progress slowly over many years [9].

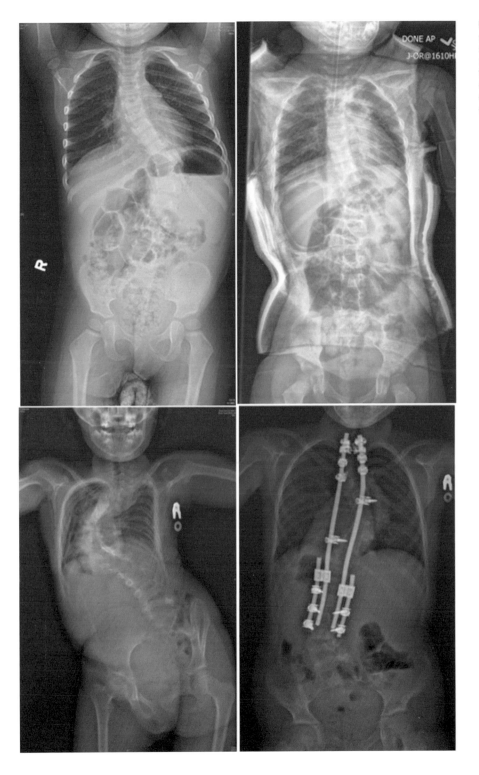

Figure 6.8 Idiopathic infantile and juvenile scoliosis treatments. Top: Child with infantile scoliosis treated with serial casting (every 2 to 3 months). Bottom: Child with juvenile scoliosis treated with growing rods, which were elongated every 6 months using a small incision over the domino connector and subsequent elongation of the rods.

Treatment focuses on maintaining curve size below 40°. Options include braces and surgery.

Braces –– Braces are used for curves for a Cobb angle of 20°–40° and with significant remaining growth, e.g. SpineCor and Boston-style thermoplastic devices. A lower chance of curve control with brace treatment occurs for curves >40°, correction of <50% in brace (X-ray with and without the brace), braces worn less than 16 hours per day and boys.

Surgery –– Surgery aims to reduce the Cobb angle of the curve and involves spinal fusion with instrumentation. Modern pedicle screw-based instrumentation has dramatically improved the ability of the surgeon to derotate the spine and translate the apex toward the midline. Most systems are built around the use of two precontoured rods, with segmental fixation of the spine with hooks and screws. These implants are sequentially connected to the rods, allowing gradual deformity correction prior to a bony fusion. The vast majority of procedures are now performed posteriorly as a result of these techniques.

Anterior surgery is generally reserved for thoracolumbar scoliosis with an apex at or below T12, whereby preservation of mobile levels at L3/4 and L4/5 can sometimes be maintained preferentially over posterior surgery. This is usually achieved via a thoraco-abdominal approach, which requires temporary detachment of the diaphragm.

Surgery enables a significant reduction in the size of the curve, and commensurate improvement in the cosmetic appearance of the trunk. On average, an improvement in 50% of the Cobb angle and apical trunk rotational angle is seen.

Complication rates for posterior surgery are about 5–10%, with infection and pain being most common. With modern implant design, loss of correction is rare and the incidence of revision surgery is low. The risk of paralysis following surgery in an adolescent scoliosis patient with a normal MRI scan is in the region of 1:800.

Syndromic and neuromuscular

Treatment in these patients is dependent upon the underlying diagnosis and ambulatory status. The principles, however, are the same for both groups.

In ambulant patients, pelvic obliquity is rare, and treatment is aimed at maintaining ambulation and preventing progression. Treatment is similar to that for idiopathic scoliosis; hence, it depends on age, remaining growth, progression rate and comorbidities.

In non-ambulant patients, the aim is to maintain sitting function. The long C-shaped curves that are commonly seen can lead to pelvic obliquity and associated postural difficulties. These curves are often well tolerated and agreement with the patients' carers for observation alone is sufficient.

In some cases, however, the degree of curvature, pelvic obliquity and imbalance, leads to pain and poor quality of life. In this scenario, posterior fusion of the entire spine, usually incorporating the pelvis, is possible. Major improvements in comfort, eating, sleeping and sitting can be achieved, but at the risk of major complications, such as infection, wound problems, and prolonged paralytic ileus. Mortality can be as high as 5%.

Combined anterior and posterior surgery is reserved for the worst cases, with stiff deformed spines. This can be undertaken either as a single or staged procedure, and involves some form of release anteriorly, by removing either discs or whole vertebrae, prior to a posterior fixation.

Kyphosis

Posterior corrective surgery can be undertaken either for cosmesis, as in Scheuermann's kyphosis, or to correct future or present neurological problems, when a significant kyphotic deformity is present.

Long posterior constructs are required to give stable fixation and balance, without the risk of implant failure. Careful attention must be paid to the overall sagittal balance, and posterior-based osteotomies are often performed.

The risks are similar to scoliosis in most cases, and depend predominantly on the size of curve and patient comorbidities. The major difference is in neurological risk. For Scheuermann's kyphosis, the risk of paralysis is about 1%, while for a complex kyphosis requiring osteotomies, in a patient with pre-existing neurological abnormalities, the risks can escalate to 20%.

Summary

When presented with a question regarding spinal deformity at the FRCS (Tr & Orth) exam, the main aim is to show a logical approach to a complex and largely specialist area.

A clear description of the presenting problems from the patient's perspective and an understanding of the types of deformity will suffice.

An ordered exposition of the classification of scoliosis, with a logical order of either congenital or acquired, with some recognition of prevalence, is helpful.

With regards to presentation, appearance is the commonest problem in idiopathic forms of spinal deformity, although with increasing severity of risk for cardiopulmonary restriction with earlier onset.

Untreated, the neurological risk is generally low for scoliotic deformities, with increased incidence seen in angular kyphosis, in particular congenital kyphosis.

In non-idiopathic curves, the cardiorespiratory risk may be higher, and function becomes more important with regards to pelvic obliquity and sitting.

Clinical assessment is aimed at excluding underlying causes, such as syndromes, in particular neurofibromatosis, and spinal dysraphism. A description of alignment and balance when standing and of the forward bend tests demonstrates the deformity. Neurological examination must include abdominal reflexes.

Investigations begin with plain full-length weight-bearing X-rays, with CT generally reserved for complex deformities. MRI is performed on all ambulant patients undergoing surgery and in any case with abnormal neurological signs or a higher incidence of anomaly, such as congenital or juvenile curves.

Treatment, as with all conditions, is based around an understanding of the natural history of the deformity in question, including the present and future functional or cosmetic issues.

Bracing has a limited role, but may be helpful in delaying progression sufficiently to prevent early growth-restrictive surgery. Surgery is limited to the more severe curves with risk of future progression or functional limitation. The majority of surgery is currently performed via a posterior approach, with pedicle screw instrumentation.

Infection

Aetiology and definition

Usually younger children, of 2–8 years old are affected. The aetiology is usually haematogenous spread and is thought to be due to the good blood supply to the vertebral bodies and the cartilaginous vertebral endplates. Direct invasion from a local infection may also occur. The lumbar spine is the commonest site.

There are four general groups:

Pyrogenic: The most common (>90%) is *Staphylococcus aureus*.

Tuberculosis.

Iatrogenic: Usually after instrumented spinal deformity corrections. Idiopathic scoliosis, 1%; neuromuscular scoliosis, 4%.

Fungal: *Aspergillus, Cryptococcus, Candida*.

Classification

There is no accepted classification but in children, the vertebra or disc can be involved, resulting in:

- Discitis,
- Vertebral osteomyelitis,
- Paraspinal abscess, e.g. psoas,
- Epidural abscess.

Natural history

Low-virulence infections in non-immunocompromised patients may resolve spontaneously but, in general, progression is expected with vertebral body destruction or abscess formation.

Clinical presentation

The lumbar spine is the commonest place. Presenting symptoms include:

- Back pain (50%),
- Limp,
- Abdominal pain,
- General malaise,
- Fever.

Always consider this diagnosis in a young child who is limping or unable to bear weight. A thorough history is essential, as suspicion of tuberculosis or any immunosuppression (HIV, chemotherapy, long-term steroids) may raise the possibility of a non-staphylococcal cause.

Examination may reveal spinal tenderness or evidence of paraspinal muscle spasm. Neurological deficit is very rare and due to:

- Epidural abscess,
- Vertebral destruction with kyphosis.

Investigation

Blood tests

White cell count (WCC), erythrocyte sedimentation rate (ESR) and C-reactive protein (CRP) levels are likely to be raised with spinal infection but could also be raised with infection elsewhere or malignancy.

Blood cultures

These are positive in approximately 50% of cases and should be repeated with temperature spikes.

Plain radiographs

These may be normal in early infection although 75% show disc height loss, irregular endplates, or bone destruction or collapse.

Isotope bone scan

This is a useful screening investigation in a child who presents with diffuse back pain, to try to localize the exact site for further investigations, e.g. MRI. A chronic low-grade postoperative infection presenting with back pain can be detected with a bone scan.

MRI

This is the investigation of choice, as it shows pus, granulation tissue and oedema very clearly (Figure 6.9). With disc involvement, this is usually diagnostic although low-virulence infections may be difficult to distinguish from Scheuermann's changes. Vertebral involvement may raise the possibility of tumours, including leukaemia or lymphoma. Vertebral

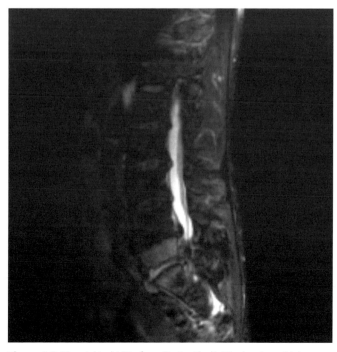

Figure 6.9 T2 weighted MRI of a patient with discitis, showing a high signal in the L5/S1 disc and pus collecting anterior to the disc.

collapse, especially vertebra plana, may raise the possibility of histiocytosis or eosinophilic granuloma. Vertebral body changes may suggest SAPHO (synovitis, acne, pustulosis, hyperostosis and osteitis).

MRI findings always lag behind the clinical picture, making it a poor modality for monitoring response to treatment. Consider including the sacroiliac joints if clinically indicated, as infection or inflammation (ankylosing spondylitis) may occur.

Biopsy

There is less need for biopsy in children than in adults, except in older teenagers. Biopsies should be sent to the microbiology and histology departments for analysis. Prolonged culture should be requested and the possibility of fungal infections considered.

Indications for biopsy include:

- Vertebral osteomyelitis, where other diagnoses need to be excluded.
- Failure of clinical and blood test improvement on flucloxacillin. The antibiotics should ideally be stopped for 1 week.
- Suspicion that the infection may not be *Staphylococcus aureus* – immunosuppression, possible tuberculosis, sickle cell disease, long indolent course suggestive of possible fungal infection.

QuantiFERON

This is indicated if tuberculosis is suspected. Beware false positives in other mycobacterium infections. There are limited data for this test in children.

Management

The treatment aims are to eradicate infection and prevent or minimize spinal deformity. This is achieved by:

1. A short period of bed rest, usually a few days.
2. Peripherally inserted central catheter.
3. Intravenous flucloxacillin initially for 7–14 days; depending on clinical and blood test improvement, this can be changed to oral antibiotics for 4–6 weeks.
4. Weekly monitoring of white cell count (WCC), erythrocyte sedimentation rate (ESR) and C-reactive protein (CRP). The CRP level settles faster than the ESR.
5. The requirement for bracing is controversial. Brace immobilization may help with 'instability'-type pain. Thoracolumbar braces are unlikely to prevent deformity. Hard cervical collars may prevent kyphosis.
6. If persistent or worsening pain or failure of inflammatory marker improvement, consider stopping antibiotics for 1 week and biopsy.
7. Plain radiograph at 12 months to document restoration of disc height, loss of disc height or fusion.

Tuberculosis infections

These infections can affect multiple vertebral bodies, leading to anterior abscess formation, and cause anterior collapse, resulting in deformity or neurological deficit.

Anterior abscesses in the cervical or upper thoracic spine can cause respiratory compromise in children. A biopsy is required for diagnosis and antibiotic sensitivity, as resistant strains are becoming more common. In the absence of an abscess, bony destruction or collapse, the treatment is non-surgical using appropriate antibiotics.

The aims of surgical treatment are to eradicate the infection and stabilize the spine to achieve a fusion and prevent late progressive deformity that may result in paraplegia.

An abscess with minimal bone involvement should be surgically drained (often by a costotransverse approach) to prevent it spreading and involving more vertebrae.

An anterior abscess with significant bony involvement and no neurological deficit should be drained and the bone debrided by an anterior or posterolateral approach. The cavity should be supported with a rib strut graft, which can be oversized to improve any deformity.

Where there is neurological deficit, the spinal cord should be decompressed and the spinal column reconstructed and stabilized.

If the cord compression is due to acute bony collapse or pus, the neurological outlook is good. However, if the compression is caused by chronic deformity with organized fibrosis, the neurological outlook is poor. In the lumbar spine and lumbosacral junction, it is important to prevent a localized kyphosis to reduce the risk of late back pain.

Indications for surgery

Neurological deficit may result from an epidural abscess, especially at spinal cord level. This is treated by laminectomy or multiple laminectomies, using a small catheter to wash out the abscess. Pre-operative MRI with contrast is good for distinguishing pus from infected granulation tissue that cannot be washed out (enhancing rim with contrast). A costotransverse approach can be used to drain a thoracic epidural abscess, especially in tuberculosis infection.

Occasionally, bone loss may cause severe deformity requiring surgical reconstruction. The aims of surgery are:

1. Decompression of compressed neurological elements,
2. Biopsy (if required),
3. Thorough debridement,
4. Stabilization,
5. Fusion (usually spontaneous, no requirement to bone graft).

Iatrogenic spinal infections are usually treated with a thorough washout and debridement, as the infection often follows posterior instrumentation. Multiple tissue samples should be taken before any antibiotics are given. These should be sent to the microbiology department for immediate processing and prolonged culture.

Mildly infected wounds can be closed primarily and broad-spectrum antimicrobial therapy started initially; this should be narrowed once culture results are available. Unless the metalwork is loose, it should be left *in situ*. Bone grafts should probably be removed and discarded. There should be a low threshold for further washouts if the wound is leaking or inflammatory markers do not settle.

Heavily infected wounds may be treated with vacuum therapy after initial washout and debridement, with a planned second return to theatre for re-debridement and closure. Intravenous antibiotics should be given for at least 2 weeks followed by oral antibiotics for 3 months. If infection persists (or presents very late after surgery and is low grade) it can be suppressed with antibiotics until the spine has fused, so long as the instrumentation is not loose. The instrumentation can then be removed.

Removal of instrumentation for suspected low-grade or chronic infection will usually settle the infection. Samples should be taken at the time of surgery. The link between postoperative pain and low-grade infection is not well established although *Propionibacterium*, a low-virulence skin organism, is a common cause.

Tumour

This section provides an overview of spinal tumours. A detailed description of individual tumours is covered in Chapter 12, but intradural spinal tumours or spinal dysraphism are not considered. In children, 70% of primary bony tumours are benign. Generally, most cervical vertebrae tumours are benign, while thoracic and lumbar tumours are more commonly malignant. The following tumours are known to affect the spine:

1. Benign:
   a. Osteoid osteoma,
   b. Osteoblastoma,
   c. Aneurysmal bone cyst,
   d. Giant cell tumour,
   e. Eosinophilic granuloma,
   f. Osteochondroma,
   g. Neurofibroma.

2. Malignant:
   a. Ewing's sarcoma,
   b. Osteosarcoma,
   c. Chondrosarcoma,
   d. Leukaemia,
   e. Lymphoma,
   f. Metastasis.

Figure 6.10 summarizes the predilection of spinal tumour.

Clinical presentation

Worrying symptoms include:
- Severe pain requiring regular analgesia,
- Waking up at night in pain,
- Pain that prevents engagement in enjoyable activities,
- Fever (pyrexia),
- Neurological symptoms, including bladder or bowel dysfunction,
- Rapid new-onset deformity, especially if associated with pain.

Investigation

Blood tests

Full blood count (including film) and erythrocyte sedimentation rate are useful screening investigations, as the child will probably present with back pain.

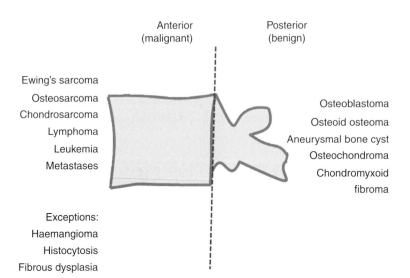

Anterior (malignant)   Posterior (benign)

Ewing's sarcoma
Osteosarcoma
Chondrosarcoma
Lymphoma
Leukemia
Metastases

Osteoblastoma
Osteoid osteoma
Aneurysmal bone cyst
Osteochondroma
Chondromyxoid fibroma

Exceptions:
Haemangioma
Histocytosis
Fibrous dysplasia

Figure 6.10 Predilection of spinal tumour.

Plain radiographs

These may show bone destruction or collapse. An absent pedicle is a classic sign.

Bone scan

As with spinal infection, this can be useful in localizing tumours and is a good screening tool in children who would require a general anaesthesia or sedation for MRI where the level of clinical suspicion is low. Bone scans are also useful for defining multiple tumours or metastatic disease.

MRI

This is excellent for diagnosis and assessing neurological involvement. It is also useful for defining anatomical location:

- Intradural, intramedullary,
- Intradural, extramedullary,
- Extradural,
- Bone.

CT

This is useful for evaluating bony involvement and can be used to diagnose for osteoid osteoma (central nidus with surrounding lytic area). It is essential to stage malignant tumours with CT of the chest, abdomen and pelvis.

Biopsy

Biopsy may be excisional or incisional. An incisional biopsy track must be excisable if en-bloc (potential curative) resection is planned.

Management

In the spine, surgical treatment consists of:

1. Decompression, with some intralesional tumour removal aimed at decompressing neurological elements, obtaining a biopsy and achieving some local control. Stabilization may be required if spinal instability exists or results from the surgical decompression. This is often emergency treatment, when there is spinal cord compression and tumours are usually high grade. Surgery is supplemented with chemotherapy or radiotherapy (or both). Outcome is not always poor, e.g. lymphoma.
2. Intralesional excision aimed at removing all macroscopic tumours. This is often performed for benign tumours and has a low recurrence rate. Stabilization is rarely required.
3. Marginal, en-bloc resection. This is rarely possible in the spine and involves removal of the whole vertebra (vertebrectomy), attempting to remove the tumour with a wide margin of resection.

Trauma and other cervical spine problems
General considerations

The initial management of a child with a suspected spinal column injury is the same as for an adult. A paediatric spinal board should be used in children aged <8 years to avoid neck flexion due to their relatively large heads. In younger children, injury is more common in the upper cervical spine, while after the age of 8, the midcervical spine is more commonly injured.

The odontoid ossification centre fuses to the C2 body ossification centre between ages 3 and 6. By 8 years of age, the only important ossification centre not to have appeared and fused is the apical odontoid epiphysis, which usually only appears between ages 8 and 12. There is often slight wedging of the cervical vertebral bodies until about age 10.

Spinal cord injury

Spinal cord injury without radiological abnormality (SCIWORA) is rare. Physeal injuries (separation of the vertebral endplate from the vertebral body) that are not easily visible radiologically can result in spinal cord injury and inappropriately applied traction can result in spinal cord injury. SCIWORA is more common in the cervical spine and in younger children. Complete cord injury has a poor prognosis, while incomplete cord injury often results in a good functional recovery. The onset of SCIWORA can be delayed, with most patients recalling transient neurological symptoms at the time of injury. A Frankel grade is used to determine the severity of neurological involvement and any recovery:

Frankel A: Complete paralysis

Frankel B: Sensory function only below the injury level

Frankel C: Incomplete motor function (grade 1–2/5) below the injury level

Frankel D: Fair to good motor function (grade 3–4/5) below the injury level

Frankel E: Normal motor function (grade 5/5)

Pseudosubluxation

Anterior subluxation of C2 on C3 of up to 4 mm is considered normal in children up to 8 years of age. Occasionally, C3/C4 may be involved. Radiographs may also reveal the absence of soft-tissue swelling and normal alignment of the posterior spinolaminar line (Figure 6.11).

Occipital-atlantal dislocation

This is a rare injury but is more common in younger children because of the tendency for upper cervical spine injuries. These injuries are usually fatal.

Atlantoaxial rotatory subluxation

Although this can be traumatic, it is usually secondary to an upper respiratory tract infection (Grisel's syndrome). Patients usually present with a torticollis and often have pain. Diagnosis is made with dynamic CT, with the head rotated to the left and right. The Fielding and Hawkin classification is used (Figure 6.12).

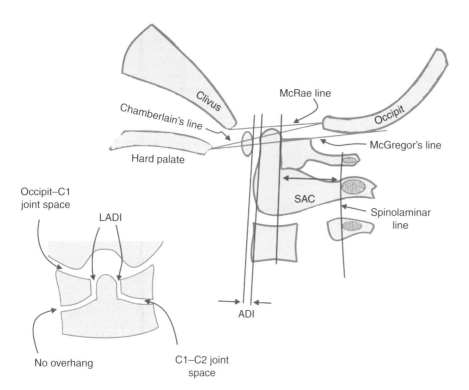

Figure 6.11 Craniospinal junction radioanatomy, showing extremely important radiological measurements. ADI (anterior atlantodens index), <3–5 mm; SAC (space available to the cord, also called the posterior atlantodens index, >13 mm; LADI (lateral atlantodens index, 2–3 mm, symmetrical on both sides); O–C1 and C1–C2, 1–2 mm). McRae's line defines the opening of the foramen magnum: the tip of the dens may protrude slightly above this line, but if the dens is below this line then impaction is not present. McGregor's line is a line drawn from the posterior edge of the hard palate to the caudal posterior occiput curve; cranial settling is present when the tip of dens is more than 4.5 mm above this line. Chamberlain's line (an Englishman between two Scots) is a line from the dorsal margin of the hard palate to the posterior edge of the foramen magnum: this line is often hard to visualize on standard radiographs; a dens >6 mm above this line is consistent with impaction.

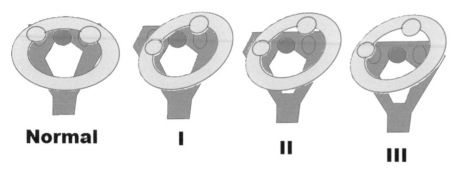

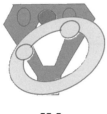

Figure 6.12 Fielding and Hawkin classification. Type I: Rotation without anterior displacement of the C1 (transverse ligament intact). Type II: Rotation with 3–5 mm anterior translation (transverse ligament deficient). Type III: Rotation with >5 mm anterior translation. Type IV: Rotation with posterior translation due to deficient odontoid.

Normal   **I**   **II**   **III**

IV

Treatment

If detected early, 1–2 weeks in a soft cervical collar with analgesia usually results in resolution. If this fails, halter or halo traction (depending on the age of the patient) for 1–2 weeks followed by 8 weeks in a halo vest may be required. Fusion of the C1/2 is required if the initial management fails or the diagnosis is made after 1 month.

C1/2 instability

The normal atlantodens interval is up to 4.5 mm. Causes of instability include:

1. Previous or acute trauma,
2. Down's syndrome,
3. Juvenile rheumatoid arthritis,

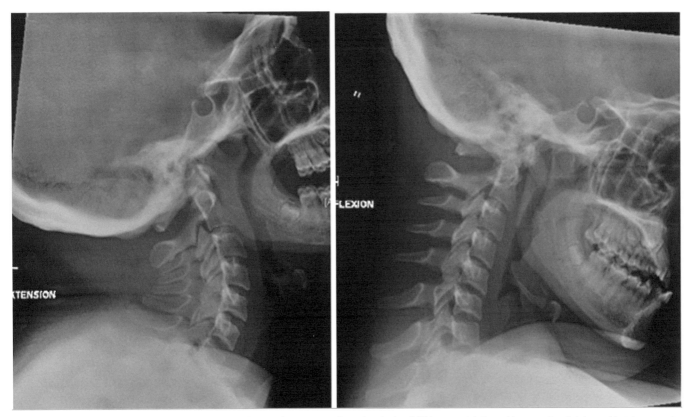

Figure 6.13 C1/2 instability in a child with Down's syndrome. The anterior atlantodens index (ADI) is normal (<3 mm) in extension (left image) but increases to 5 mm in flexion (right image).

4. Spondyloepiphyseal dysplasia,
5. Kniest syndrome,
6. Mucopolysaccharidoses.

Surgery in the form of C1/2 fusion is required in the presence of neurological symptoms or if the space available for the spinal cord is less than 14 mm. Ideally, lateral mass screws are inserted in C1 and pedicle screws in C2 (Figure 6.13).

Basilar impression

Basilar impression or invagination is thought to be due to a bony abnormality at the base of the skull, causing cephalad migration of the odontoid into the foramen magnum and narrowing the space available for the spinal cord at the craniocervical junction. Patients will usually present with headaches, lower cranial nerve abnormalities, nystagmus and cervical myelopathy. On X-ray or MRI, the tip of the odontoid peg should not be above the line joining the clivus with the posterior rim of the foramen magnum (McRae's line). Treatment is difficult but usually requires a craniocervical decompression and instrumented fusion from the occiput (C0) to the midcervical spine.

Os odontoideum

It is uncertain whether this is a failure of fusion or an old fracture at the base of the odontoid. Occasionally, patients will present with spinal cord injury after relatively mild trauma.

Treatment is non-operative; however, if C1/2 instability is observed in lateral radiographs on flexion or extension, a C1/2 posterior fusion is advised, even if the patient is asymptomatic.

Torticollis

Torticollis is a tilting of the head to the affected side and rotation toward the unaffected side. That is, in a right-sided torticollis, the head will tilt to the right and rotate anticlockwise to the left.

Patients can present at any age. Torticollis can be classified as follows:

- Congenital:
  - Congenital muscular torticollis (commonest cause);
  - Vertebral anomalies;
    - Failure of segmentation – occipitalization of C1;
    - Failure of formation – congenital hemi-atlas;
    - Combined.
  - Ocular.
- Acquired: painful:
  - Traumatic – C1 fracture;
  - Inflammatory – atlantoaxial rotatory subluxation, juvenile rheumatoid, infection;
  - Tumour – osteoid osteoma, eosinophilic granuloma.

119

- Acquired: non-painful;
- CNS tumour – posterior fossa, acoustic neuroma, cervical cord;
- Syringomyelia;
- Ligamentous laxity – Down's syndrome, spondyloepiphyseal dysplasia.

Congenital muscular torticollis is the commonest type. The cause is unknown, though it is thought to be due to abnormality of the sternomastoid muscle. If the history dates back to birth, there is a palpable 'tumour' in the sternomastoid muscle (disappears by 4 months of age), and the sternomastoid feels tight (often difficult to be sure in a baby), a diagnosis of congenital muscular torticollis can be made. This is treated with stretches and postural encouragement (the baby is encouraged to rotate its head to the tight side).

If stretching fails to improve the condition (<10%), or presentation is abnormal, other causes should be considered. In practice, this means an ophthalmic examination, CT of the cervical spine and MRI of the cervical spine and head.

Other causes should be treated as required. Congenital muscular torticollis should be treated around 6 years of age, if it is still significant. This involves a unipolar (distal release of clavicular head and z-lengthening of the sternal head) or bipolar (as for unipolar and proximal release just below mastoid attachment) release. Bipolar release produces better results but the proximal release has a risk of accessory nerve injury. Other causes should be treated based on the aetiology.

Chance fracture

These are common following road traffic accidents, with the commonest mechanism being a lap-belt injury (hyperflexion), and are often associated with intra-abdominal injury. Spinal cord injury is common and bony chance fractures are more common in children than in adults (bones weaker, ligaments more lax) (Figure 6.14).

Spondylolysis and spondylolisthesis
Definition and aetiology

Spondylolysis is a stress fracture of the pars intra-articularis. It is most common at L5 but does occur in other lumbar segments. It is caused by repetitive trauma to the pars from the inferior L4 facet in extension; sporting activities involving lumbar spine extension are known risk factors. Approximately 5% of 5 year olds and 6% of adults have a lumbar spine spondylolysis.

Spondylolisthesis is where a cranial vertebra slips anteriorly on the caudal vertebra. The opposite of this is called a retrolisthesis.

Classification

Spondylolisthesis can be described by cause (Table 6.1).

The degree of slip is graded by dividing the superior endplate of S1 into quarters and observing how far the

Table 6.1 Spondylolisthesis classification [10]

Type	Age	Pathology/Other
I: Dysplastic	Child	Congenital dysplasia of S1 superior facet
II: Isthmic	5–50 years	Predisposition leading to elongation/fracture of pars (L5–S1)
III: Degenerative	>40 years	Facet arthrosis leading to subluxation (L4–L5)
IV: Traumatic	Any age	Acute fracture other than pars
V: Pathological	Any age	Incompetence of bony elements
VI: Postsurgical	Adult	Excessive resection of neural arches or facets

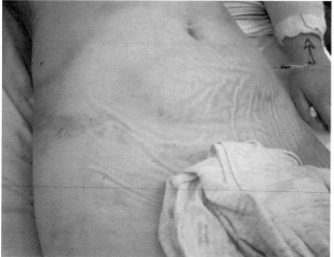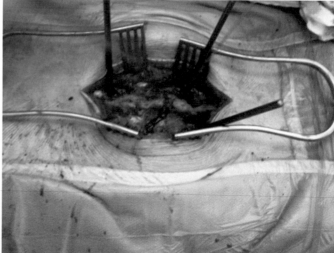

Figure 6.14 Chance facture. This 16-year-old girl was a seat-belted passenger involved in a front impact car collision. Left: There are seat-belt bruises. Right: The torn supraspinous and interspinous ligament caused by flexion distraction injury.

posteroinferior corner of the L5 vertebral body slips forward onto S1 [11] such that:

Grade 1: 0–25% slip,

Grade 2: 25–50% slip,

Grade 3: 50–75% slip,

Grade 4: 75–100% slip,

Grade 5: >100% slip = spondyloptosis (not in the original description).

Natural history

Many patients remain asymptomatic and management depends on symptoms. Reported risk factors for progression include:

1. Young age (10–15),
2. Female,
3. Dysplastic spondylolisthesis,
4. Spondylolisthesis above L5–S1,
5. Slip angle >10° or sacral inclination >30°,
6. High grade >50%,
7. Dome shape,
8. Flexion type.

Clinical presentation

In childhood, spondylolysis usually presents with low back pain, gait abnormalities and occasional leg pain secondary to L5 root irritation, which lies just below the pars in the L5/S1 foramen.

Spondylolisthesis is usually secondary to spondylolysis (lytic spondylolisthesis) although occasional cases of dysplastic spondylolisthesis are seen. Both will present with back pain and L5 radicular leg pain, with the L5 nerve root compressed in the foramen at L5/S1. In dysplastic spondylolisthesis, the S1 roots are also commonly compressed in the lateral recess at L5/S1.

On examination, straight leg raise is usually decreased due to bilateral hamstring tightness. Neurological findings are usually normal and any weakness or other neurological abnormality should raise questions as to whether the spondylolysis or spondylolisthesis is just an incidental finding and there is another cause for the patient's symptoms.

Investigation

Plain X-radiographs show a spondylolysis in 40–60% of cases. The radiation doses of oblique radiographs of the lumbosacral junction are higher than for CT so should no longer be performed. A lateral standing radiograph will show the degree of slip and comparison with supine investigations (CT or MRI) will demonstrate whether the spondylolisthesis is mobile. The sagittal plane alignment of the spine is thought to be important. Full-spine standing lateral radiographs including the hips will allow an overall assessment of sagittal balance and measurement of pelvic incidence and sacral slope, which may be clinically significant when managing high-grade (3 and 4) spondylolisthesis.

CT is diagnostic showing the spondylolysis and any spondylolisthesis. Sagittal reconstructions are the best images to view. MRI shows any nerve root compression and any degenerative change in the discs (Figure 6.15).

Management

Spondylolysis

- Reassurance and analgesia.
- Stop any sporting activity, especially sport involving extension.
- Physiotherapy but avoiding extension exercises.
- Reintroduce activities at 3 months if the pain has settled.
- If unsuccessful, try a pars injection (steroid + local anaesthetic) followed by further physiotherapy.
- If unsuccessful then uninstrumented fusion (supported by long-term follow-up evidence of fusion versus lysis repair). Bilateral Wiltse approach, iliac crest graft and 3 months in a lumbosacral orthosis. This would be at L5/S1 for an L5 spondylolysis. Consider pars repair (Buck's fusion with a 3.5 mm lagged cortical screw and bone grafting) for unilateral spondylolysis.

Low-grade spondylolisthesis (Grades 1 and 2)

The initial treatment is the same as for spondylolysis. Pars injections are rarely beneficial but may have a role in diagnosing the source of back pain.

If non-operative measures fail to relieve back pain, an uninstrumented fusion is advised. This has a 70% chance of improving back pain.

If the main symptom is radicular leg pain and there is nerve compression in the foramen, an instrumented fusion and L5 decompression through a midline approach and using an iliac crest graft is the best option. The L5 root decompression is in the foramen at L5/S1, rather than the lateral recess at L4/5.

High-grade spondylolisthesis (Grades 3, 4 and 5)

High-grade spondylolisthesis is likely to progress. If the presentation is back pain only, an *in-situ* L5/S1 instrumented fusion with iliac crest graft through bilateral Wiltse approaches is advised.

If there is significant radicular leg pain with or without back pain, a midline approach with L5/S1 instrumented fusion and L5 decompression should be performed.

Reduction of high-grade spondylolisthesis is sometimes performed in children and involves a posterior instrumented fusion from L4 to S1 and total removal of the L5/S1 disc, usually from a posterior approach with interbody fusion. This procedure has the advantage of improved cosmesis and a high fusion rate but is a much more complex procedure and has a 10% chance of neurological injury (L5 = foot drop).

Back and radicular pain

Back pain is a common presentation in childhood, with an incidence of approximately 40% in teenagers. In general, back

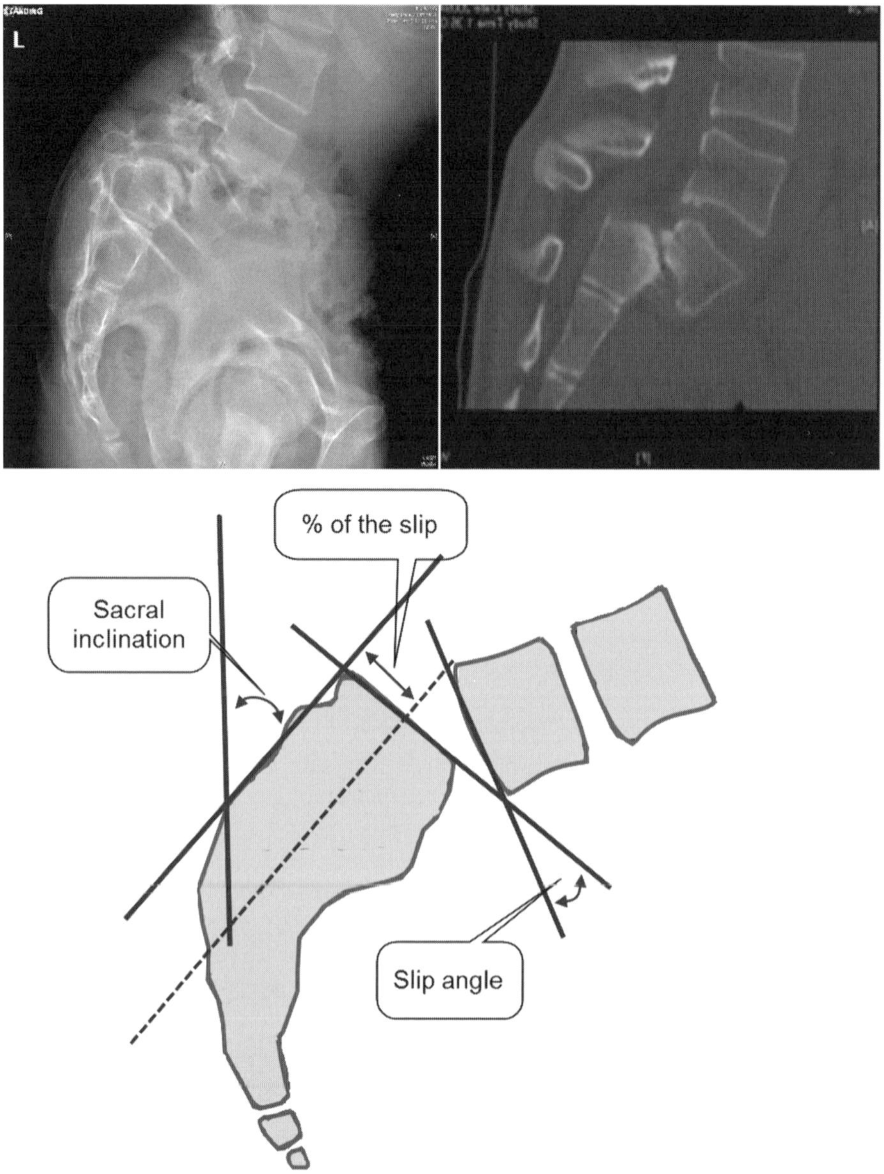

Figure 6.15 Spondylolisthesis.

pain in patients younger than 10 is likely to be pathological while the opposite is true in those older than 10. The various causes of back pain have been considered already. Sinister causes of back pain tend to have a relatively short history and the pain will be continuous and worsening. In addition, the pain interferes with activities that the child likes and is present at night, preventing sleep. Regular analgesia is usually required. A history of pyrexia is suspicious. Neurological symptoms or signs are obviously significant.

Investigative blood tests (full cell count and erythrocyte sedimentation rate (ESR)) should be performed in all children with persistent back pain. Plain X-radiography may be considered if there is suspicion of tumour, deformity, spondylolysis or spondylolisthesis.

Bone scan or MRI (or both) should always be performed in children younger than 10 with back pain and should be considered in older children with sinister features or who fail to resolve with physiotherapy.

Lumbar disc protrusions are rare in children and will often present with just back pain although some will present with radicular pain. Straight leg raise is usually restricted. MRI is diagnostic. The initial treatment is physiotherapy and nerve root injections may be considered for radicular pain, although the success is only about 50%. Chemonucleolysis with chymopapain although a successful treatment is no longer available. Lumbar discectomy will usually improve back and leg pain but there is a high incidence of recurrence and many patients have chronic low back pain and require further surgery.

References

1. Mehta MH (1972) The rib-vertebra angle in the early diagnosis between resolving and progressive infantile scoliosis. *J Bone Joint Surg Br* **54**(2):230–43.

2. Dearolf WW 3rd, Betz RR, Vogel LC *et al.* (1990) Scoliosis in pediatric spinal cord-injured patients. *J Pediatr Orthop* **10**(2):214–18.

3. Sachs B, Bradford D, Winter R *et al.* (1987) Scheuermann kyphosis. Follow-up of Milwaukee-brace treatment. *J Bone Joint Surg Am* **69**(1):50–7.

4. King HA, Moe JH, Bradford DS and Winter RB (1983) The selection of fusion levels in thoracic idiopathic scoliosis. *J Bone Joint Surg Am* **65**(9):1302–13.

5. Lenke LG, Betz RR, Harms J *et al.* (2001) Adolescent idiopathic scoliosis: a new classification to determine extent of spinal arthrodesis. *J Bone Joint Surg Am* **83-A**(8):1169–81.

6. Mehta MH (2005) Growth as a corrective force in the early treatment of progressive infantile scoliosis. *J Bone Joint Surg Br* **87**(9):1237–47.

7. Dubousset J, Herring JA and Shufflebarger H (1989) The crankshaft phenomenon. *J Pediatr Orthop* **9**(5):541–50.

8. Luque ER (1982) Paralytic scoliosis in growing children. *Clin Orthop Relat Res* **163**:202–9.

9. Weinstein SL, Dolan LA, Spratt KF *et al.* (2003) Health and function of patients with untreated idiopathic scoliosis: a 50-year natural history study. *JAMA* **289** (5):559–67.

10. Wiltse LL, Newman PH and MacNab I (1976) Classification of spondylosis and spondylolisthesis. *Curr Orthop Pract* **117**:23–9.

11. Meyerding HW (1932) Spondylolisthesis. *Surg, Gynecol and Obstet* **54**:371–7.

The shoulder

Om Lahoti and Matt Nixon

Obstetric brachial plexus injury

Aetiology

The incidence of obstetric brachial plexus birth injury (OBPI) is around 1 per 1000 live births. Around 25% of patients are left with permanent disability without intervention. The shoulder is the most commonly affected joint and, owing to the subsequent imbalance of musculature, the abnormal deforming forces cause dysplasia of the glenohumeral joint. In the growing child, this presents with a changing pattern of pathology, which requires a multidisciplinary approach and a broad range of treatment modalities to optimize function.

A common cause is a traction injury to the brachial plexus during the later stages of vaginal delivery when the head is pulled away from the shoulder. The mechanism of injury is a forced lateral flexion of the cervical spine, resulting in injury initially to the upper cervical roots (C5–C7), causing an Erb's palsy, and, in more severe cases, the entire brachial plexus (C5–T1). With this mechanism, isolated lower root injuries (C8–T1, Klumpke's palsy) do not tend to occur in OBPI. Other rare causes are abnormal forces on the shoulder over the sacral promontory or abnormal forces in an abnormal uterus, such as a bicornuate or fibroid uterus.

The following are risk factors:

1. Large babies (>4 kg),
2. Difficult labour,
3. Abnormal fetal presentation, such as breech delivery or shoulder dystocia,
4. Multiple pregnancies,
5. A previous child with OBPI.

Typical scenarios involve large babies (birth weight more than 4 kg) with cephalic presentation and shoulder dystocia, requiring excessive force to deliver the shoulder, resulting in traction to the C5 and C6 roots or small babies – weighing under 3 kg – with breech presentation requiring manipulation of the neck to deliver the arms and head, resulting in traction on the upper and lower roots. This mechanism may be associated with nerve root tearing or avulsion of nerve roots.

Anatomical (Narakas)

The severity of injury has been classified by Narakas into four prognostic grades:

Grade 1: This involves only the C5/6 roots and presents with weakness of shoulder abduction and elbow flexion.

Grade 2: The C7 nerve root is also involved with associated wrist drop. These groups have a higher rate of spontaneous recovery.

Grade 3: Complete paralysis.

Grade 4: This is also associated with Horner's syndrome.

Narakas Grade 3 and 4 patients have a significantly worse prognosis.

Erb's palsy

OBPI lesions involving the upper roots in isolation (Narakas Grades 1 and 2) cause weakness to the supra- and infraspinatus muscles (due to involvement of the suprascapular nerve) and the rhomboids (dorsal scapular nerve palsy), leading to weakness of external rotation and abduction, with unopposed action of the subscapularis (supplied by the upper and lower subscapular nerves) leading to an internal rotation contracture. Shoulder abduction and deltoid function are often abnormal in these patients. The axillary nerve is supplied from multiple levels and the deltoid muscle belly often appears healthy at the time of surgery. It is more likely that deltoid dysfunction is a result of lack of synergistic function of the supraspinatus. The teres minor (supplied by the axillary nerve) may have some function in Narakas 1 or 2 injuries, but it is too weak to oppose the action of the subscapularis. The pectoralis muscles may also be weak, but their supply from both the medial and lateral pectoral nerves ensures that some function remains in isolated upper root injuries.

The resulting muscle imbalance leads to progressive flattening and retroversion of the humeral head. The glenoid becomes biconcave, with a false postero-inferior facet, which is lined by hyaline cartilage. With time, the humerus dislocates posteriorly, creating a pseudoglenoid.

Postgraduate Paediatric Orthopaedics, ed. Sattar Alshryda, Stan Jones and Paul A. Banaszkiewicz. Published by Cambridge University Press.
© Cambridge University Press 2014.

Secondary adaptive changes occur with overgrowth of the acromion and lateral clavicle. The coracohumeral and coracoacromial ligaments become elongated and tight, further restricting external rotation.

Total plexus injuries

In total plexus injuries (Narakas Grades 3 and 4), the lower root involvement leads mainly to hand weakness, but also to increased weakness of the deltoid, subscapularis and pectoralis muscles. This results in a flail shoulder, but with less internal rotation contracture.

Types of neuronal injury

Seddon's classification (neurapraxia, axonotmesis and neurotmesis) is important in determining the type of injury and, hence, recovery; however, it can be difficult to determine which type of injury has occurred, and by the time this is known it may be too late to perform primary reconstructive surgery to the damaged nerve roots.

The binding of the nerve roots to the axial skeleton by connective tissue is important. This is greater in the upper roots, resulting in a more distal, postganglionic nerve rupture compared with the preganglionic avulsion, directly from the spine, seen in the lower roots. Surgically, this is important as the presence of a root stump facilitates nerve grafting in the neonatal period (Figure 7.1). This has connotations for surgical options and prognosis.

Assessment

Examination of the infant should focus on the whole child, including all four extremities, to confirm that lower limbs are not involved – involvement of all four limbs or of one upper and one lower limb suggests other neurological causes, such as infantile diplegia or quadriplegia.

Horner's syndrome is a consequence of sympathetic neuron involvement at the T1 level. It signifies a severe total plexus injury and is associated with dry skin, miosis, ptosis and enophthalmos. The phrenic nerve may also be involved. This poses a higher anaesthetic risk and also limits the use of intercostal nerves as potential nerve donors (Figure 7.2).

In the infant, the differential diagnosis of a flail limb includes clavicle or humeral fracture and septic arthritis. An isolated clavicle or humerus fracture without concomitant brachial plexus injury causes pseudoparalysis of arm but the arm does not adopt the typical posture of a brachial plexus injury and spontaneous contraction in the deltoid and biceps is observed after 24 to 48 hours.

Surgical planning

The Toronto score assesses neonatal shoulder abduction, elbow flexion and wrist, digit and thumb extension, with normal function scoring 2, reduced function, 1, and no function, 0.

In older children (>2 years), the Mallet score (Figure 7.3) is a more comprehensive clinical assessment of shoulder function (abduction, external rotation, hand to head, hand to back and hand to mouth) with normal function scoring V and no function scoring I.

Assessment for surgical planning includes differentiation between supra- and infraclavicular involvement, to guide the surgical approach. In all cases, access to the upper roots is required, utilizing a supraclavicular approach. In more severe total plexus injuries, an extended approach involving an additional infraclavicular approach is also required. Differentiating between pre- and postganglionic injuries clinically is difficult at the best of times, and even more so in neonates. Awareness of the common patterns of injury is

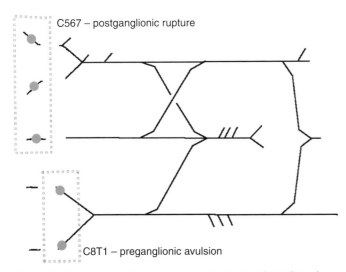

Figure 7.1 The patterns of pre- and postganglionic injury depends on the nerve root level.

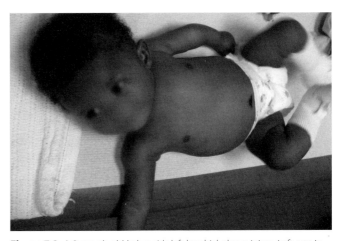

Figure 7.2 A 3-month-old baby with left brachial plexus injury. Left arm is lying by the side of the body (adducted) in internally rotated position, elbow is extended and fingers are flexed. Child has brachial plexus birth palsy (obstetric palsy) involving upper trunk of brachial plexus (Erb's palsy). Eyes appear to be symmetric without evidence of Horner's syndrome, so it is a postganglionic lesion.

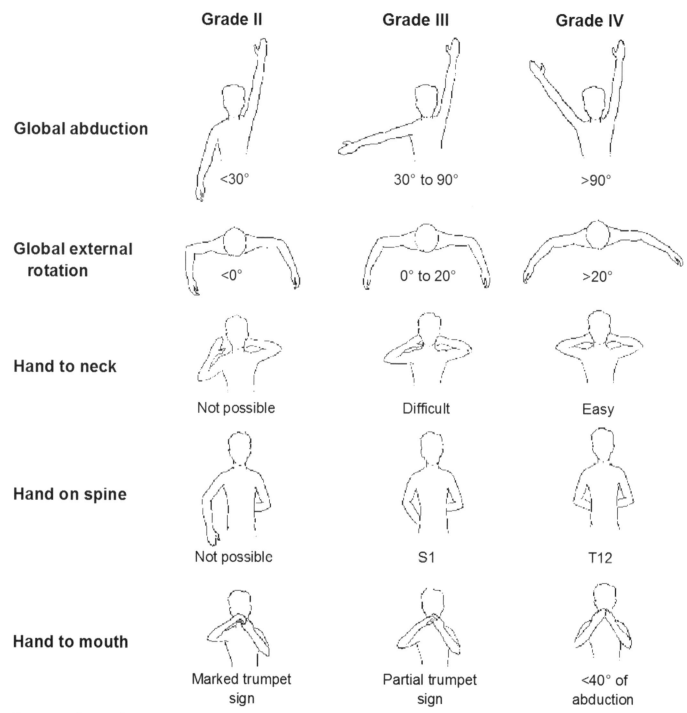

Figure 7.3 Mallet score. This requires the child's cooperation (useful after the age of 2 years). Grade I represents no ability while Grade V is normal. The 'trumpet sign' is named after the method of holding the trumpet (almost 90° abduction of affected arm when bringing hand to the mouth).

important – isolated upper plexus injuries (Narakas Grades 1 and 2) are usually postganglionic (and so graftable), whereas total plexus (Narakas Grade 3), particularly if Horner's syndrome is present (Narakas Grade 4) is more likely to be preganglionic, and need extraplexus nerve transfers. With this in mind, it is important to assess muscle function from potential donor nerves (such as spinal accessory nerve and the intercostal nerves).

Investigations

Dynamic chest fluoroscopy can be used to assess phrenic nerve function. Electromyography and CT myelography attempt to assess involvement of the dorsal root ganglia but are frequently unhelpful. Surgical exploration is more beneficial as it enables direct assessment of the injury and nerve stimulation, and is often combined with neurolysis

Table 7.1 Summary of key problems and management principles

Age	Pathology	Potential problems	Management
0–3 months	Neuropraxia vs neurotmesis	Awareness Differential diagnosis Prevent contractures	Refer to specialist Exclude infection or fracture Physiotherapy
3–24 months	Irreversible neurological injury	Window of opportunity Surgical planning	Surgical exploration, neurolysis and repair Assess donors and approach
1–3 years	Internal rotation imbalance	Contracture	Examination under anaesthesia + arthrogram Arthroscopic release
3–8 years	Glenoid dysplasia	Recurrent dysplasia	Arthroscopic release + lateral latissimus dorsi transfer
>8 years	Glenohumeral joint (GHJ) dislocation	Severe dysplasia Less remodelling potential	Glenoplasty

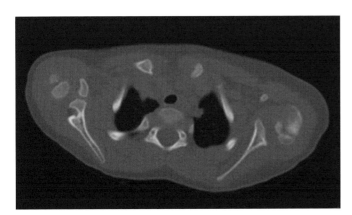

Figure 7.4 Glenohumeral dysplasia of the shoulder in a child with OBPI. Cross-section CT showing a posterior subluxation of the humeral head with flattening of the posterior half of the glenoid.

and primary nerve reconstruction. Total plexus involvement, preganglionic injury, Horner's syndrome or a Toronto score of less than 4 at 3 months are all indications for surgical exploration. Return of biceps function at 3 months is an often-quoted good prognostic sign; however, it is falsely positive in 12% of cases.

In a child under 18 months, owing to the lack of ossification of the proximal humerus, clinical examination is the most useful tool for assessment of the shoulder. Ultrasound provides dynamic assessment of instability, but is not useful for the assessment of dysplasia, which is better evaluated by arthrography and examination under anaesthesia.

CT and MRI are the best imaging modalities in the older child, although the former carries the risk of ionizing radiation. Using axial CT, glenoid version can be measured relative to the spine of the scapula and is normally 10°–20° retroverted (Figure 7.4). Joint reduction may be assessed using the posterior humeral head articulation (PHHA) – a measure of the percentage of the humeral head anterior to the middle of the glenoid fossa.

Management

Microsurgical options in the neonatal period include neurolysis and repair of the injured nerve to its original or an alternative nerve stump (direct and indirect neurotization). Potential donor nerves must be functional and expendable and may be either intraplexus (the C5–7 stumps, if intact) or extraplexus (spinal accessory nerve, intercostal nerves and even the contralateral C7 root). Neurotization may be facilitated with sural, saphenous or artificial nerve grafts.

A typical nerve transfer in Erb's palsy involves using a branch of the spinal accessory nerve to reconstruct the suprascapular nerve with nerve grafting of the upper and posterior trunks to the C5/6 stumps.

After the age of 2 years, the results of nerve transfer procedures are poor and a different approach to management is required. The aim is to reduce the glenohumeral joint and rebalance the shoulder to promote remodelling and restore function. The fundamental principles are to release tight anterior structures, ensure a concentric reduction and restore external rotation power.

The primary structure causing anterior tightness is the subscapularis muscle with secondary contractures of the MGHL (middle glenohumeral ligament), IGHL (inferior glenohumeral ligament) and the rotator interval. The most commonly transferred muscle is the latissimus dorsi (with or without the teres major), which is brought from its distal anterior insertion to a proximal posterior position onto the greater tuberosity, thereby counteracting the internal rotation force of the subscapularis and depressing the humeral head in a similar fashion to the supraspinatus.

A number of bony procedures have been described to address established glenohumeral dysplasia, which may occur despite early neurological reconstruction. These are usually performed in an older child in whom there is a fixed deformity associated with torsional deformities of the humerus or dysplasia of the humeral head or glenoid.

The main problems in the humerus are flattening of the humeral head and excessive retroversion. It is difficult to refashion the shape of the head; hence, it is advisable to maintain the humeral head in a concentric articulation from an early age to allow remodelling to occur. A proximal derotation osteotomy is indicated in cases of >40° retroversion. This is summarized in Table 7.1.

Sprengel's deformity

This is a rare congenital anomaly and is the result of failure of descent of the scapula from the fetal position in the neck. The scapula remains hypoplastic and elevated (Figure 7.5). In 70% of cases, it is associated with other abnormalities. The muscles that attach the scapula to the spine and chest wall, such as the rhomboids, trapezius and elevator scapula, show varying degrees of hypoplasia or aplasia. Bony abnormalities include

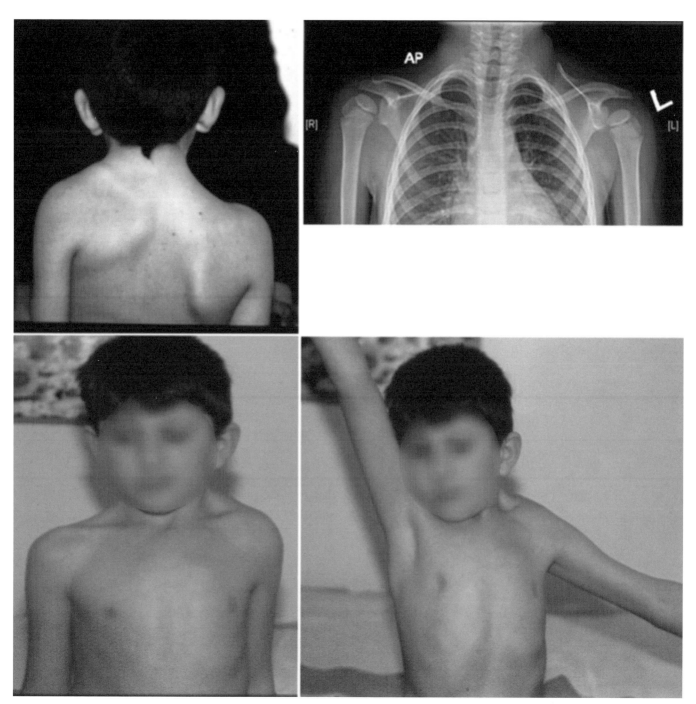

Figure 7.5 Sprengel's shoulder.

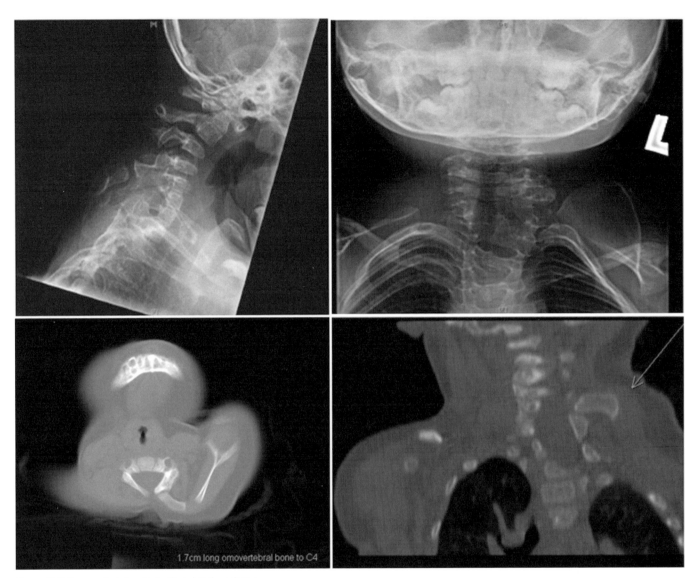

Figure 7.6 Sprengel's deformity in Klippel–Feil syndrome.

cervical hemivertebra with or without scoliosis, hypoplasia of the clavicle and Klippel–Feil syndrome. It is also associated with an omovertebral bone (Figure 7.6), which connects the superior border of the scapula to the spinous processes or lamina of the lower cervical vertebra, thus severely restricting scapular movement. A short humerus or femur, or longitudinal deficiency of the radius or tibia may be associated. Cardiac and kidney anomalies are also seen.

Treatment

Parents seek medical attention for two main reasons – cosmetic and variable loss of shoulder function.

The primary goals of treatment are to improve function and cosmesis. Disability is proportionate to the severity of the deformity. The outcome of surgery is better in early childhood, as the scapula is mobile. Cavendish has classified the deformity into four grades:

Grade I: The deformity and functional deficits are very minor and no treatment is required.

Grade II: The affected scapula is 1–2 cm higher than the normal side and the superior border of the scapula is prominent. Extraperiosteal excision of the prominent superior border of the scapula is recommended.

Grade III: The scapula is 2–5 cm higher. Lowering the scapula improves cosmesis dramatically and function also improves.

Grade IV: The scapula is high in the neck, very near the occiput, and shoulder function is severely restricted. Surgical release and reposition of the scapula improves appearance but there is often very little improvement in function in this group.

Several surgical procedures have been described:

- The Woodward procedure (or its modifications) involves release of trapezius and rhomboid muscles through a midline incision, excision of omovertebral bone when present and repositioning of the scapula.
- The modified Green scapuloplasty procedure involves two staged operations; with the patient supine, a clavicle osteotomy is performed to protect the brachial plexus. Then the patient is positioned prone. Muscles are detached from their scapular insertion subperiosteally and the omovertebral bone, if present, is excised. The supraspinous fossa of the scapula is resected. The scapula is then displaced distally down to the level of the normal side. The muscles are reattached in a certain order.
- König described an osteotomy within the scapula with the lateral portion pulled down to restore the shoulder joint to its appropriate position (Figure 7.7).
- The Mears partial scapular resection (Figure 7.8) involves excision of the suprascapular fossa and a diagonal osteotomy from the superior border to the lateral border of the scapula. The shoulder is passively abducted fully

and the overlapping part excised from the body of the scapula. The two parts can then be sutured together and the layers are closed on top.

Clavicle pseudarthrosis

Congenital pseudarthrosis of the clavicle is a rare condition and invariably seen on the right side. Left-sided clavicle pseudarthrosis is only associated with dextrocardia. Bilateral cases are very rare.

The clavicle develops from the fusion of two cartilaginous masses during the seventh week of life. Congenital pseudarthrosis arises as a result of failure of fusion of these two cartilage masses. With the heart on the left side, the subclavian artery is high on the right side and it is postulated that pulsations of the high subclavian artery hinder the fusion of the two cartilage anlages, resulting in pseudarthrosis. The situation reverses in dextrocardia.

Surgery is indicated for pain and shoulder deformity interfering with function. Reduction and internal fixation with or without bone graft is usually successful in achieving union (in contradiction with pseudarthrosis associated with neurofibromatosis) (Figure 7.9).

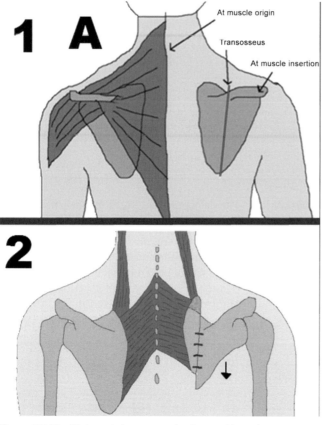

Figure 7.7 The König vertical osteotomy involves a midscapula osteotomy and advancing the lateral scapula distally.

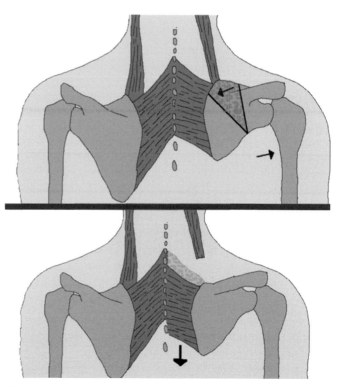

Figure 7.8 Mears partial scapular resection and Woodward operation for Sprengel's deformity. The Mears osteotomy is a closing wedge osteotomy to modify the arc of motion of the glenohumeral joint.

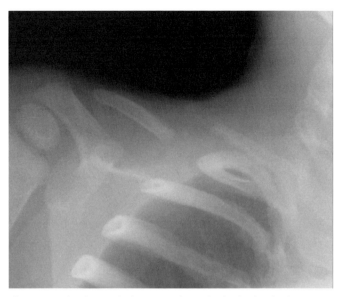

Figure 7.9 Clavicle pseudarthrosis. X-radiograph of right clavicle shows discontinuity in the middle third of the clavicle; the adjoining ends of the clavicle are rounded off. This is a case of congenital pseudarthrosis of the right clavicle.

Upper-limb cerebral palsy

Children with cerebral palsy can have well-described patterns of upper-limb involvement.

In the shoulder, there may be an adduction – an internal rotation contracture, with a flexion contracture at the elbow. In the wrist, there is most commonly a flexion–pronation contracture, although extension deformities may also be seen. In the hand, a thumb-in-palm deformity may be due to intrinsic or extrinsic muscle contracture; attempts to counteract wrist flexion by recruitment of long finger extensors may result in a swan neck deformity; alternatively, the fingers may become clasped or develop lumbrical tightness. Together, these problems prevent accurate positioning of the hand in space, appropriate grip and release.

In addition to restriction in function, other encountered upper-limb problems include pain, spasticity, hygiene and concerns about the appearance of the hand. This last problem is frequently overlooked, despite recent studies suggesting that patient satisfaction is more dependent on cosmetic appearance than functional outcome.

Function in patients with cerebral palsy can be assessed by a number of methods. In the lower limb, the most commonly used classification is the Gross Motor Functional Classification System (GMFCS), which is principally a measure of ambulation ability. A similar five-part scale for upper-limb function is the Manual Ability Classification System (MACS). This assesses a patient's ability to complete manual tasks with or without appropriate adaptations.

Treatment principles

Patients younger than 12 years carry the risk of overcorrection of deformity and are treated more conservatively, those over 12 years are more suitable for definitive contracture correction.

Functional contractures (such as thumb-in-palm or wrist flexion deformities) should be treated early to maintain function, while other contractures may be treated if these pose a problem in the older child.

High-functioning patients with correctable contractures are best treated with rebalancing procedures, while those with low function or fixed contractures are best treated with stabilizing procedures, such as arthrodesis.

Facioscapulohumeral dystrophy

This is an autosomal dominant muscular dystrophy. It selectively affects the muscles of the face and shoulder girdle. Clinically, this manifests as a Bell's-palsy-type droop to the face, with the classical sign of being unable to whistle.

In the shoulder, the scapula cannot be stabilized during abduction, preventing arm elevation despite good deltoid function. Marked winging is usually obvious. The treatment is scapulothoracic fusion using a plate and cerclage wiring technique.

The differential for winging in children includes localized nerve palsies (long thoracic and spinal accessory nerve), shoulder instability (scapula dyskinesia) and scoliosis.

Adolescent shoulder instability

Instability may be divided into three Stanmore types:
- Traumatic structural pathology (such as a Bankart's defect),
- Atraumatic structural pathology (such as capsular laxity),
- Abnormal muscle patterning.

The incidence of instability is poorly described in the paediatric population, although traumatic shoulder dislocation has been described in infants as young as 2 years old and, with increased participation in contact sports, the incidence is increasing. It is widely acknowledged that younger patients have a higher risk of recurrence if treated non-operatively (up to 100% in some studies), with rates highest in boys and usually occurring within 2 years of the initial dislocation.

The high risk of further dislocations is caused by disruption of the surrounding structures during the initial event, such as tears to the joint capsule or the glenoid labrum, or damage to the glenoid or humeral head. Adolescents are at higher risk, owing to both their enthusiasm for re-participating in high-risk activities (such as contact sports) and adolescent hyperlaxity. Recurrent shoulder dislocation in adolescence can go on to cause particular problems, such as glenohumeral joint degeneration, later in life.

Results for arthroscopic reattachment of the damaged labrum to reconstitute the inferior glenohumeral ligament are reasonable in adults. Adolescents have a higher early re-dislocation rate following arthroscopic stabilization (up to a third), although this is lower than when managed non-operatively, and their satisfaction and return to sports is good. Such patients may be more suitable to have a primary coracoid transfer procedure if they wish to return to contact sports.

Bibliography

1. Herring JA (2008) *Tachdjian's Pediatric Orthopaedics*, 4th edition, volume 1. Philadelphia: Saunders Elsevier.

2. Waters PM and Bae D (2012) *Pediatric Hand and Upper Limb Surgery: A Practical Guide.* Philadelphia: Lippincott Williams & Wilkins.

3. Nixon M and Trail I (2013) Management of shoulder problems following obstetric brachial plexus injury. *Shoulder & Elbow* doi: 10.1111/sae.12003.

4. Gilbert A (2001) *Brachial Plexus Injuries.* London: Martin Dunitz.

5. Nixon M (2012) *Paediatric Orthopaedics* Raleigh, NC: Lulu Publishing.

The elbow

Om Lahoti and Matt Nixon

Radioulnar synostosis

Radioulnar synostosis may be either congenital or post-traumatic. The precise cause of congenital synostosis is unknown.

Embryologically, the elbow forms from the three cartilaginous parts representing the humerus, radius and ulna. A programmed cavitation process leads to the formation of the elbow joint; if this process fails, enchondral ossification results in a bony synostosis. Because the forearm bones differentiate at a time when the fetal forearm is in pronation, almost all forearm synostoses are fixed in this position. Moreover, this process occurs at a time when all organ systems are forming, hence synostosis is seen in conjunction with, for example, Apert syndrome (acrocephalosyndactyly), Carpenter syndrome (acropolysyndactyly), arthrogryposis and Klinefelter syndrome.

Congenital radioulnar synostosis is bilateral in 60% of cases. Like tarsal coalition, although it is a prenatal condition and present at birth, it is often undetected until early childhood, when lack of forearm rotation, i.e. pronation or supination, is observed in day-to-day activities. In severe cases there is hyperpronation with a 'back-handed grasp'. In these situations, early realignment is indicated to allow proper hand development. In minor cases, minor trauma is often blamed for restriction but the X-ray findings are typical. Occasionally, synostosis may be post-traumatic, secondary to abnormal healing of combined radius and ulna fractures.

X-ray is required to assess:

- The degree and type of synostosis. Radiographs show loss of radial head contour and fusion of the radius and ulna proximally and extending to a variable distance distally (Figure 8.1).
- Associated radial head dislocation.

There may be associated radiocapitellar dislocation, which can cause a prominent lump.

Treatment

Options for treatment include conservative management and excision of the synostosis with or without realignment osteotomy.

In unilateral cases, the disability is often minimal and surgery is not indicated.

In bilateral involvement, the disability may be sufficiently significant to warrant surgical treatment. Excision of the synostosis alone is not advised, as it recurs and is associated with a poor outcome. However, in post-traumatic cases with significant functional impairment, excision and interposition of vascularized fat graft has been undertaken with some success in preventing recurrence.

Rotational realignment osteotomy of the radius fixes the forearm in the desired position to improve function and is a relatively simple procedure. There is some debate about the optimal functional position. Traditional texts advise that in bilateral cases the dominant forearm should be placed in 30°–45° supination, although with modern tasks requiring pronation for keyboard activities, etc., the dominant hand is better in midpronation and the non-dominant hand in neutral. In unilateral cases, the forearm is fixed in neutral rotation.

If the correction required is greater than 45°, osteotomy of both the radius and ulna is advised. Post-operatively, the limb is closely monitored for neurovascular compromise and compartment syndrome.

Non-traumatic radial head dislocation

Children with congenital radial head dislocation usually have reasonable elbow function and satisfactory supination and pronation with pain-free movement of the elbow. A click may be audible and a prominent palpable lump observed (radial head).

There are a number of associated syndromes, such as Larsen syndrome and nail-patella syndrome, in which other joints are also dislocated, so a thorough assessment is required.

It is important to differentiate between congenital and post-traumatic cases (Monteggia fracture); the former is usually managed conservatively, while the latter usually requires reconstructive surgery to restore anatomy.

Postgraduate Paediatric Orthopaedics, ed. Sattar Alshryda, Stan Jones and Paul A. Banaszkiewicz. Published by Cambridge University Press.
© Cambridge University Press 2014.

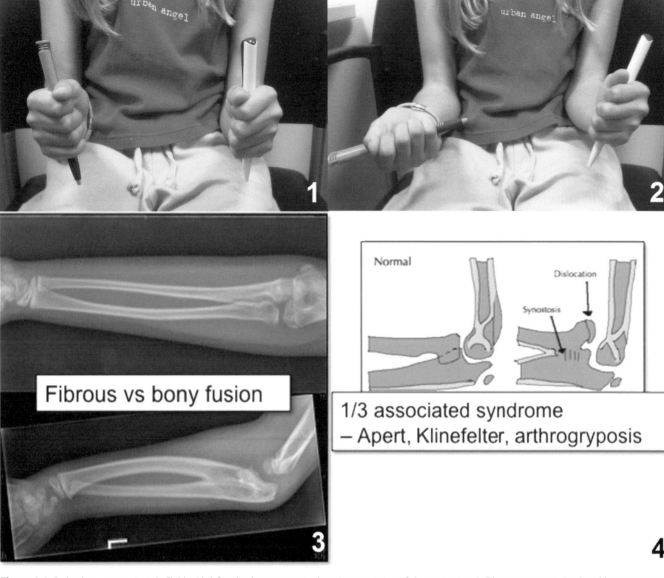

Figure 8.1 Radioulnar synostosis. 1, 2: Child with left radioulnar synostosis; there is a restriction of the supination. 3: Fibrous synostosis (top) and bony synostosis (bottom). 4: Diagrammatic features of synostosis with and without radial head dislocation.

The focus of history and examinations is on:

- Distinguishing between congenital and post-traumatic cases,
- Functional compromise,
- Associated syndromes.

Radiology

Radiography can be used to assess:

- Shape of the radial head,
- Direction of dislocation.

Radiographs confirm the diagnosis but also differentiate between congenital and post-traumatic cases. In congenital cases, the radial head loses its concave shape and becomes round. In addition, the capitellum and proximal ulna are convex. In some cases, it may be necessary to take comparison X-rays of the other elbow.

Treatment

There are three main treatment options:

- Non-operative,
- Radial head excision,
- Radiocapitellar joint reconstruction.

Most congenital cases are treated non-operatively; however, radial head excision may be undertaken at skeletal maturity if pain develops. This will also improve pronation, supination and extension. Radial head excision is not advised in young children, as it leads to proximal migration of the radius, secondary wrist pain and cubitus valgus.

Radiocapitellar joint reconstruction is often reserved for post-traumatic Monteggia cases. Options include:

- Soft-tissue reconstruction with osteotomy,
- Radial shortening or ulnar lengthening.

Results can be unpredictable.

Madelung's deformity

Madelung's deformity results from inadequate development of the distal radial epiphysis. It is caused by asymmetric growth arrest of the volar and ulnar aspects of distal radial physis and is thought to be due to an abnormal band between the radius and lunate, called the Vickers ligament.

This results in increased volar and ulnar tilt. The ulna grows normally, thus becoming longer than the radius. This causes the ulnar head to be prominent and the carpus migrates proximally into the gap between the radius and ulna. In addition, the forearm is shorter than normal (Figure 8.2).

The most common form is an autosomal dominant hereditary disorder affecting adolescent girls, usually bilaterally. A similar deformity is seen in multiple epiphyseal dysplasia, Ollier disease, post-traumatic or infective growth arrest. Multiple hereditary exostoses causes a pseudo-Madelung's deformity in which growth arrest in the ulna tethers the radius and pulls it round into a similarly abnormal position (see later for details).

Radiographs confirm the diagnosis but also help determine the degree of deformity and assess the remaining growth potential. The ulna is normal in Madelung's but abnormal in pseudo-Madelung's (Figure 8.2). The radius is in ulnar and volar deviation with increased inclination and proximal migration of the lunate and other carpal bones. MRI may also be used to assess the degree of physeal arrest.

Many patients with Madelung's deformity have good wrist function and very little pain and the main concern is cosmetic. However, the wrist can become painful after skeletal maturity.

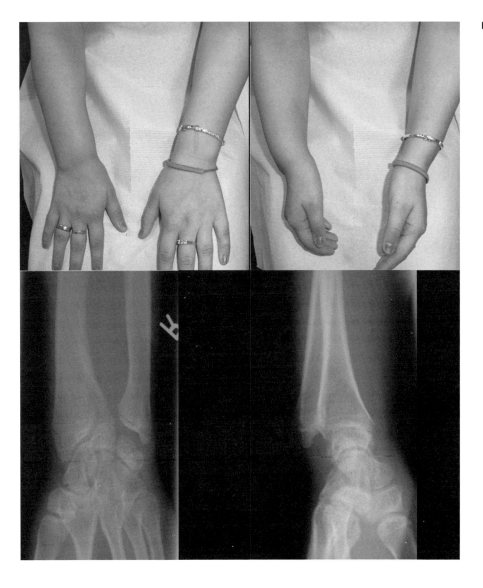

Figure 8.2 Madelung's deformity.

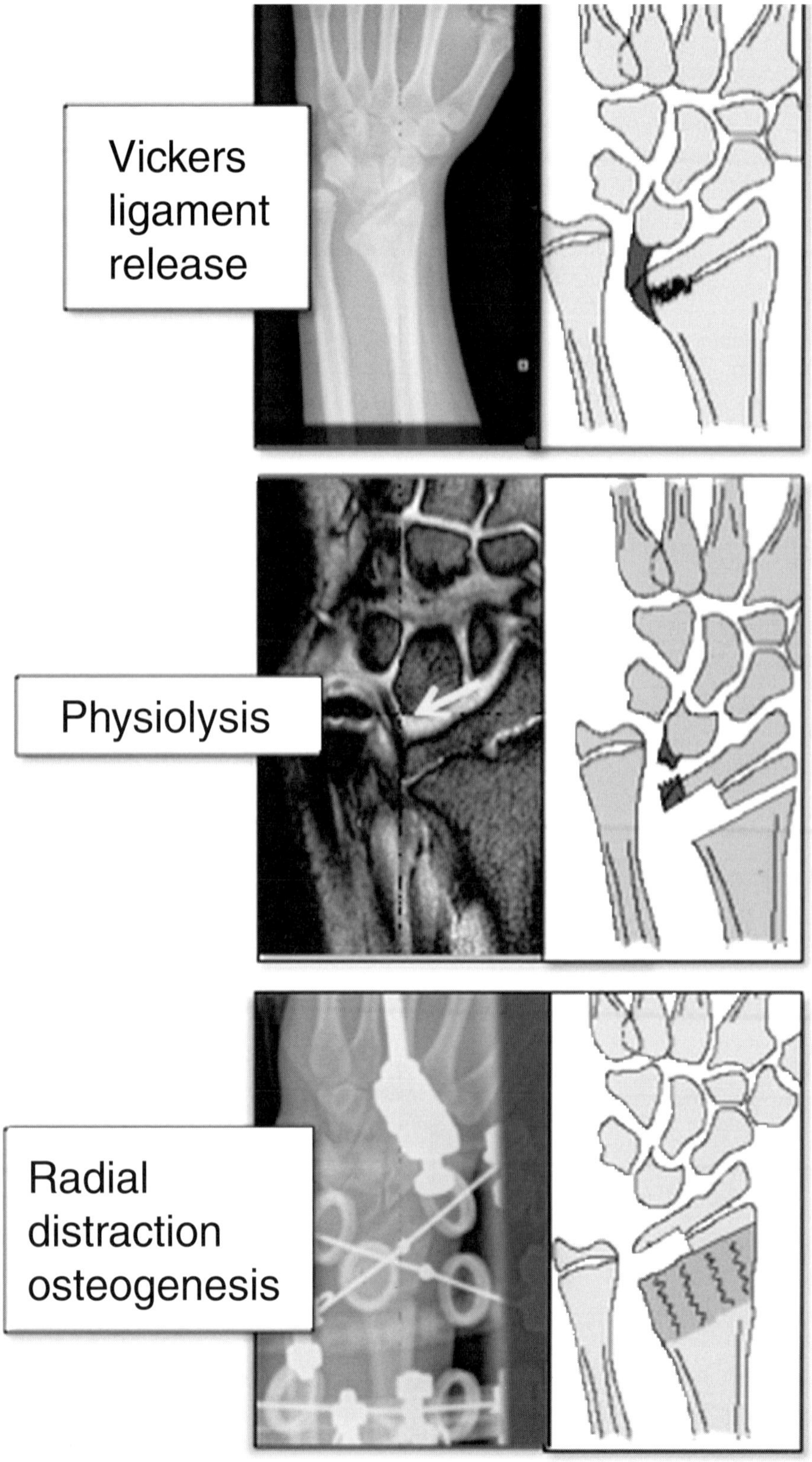

Vickers
ligament
release

Physiolysis

Radial
distraction
osteogenesis

Figure 8.3 Madelung's deformity treatment options.

Treatment (Figure 8.3) can be divided into:

- Skeletally immature vs skeletally mature,
- Radius vs ulna,
- Salvage procedures.

In the skeletally immature, growth can be restored by releasing the Vickers ligament and physeal bar, and combining this with epiphysiodesis of the ulna.

In the skeletally mature, the radial deformity can be acutely corrected with a radial osteotomy and the length discrepancy treated with ulna shortening. Alternatively, the ulna can be neglected and the radius lengthened and realigned with Ilizarov distraction osteogenesis. Both these strategies aim to restore normal anatomy at the distal radial ulnar joint.

Salvage procedures, including excision of the distal end of the ulna (Darrach procedure), fusion of the distal ulna to the radius and excision of a segment proximal to the fusion (Sauve–Kapandji procedure), are appropriate. These, however, address the wrong bone (i.e. the ulna, which is non-pathological).

Longitudinal deficiency (radial and ulna dysplasia)

This is described in Chapter 9.

Fractures around the elbow

Background

Paediatric elbow fractures are peculiar because of the unique anatomy of the elbow and the high potential for complications. Improper management of these injuries may result in long-term disability. One frequent problem is in distinguishing fractures from the six normal secondary ossification centres. The mnemonic CRITOL is helpful in remembering the order of radiographic appearance of these centres:

Capitellum:	1–2 years,
Radial head:	3–5 years,
Internal (or medial) epicondyle:	5–6 years,
Trochlea:	7–8 years (often appears fragmented, owing to being bi- or tripartite),
Olecranon:	9–10 years,
Lateral epicondyle:	11–12 years.

In general, the capitellum appears radiographically at around 1 year of age, and the remaining ossification centres appear sequentially every 2 years. Girls mature earlier than boys; hence, their ossification centres appear earlier, although the sequence remains constant. The three epiphyseal ossification centres of the distal humerus (capitellum, lateral epicondyle and trochlea) fuse as one unit and then fuse later to the metaphysis. The medial epicondyle is the last to fuse to the metaphysis.

An important clinical application of this is a displaced intra-articular medial epicondyle fracture in a child older than 6 years. The absence of the medial epicondyle ossification centre in its normal position in a child of this age should suggest a displaced fracture fragment, most probably in the elbow joint.

Most of the intra-osseous blood supply of the distal humerus comes from the anastomotic vessels situated posteriorly. Although the vessels communicate with one another within the ossific nucleus, they do not communicate with vessels in either the metaphysis or the non-ossified chondroepiphysis. Thus, for practical purposes, they act as end vessels. Only a small portion of the lateral condyle (posterior aspect) is both non-articular and extracapsular.

The trochlea is covered entirely by articular cartilage and lies totally within the articular capsule. The vessels that supply the ossific centres of the trochlea must therefore traverse the periphery of the physis to enter the epiphysis. These vessels are susceptible to injury after fractures or surgical treatment causing capitellum avascular necrosis (AVN) or fishtail deformity of the distal humerus.

Supracondylar fracture

These account for 50–70% of all elbow fractures and are seen most frequently in children between the ages of 3 and 10 years. The high incidence of residual deformity and the potential for neurovascular complications make a supracondylar humeral fracture a serious injury.

Many children hold their elbows hyperextended as they fall onto their outstretched hands. This elbow hyperextension causes the olecranon process to act as a fulcrum in the olecranon fossa, resulting in extension-type fractures. A posteriorly applied force with the elbow in flexion creates a flexion-type injury (2–5% of cases).

Nerve injuries occur in about 10–15% of cases. The anterior interosseous nerve is most commonly injured. However, the radial nerve is most commonly injured when the distal fragment is displaced posteromedially. Nerve injury may be a consequence of the fracture itself or secondary to compartment syndrome.

Radiology

This includes AP and lateral views of the elbow (humerus). Oblique views of the distal humerus may occasionally be helpful in differentiating a supracondylar fracture and condylar fracture. Comparison views may occasionally be needed to evaluate an ossifying epiphysis (Figures 8.4 and 8.5).

Wilkins' modification of the Gartland classification is:

I. Undisplaced. In the absence of a clear fracture line, a posterior fat pad sign is indicator of an occult intra-articular or supracondylar fracture. Very young children may have severe injuries with very little bony abnormality, owing to the lack of ossification.
II. Angulated with intact posterior cortex (IIA, angulation only; IIB, with rotation).
III. Complete displacement (IIIA, posteromedial; IIIB, posterolateral).

Treatment

Treatment should aim to reduce and stabilize all displaced fractures. Fractures should be reduced so that, on a lateral radiograph, the anterior humeral line intersects the capitellum. Particular attention should be paid to any medial

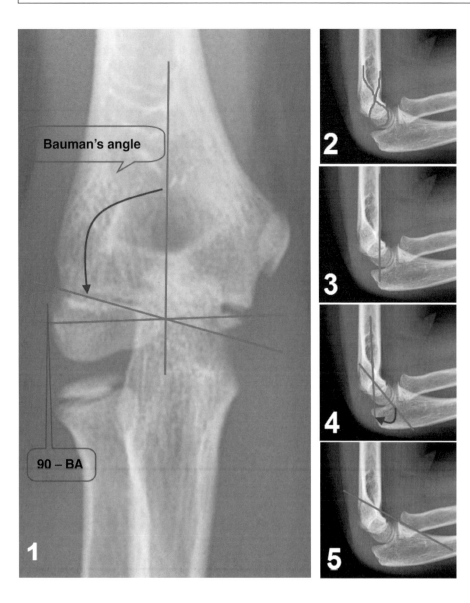

Figure 8.4 Radiological assessment of supracondylar fracture. 1: Bauman's angle (BA) formed by the capital physeal line and the long axis of the humerus (normally, 75°–80°); Bauman believed that the reciprocal angle (90° − BA) equalled the carrying angle. 2: Teardrop or hourglass; the narrow part represents the coronoid fossa. The inferior portion of the teardrop is the ossification centre of the capitellum. On a true lateral projection, this teardrop should be well defined (a useful sign of true lateral projection). 3: The anterior humeral line drawn along the anterior border of the distal humeral shaft; this should pass through the middle third of the ossification centre of the capitellum. 4: The shaft-condylar angle is the angle between the long axis of the humerus and the long axis of the lateral condyle (normally 40°). This can also be measured by the flexion angle of the distal humerus, which is calculated by measuring the angle of the lateral condylar physeal line with the long axis of the shaft of the humerus. 5: The coronoid line, which is directed proximally along the anterior border of the coronoid process, should barely touch the anterior portion of the lateral condyle.

comminution or collapse, as this may be a sign of rotational malalignment, which is a risk of further displacement and malunion.

- Stable fractures (Types I and IIA) can be treated by immobilization in a flexed above-elbow cast for 3–4 weeks. Although, flexion of >90° provides extra stability of extension-type fractures, this may comprise the circulation, and clinical judgement should be exercised.
- Displaced fractures should be treated surgically by manipulation under anaesthesia and K-wire stabilization.

Closed reduction of extension-type fractures is undertaken by applying traction followed by correction of the varus or valgus displacement and then with pressure on the olecranon, flexing the elbow.

Pin placement may use either cross wires or twin lateral wires. The former is probably a more stable construct for unstable fractures but carries the risk of ulna nerve injury. This can be minimized by placing the lateral wire first (to stabilize the fracture), extending the elbow (to move the nerve out of the way) and then performing a mini open medial wire insertion. It is imperative that the cross K-wires do not cross at the fracture site; all wires must engage the opposite cortex.

Treatment may also be undertaken by a period of overhead traction though this is not commonly practised.

Treatment algorithms for the different scenarios are.

- Undisplaced fractures should be managed in a flexed elbow cast.
- Minimally displaced and neurovascular intact injuries can be treated during the next available trauma list.
- Moderately displaced but neurovascular intact injuries are ideally treated as soon as possible. However, they may be left overnight, but need close neurovascular monitoring. Delaying treatment may carry the increased risk of needing open reduction.

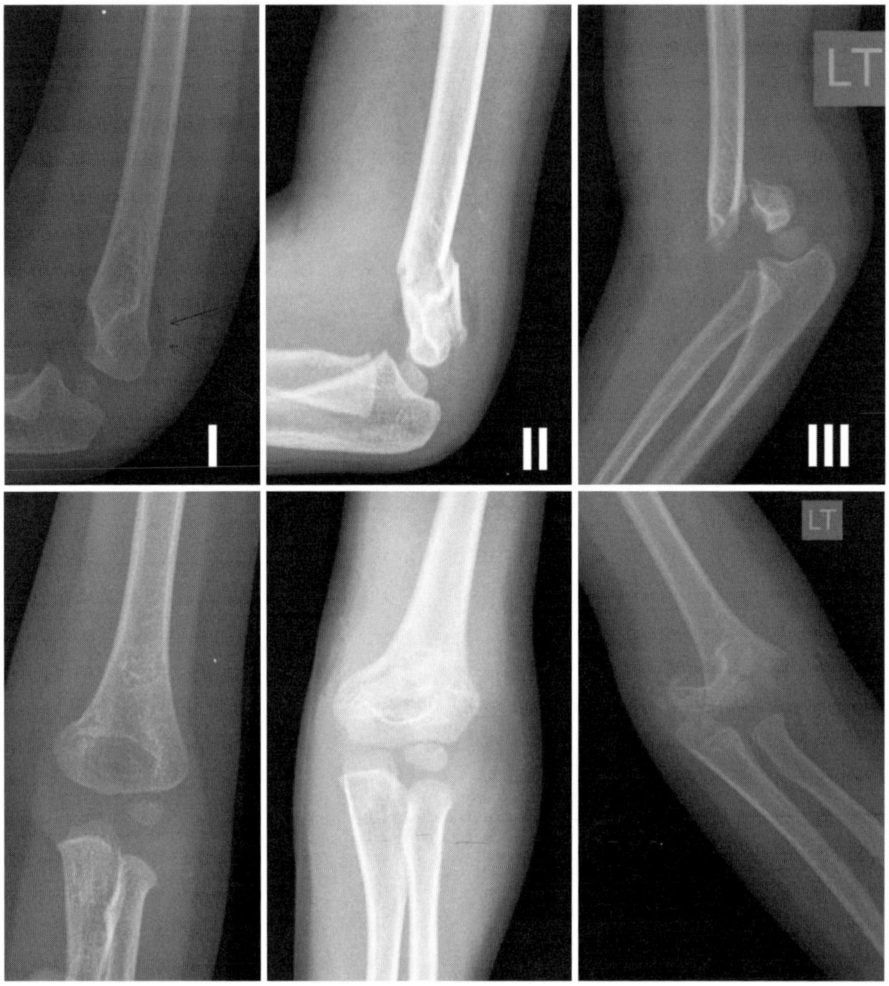

Figure 8.5 Supracondylar fracture.

- Severely displaced fractures with no neurovascular deficit should be treated as soon as possible, with close monitoring for compartment syndrome post-operation.
- Pink and pulseless limbs are at risk of compartment syndrome and require expedited closed anatomical reduction. The vascularity of the hand normally returns with fracture reduction, and can be assessed with pulse oximetry, Doppler ultrasound or regular ultrasound.
- White and pulseless limbs are a surgical emergency. Surgery should not be delayed by performing arteriograms. Though there is a reasonable chance that perfusion will be restored after closed anatomical reduction, a vascular surgeon must be informed about the case prior to surgery and be available to assist if required. The arterial insufficiency is often due to arterial spasm, but laceration or intimal flap tears may also occur. Because the median nerve lies close to the brachial artery, the presence of median nerve symptoms associated with a pulseless arm is a risk factor for arterial injury. Arterial exploration is undertaken via an anterior approach (lazy-S incision).

This exposure is also used to facilitate open reduction of the fracture (Figure 8.6).

Cubitus varus (gunstock) deformity

This is commonly caused by malunited extension-type supracondylar fractures. There is a loss of the carrying angle, which is typically associated with elbow hyperextension and internal rotation deformity (Figure 8.7). It is generally pain-less, causes little function deficit and can be left alone. It doesn't usually remodel and the deformity remains constant until skeletal maturity. The deformity is usually poorly accepted cosmetically, and parents or children frequently request correction.

Supracondylar fracture malunion usually occurs after unstable fractures with medial cortex comminution (Type IIB and III fractures), typically due to loss of reduction after inadequate fixation. Medial comminution is difficult to fix with lateral K-wires, and is better held with cross K-wires. Adequate radiographs should be obtained after fixation, including oblique column views to check for stability and reduction.

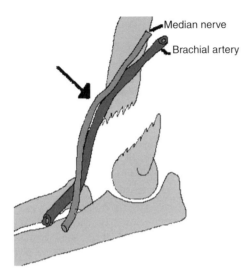

Median nerve

Brachial artery

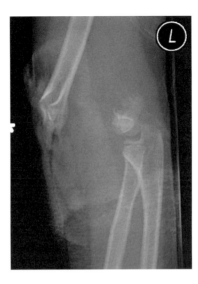

Figure 8.6 Supracondylar humeral fracture, Grade III with vascular injury.

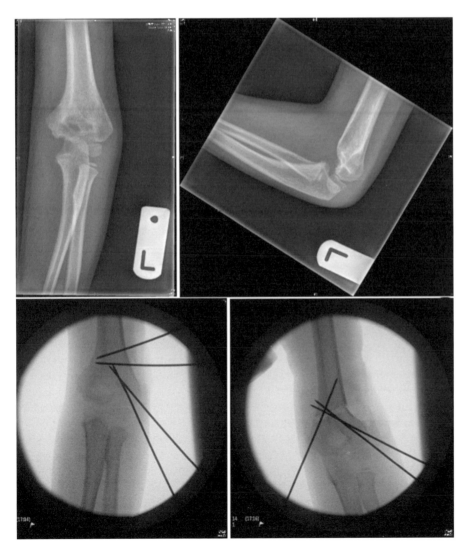

Figure 8.7 Cubitus varus deformity.

A similar deformity may occur after growth arrest of the medial column secondary to fractures or infection. This presents in a similar fashion, but may not have the hyperextension or internal rotation deformity. Unlike cubitus varus due to supracondylar fracture malunion, this deformity is often progressive until the child reaches skeletal maturity.

Management

This deformity can be managed non-operatively, but frequently the child or family request correction. Surgical correction improves the appearance and function but carries the risks of loss of fixation, elbow stiffness and nerve injury (this can be as high as 25%). Many different techniques have been described to correct some or all components of the deformity.

Essentially, a laterally based closing wedge osteotomy (to correct cubitus varus) with medial displacement of the distal fragment (to reduce the lateral prominence) and fixation in a degree of flexion (to correct hyperextension) should restore anatomy.

Fixation is with K-wires in young children and with a plate and screws in older children. An alternative method is gradual correction by distraction osteogenesis, using Ilizarov techniques.

Management of the deformity due to medial growth arrest is more difficult, as it is progressive and likely to recur. Early after the injury, excision of the physeal bar to restore growth can be performed with or without fat graft interposition followed by correction of residual deformity at skeletal maturity.

Lateral condyle fractures

These fractures (Figure 8.8) are intra-articular and transphyseal and hence have a high incidence of complication (non-union and growth arrest). They are traditionally classified by Milch; most injuries are Milch Type 2, which is commonly misconceived to be a more benign Salter–Harris Type 2 injury. In fact, all lateral condyle fractures involve the growth plate and should be considered to be Salter–Harris Type 4 injuries.

Jakob classification is more useful, as it guides management:

Jakob 1: Less than 2 mm displacement,

Jakob 2: More than 2 mm displacement, but no rotation,

Jakob 3: Malrotated and displaced.

Management

Undisplaced (Jakob Type 1) injuries are usually hinged on the articular surface and are relatively stable. These can be managed non-operatively but require close monitoring, as they have a high risk of displacement and need an extended period of immobilization (up to 6 weeks). Close follow-up (weekly) is essential to detect any displacement early, along with AP, lateral and oblique radiographs. If in doubt, injuries should be treated by percutaneous K-wire fixation.

Complete fractures with more than 2 mm displacement (Jakob Type 2) but no rotation are less stable intra-articular fractures and need anatomical reduction and fixation. This can usually be done closed and with K-wires, but may require opening or an on-table arthrogram to assess reduction. If reduction is not anatomical, there is a high risk of growth arrest and complication.

Malrotated and displaced fractures (Jakob 3) are at highest risk of complication and require open reduction and fixation. Kocher's approach is advised and care must be taken not to devascularize the lateral condyle, which receives its blood supply posteriorly. Fixation is achieved with divergent wires or a single screw, again with on-table arthrography to assess reduction if needed.

All these fractures are slow to heal, so require longer K-wire fixation than a supracondylar fracture – usually 6–8 weeks. For this reason, it is worth burying the wires to enable early mobilization.

Complications

There are two major complications:

- Non-union,
- Growth arrest.

Non-union is relatively common, as the fracture is intra-articular and usually unstable. Non-union requires open reduction and screw fixation augmented with bone graft.

Growth arrest may occur due to physeal malalignment and may be medial (causing a fishtail deformity) or complete (leading to a cubitus valgus deformity). The latter carries a risk of tardy ulnar nerve palsy.

Radial neck fractures

Radial neck fractures are not that common in the paediatric age group (7% of all elbow fractures) and result from a combination of compression, angulation and rotation forces on a valgus and hyperextended elbow. They may be associated with dislocation of the elbow or a subtle olecranon fracture (Monteggia-equivalent injury).

Another variant is seen in paediatric athletes involved in throwing sports, due to repetitive compression injury to the radial head and neck ('Little League pathology').

Careful X-ray evaluation (AP and lateral views) is necessary to diagnose radial neck fractures and their displacement; this is critical to plan treatment. Oblique views of the radial head in supination and pronation may be needed.

The aim of treatment is to restore near-normal supination and pronation. The two important factors that determine the treatment are radial head angulation and displacement.

Radial head angulation <30° and <3 mm displacement is treated in a cast with the elbow at 90° flexion and forearm in neutral rotation for 2–3 weeks.

Radial head angulation >30° and >3 mm displacement is treated with closed reduction under general anaesthesia or sedation. Several closed and percutaneous techniques have

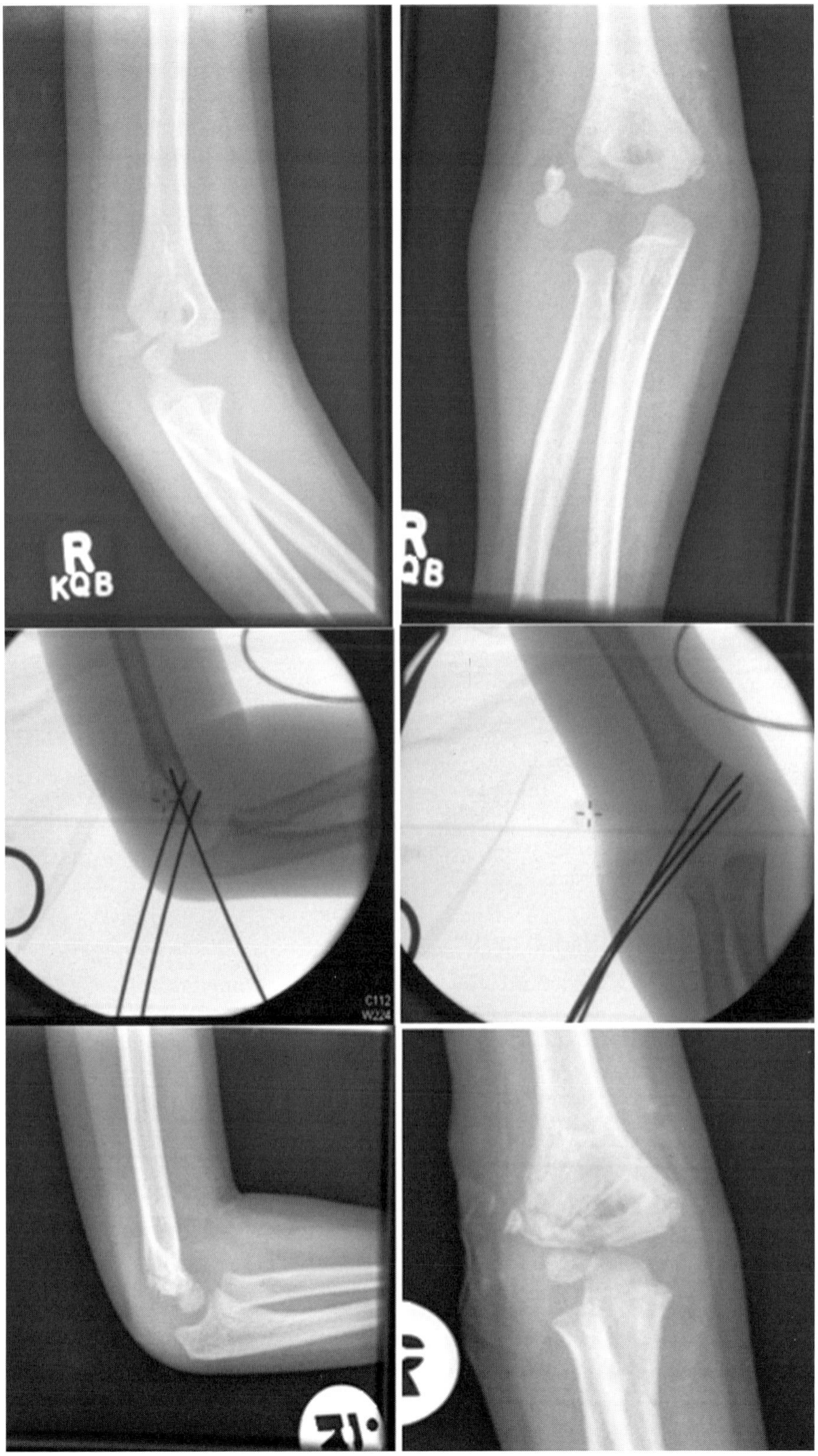

Figure 8.8 Lateral condyle fractures.

been described; the principle is to exert pressure on the displaced fragment, thus relocating it on the shaft of the radius by rotational movement, either in flexion or extension of the elbow. If closed methods are successful in obtaining satisfactory reduction, the fracture can be immobilized in a plaster cast for 2–3 weeks.

If fracture fails to reduce or is unstable after closed reduction of the fracture, percutaneous reduction and fixation with

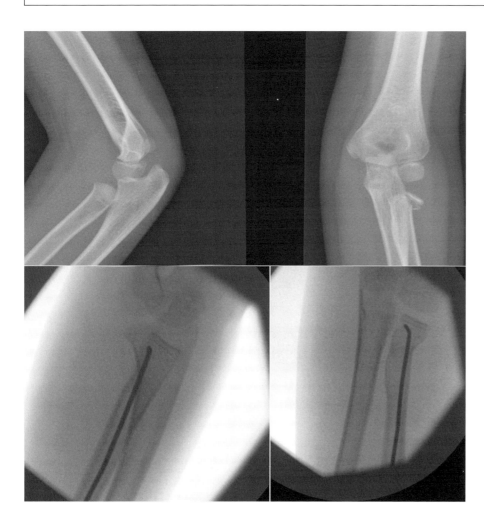

Figure 8.9 Radial neck fracture.

K-wire or elastic intramedullary nails are advised (Figure 8.9). The elbow should then be immobilized in a cast for 2–3 weeks.

Open reduction is rarely indicated and is associated with the risk of stiffness, avascular necrosis and non-union.

Complications of this fracture are common and include loss of pronation and supination and, rarely, stiffness of elbow. Avascular necrosis is associated with open reduction. Premature closure of physis can lead to cubitus valgus.

Displaced fracture of the radial neck is treated with an intramedullary elastic nail. Entry is in the distal radius proximal to the distal radial physis. The nail is used to hook the fracture to reduce and also stabilize it. The elbow is immobilized in a cast for 2 weeks.

Monteggia fracture

A Monteggia fracture is an injury to the forearm associated with radiocapitellar joint dislocation. While some injuries are obvious, others are more subtle and, if missed, can be the cause of significant long-term morbidity. As forearm fractures heal quickly in children, vigilance is required to ensure they are not missed.

The golden rules of management are:

- Always request imaging of the elbow in all forearm fractures,
- A line through the centre of the radial neck and head must intersect with the centre of the capitellum on all views, whatever the degree of flexion or extension.

Bado classified these injuries based on the direction of radial head dislocation (Figure 8.10).

Type I: Ulna fracture and anterior dislocation of the radial head,

Type II: Ulnar fracture and posterior dislocation (rare),

Type III: Ulnar fracture and lateral dislocation,

Type IV: Fracture dislocation and radius and ulna fracture.

Type I injuries are the commonest. Other variants include both bone fractures and radial column dislocation with plastic deformation but no fracture, the latter of which is particularly difficult to manage. As the posterior interosseous nerve lies anterior to the radial head, it is vulnerable to injury both with

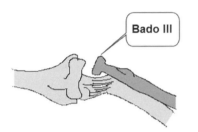
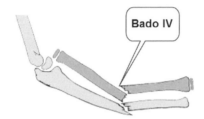
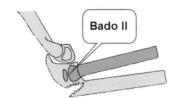

Figure 8.10 Bado classification of Monteggia fracture.

the acute injury (especially in Bado Type I injuries) and after attempted open reduction of the radial head.

Principles of management of acute injury are:

- Closed manipulation:

  - If the radial head reduces closed and the associated ulna fracture is stable, the injury can be managed in a POP (plaster-of-Paris) cast with weekly X-ray review until union.
  - If the radial head reduces closed but remains unstable, fixation of the ulna will usually stabilize the joint.

- Open reduction of the radial head. If the radial head does not reduce by closed means, open reduction is required using Kocher's approach (protecting the posterior interosseous nerve). The common cause of failed closed reduction is the head slipping out of the annular ligament. Fixation of the ulna fracture is usually required to improve stability.

- Acute ulna osteotomy is indicated in cases of plastic deformation when the radial head will not reduce by closed methods.

Missed or late-presenting Monteggia fractures are difficult to manage (Figure 8.11). The options include:

- Acute reduction,
- Gradual reduction,
- Radial head excision.

The radial head can be reduced acutely by Kocher's approach. The ulna may need to be osteotomized to facilitate this. The radial head is then temporarily held with a transcapitellar K-wire. A loop of palmaris longus is passed around the radial head to act as the annular ligament, although this often leads to stiffness, so it is better to restore bony alignment by fixing the ulna in such a position as to maintain radial head reduction. The K-wire can then be removed.

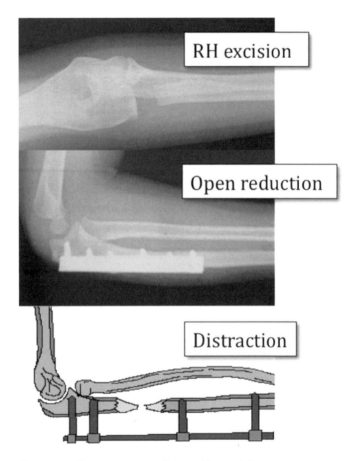

Figure 8.11 Treatment options of missed Monteggia fracture.

Acute open reduction can be difficult, owing to proximal migration of the radius, and carries the risk of posterior interosseous nerve palsy. An alternative strategy is Ilizarov distraction osteogenesis to lengthen and angulate the ulna and allow closed reduction of the radial head. This requires lengthy treatment with an external fixator and may also lead to postoperative stiffness.

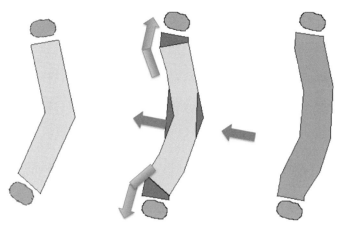

Figure 8.12 Forearm fracture.

At skeletal maturity, the dislocated radial head can be excised if the patient experiences severe pain or loss of elbow movement. Excision prior to skeletal maturity carries the risk of developing an Essex–Lopresti injury.

Forearm fractures

Forearm fractures are the most common paediatric fracture requiring surgery. The incidence is 1:100 children per year, with a peak incidence in 12-to-14-year-old children. There is a wide scope of fractures and management options, determined by a variable amount of skeletal growth and remodelling potential. Management is evolving to correspond with patient and family expectations regarding early return to full activity.

Three questions should be asked when determining how much deformity can be accepted:

- What is normal anatomy?
- How much remodelling will occur?
- What are the clinical effects of residual deformity?

The ulna is subcutaneous and a straight bone. Malunion causes cosmetic deformity but is generally more forgiving functionally. The radius is less visible, but malunion causes impaired function, particularly pronation and supination. The normal radial bow is seen on the AP radiograph at a distance 60% along a line drawn from the bicipital tuberosity to the distal medial radius, and measuring 10% of this line.

The rotational profile is important. The ulna styloid should lie 180° opposite the coronoid process, and the radial styloid should be 180° opposite the bicipital tuberosity. One-half of 'well-healed' forearm fractures actually have restricted rotation on accurate assessment, with every 1° of rotational malunion corresponding to 1–2° loss of clinical rotation. In general, up to 10° of rotational malalignment is well tolerated. Malrotation of the radius is particularly important for loss of total range of motion, whereas malrotation of the ulna changes the arc of movement.

Fracture remodelling is influenced by remaining growth potential, type of displacement and location of fracture in the forearm. Little is really known about the physiological basis of remodelling, but it is thought to occur as the result of a combination of Wolff's law and the Hueter–Volkmann principle. Distally, there is physeal realignment, which occurs best in the plane of movement and in rapidly growing physes (distal > proximal radius). In the medulla, there is periosteal bone growth in the concavity of the deformity, with resorption from the convexity.

The general principle of management is that the younger the child, the greater the potential for remodelling. Fractures closer to the wrist – distal third fractures – remodel better than proximal third fractures because of proximity to the rapidly growing distal radial physis. Angulation in the plane of movement of the nearest joint remodels better. In practice, up to 20° of angulation in the distal third, 15° in the middle third and 10° in the proximal third are acceptable if a child has 2 years growth remaining. Translation of 100% and up to 1 cm shortening are also acceptable (Figure 8.12).

Bibliography

1. Beaty JH and Kasser JR (2006) *Rockwood and Wilkins' Fractures in Children*, 6th edition. Philadelphia: Lippincott Williams & Wilkins.

2. Pirone AM, Graham HK and Krajbich JI (1988) Management of displaced extension-type supracondylar fractures of the humerus in children. *J Bone Joint Surg Am* 70(5):641–50.

3. Walmsley PJ, Kelly MB, Robb JE, Annan IH and Porter DE (2006) Delay increases the need for open reduction of Type-III supracondylar fractures of the humerus. *J Bone Joint Surg Br* 88(4):528–30.

4. Wright JG (2009) *Evidence-Based Orthopaedics. The Best Answers to Clinical Questions*. Philadelphia: Saunders.

5. Garbuz DS, Leitch K and Wright JG (1996) The treatment of supracondylar fractures in children with an absent radial pulse. *J Pediatr Orthop* 16(5):594–6.

6. Choi PD, Melikian R and Skaggs DL (2010) Risk factors for vascular repair and compartment syndrome in the pulseless supracondylar humerus fracture in children. *J Pediatr Orthop* 30(1):50–6.

7. Sabharwal S, Tredwell SJ, Beauchamp RD *et al.* (1997) Management of pulseless pink hand in pediatric supracondylar fractures of humerus. *J Pediatr Orthop* 17(3):303–10.

8. White L, Mehlman CT and Crawford AH (2010) Perfused, pulseless, and puzzling: a systematic review of vascular injuries in pediatric supracondylar humerus fractures and results of a POSNA questionnaire. *J Pediatr Orthop* 30(4):328–35.

Chapter

9

Congenital hand deformities

Dean E. Boyce and Jeremy Yarrow

The development of the upper limb begins during the fourth week of life *in utero*, when a limb bud, consisting of undifferentiated mesenchymal cells encased in ectoderm, develops. By 9 weeks, the bud has developed into an arm and hand with identifiable digits, and by 12 weeks the digits have differentiated.

Growth and differentiation are under the control of signal regions at the tip of the developing limb with complicated interactions and feedback systems (Figure 9.1). Induction of mesenchymal cells in the 'progress zone' at the tip of the developing limb occurs under the influence of specific zones. The apical epidermal ridge (AER) is the director of growth in the proximodistal axis (excision of the AER results in a limb stump only, while transplantation may result in a duplicate limb). Differentiation in the radioulnar axis is under the control of the zone of polarizing activity (ZPA) (transplantation of the ZPA can give rise to a 'mirror hand'). Differentiation in the volardorsal axis is under the control of the dorsal ectoderm (excision and rotation of this zone causes dorsal muscles to form ventrally). Thus, there is a complicated interaction between genes and the proteins they encode, which induces the cells of the AER, ZPA and dorsal zone that drive limb developing and patterning. Anomalies in these processes result in anomalies in limb development, and may be the result of genetic mutation, interruption of a pathway at molecular level or gross insult. The aetiology of such insults can be environmental, e.g. radiation, infection or chemical (including drugs), or hereditary, as part of a syndrome.

Congenital hand deformities are traditionally classified using the 'Swanson classification':

  i. Failure of formation, e.g. phocomelia, radial longitudinal deficiency,
 ii. Failure of differentiation, e.g. syndactyly, arthrogryposis,
iii. Duplication, e.g. radial or ulnar polydactyly,
 iv. Overgrowth, e.g. macrodactyly,
  v. Undergrowth, e.g. thumb hypoplasia,
 vi. Constriction ring syndrome,
vii. Generalized skeletal abnormalities.

This is the standard classification but it is by no means perfect. For example, is a central polysyndactyly (Figure 9.2) a failure of differentiation or a polydactyly? Some conditions, such as polydactyly, are relatively common, whereas a cleft hand is rarely encountered. The commonest and most important congenital conditions are described in this chapter.

Polydactyly

Polydactyly translates literally as 'many fingers' and is the most common congenital hand deformity. It presents as a wide spectrum of disorders but is best thought of as digital 'duplication', with both components often being of abnormal morphology and hypoplastic.

The pattern of transmission is autosomal dominant with variable penetrance.

Polydactyly is broadly categorized, in order of frequency, as postaxial (ulnar), preaxial (radial) or central.

Postaxial polydactyly

Postaxial polydactyly is duplication of the little finger. It is eight times more common than any other polydactyly, often **bilateral** and more common in Africans (1:150) than in whites (1:300), where it is more commonly syndromic.

Stelling classified postaxial polydactyly into three types, based on the degree of duplication. Type 1 is the most common. The most frequent site for Type 1 is the ulnar border of the little finger, at the level of the proximal phalanx.

Type 1 Soft-tissue mass, no skeletal structure,
Type 2 Duplicate digit/part digit articulating with normal/ bifid metacarpal/phalanx,
Type 3 Duplicate digit including duplicate metacarpal.

Diagnosis and examination

Careful examination should include testing the range of motion of both hands and feet. Radiographs are not mandatory for simple Type 1 duplications but are usually required for Types

Postgraduate Paediatric Orthopaedics, ed. Sattar Alshryda, Stan Jones and Paul A. Banaszkiewicz. Published by Cambridge University Press.
© Cambridge University Press 2014.

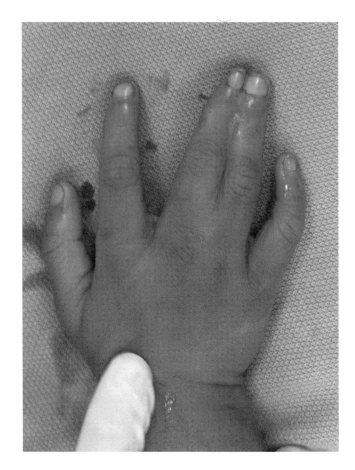

Figure 9.1 Important zones in the developing limb bud.

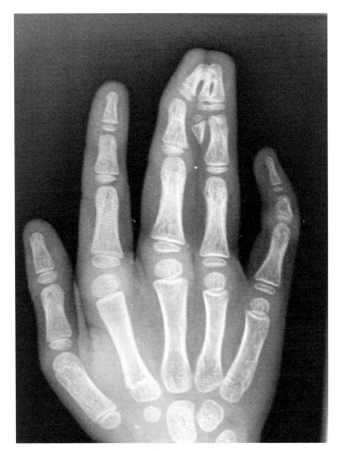

Figure 9.2 Central polysyndactyly.

2 and 3 to look for shared epiphysis, assess the morphology of 'a normal digit' and exclude symphalangism (fused phalanges), complex polysyndactyly or deformity with angulation.

Management

Type 1 duplications can be managed by excision. This can easily be performed under local anaesthetic when the child is younger than 3 months of age.

Type 2 and 3 duplications require excision and reconstruction of the functional components, including the ulnar collateral ligament (aided by a retained periosteal strip from the deleted digit) and re-insertion of the abductor digiti minimi.

Central polydactyly

Central polydactyly refers to a duplication of the index, long or ring fingers. This is the least common form. It is commonly associated with a syndactyly, only becoming apparent on pre-operative radiographs and representing a hidden central polydactyly between the syndactylized digits (Figure 9.2). Central polydactyly is frequently bilateral, with ring finger duplications being the most common, followed by the middle and index fingers.

Central polydactyly is classified using the Stelling classification, with Type 2 duplications being the most common, followed by Types 1 and 3, in reducing order.

Diagnosis and examination

Diagnosis is by clinical and radiographic assessment. Clinical assessment should include range of motion, posture and function. Classify the type and the presence and degree of syndactyly.

Management

An individualized approach is required, depending on the extent of duplication and the presence of syndactyly.

Early surgical treatment is indicated, with excision of the duplicate digit and complex bone and soft-tissue reconstruction. This varies from simple ray resection with intermetacarpal ligament reconstruction to complex redistribution of tendinous, ligamentous and skeletal elements.

Preaxial polydactyly

Preaxial polydactyly is duplication of the thumb. It has an incidence of 0.8 per 1000 live births and may have a dominant inheritance pattern. There is a female-to-male ratio of 2.5:1 and it is more common in whites.

Although a triphalangeal thumb is historically linked to maternal thalidomide ingestion, preaxial polydactyly has numerous syndromic associations, including Holt–Oram syndrome, Fanconi pancytopaenia, thrombocytopaenia absent radii (TAR), Carpenter syndrome and Bloom's syndrome. Abnormalities of the sonic hedgehog protein, which is expressed as part of radioulnar limb development and abnormal expression of other morphogens, such as the *Hox* genes, bone morphogenic protein and *GLI3* gene, have been implicated in the development of thumb duplications.

Diagnosis and examination

Clinical examination is necessary, to assess for range of movement of all fingers, as well as overall upper-limb function. Specific care should focus on the presence of thumb functional tendon units and any deformity.

In syndromic cases, the patient must be fully examined. A multidisciplinary team approach, including paediatric, cardiac and haematological investigations may be required before surgery can be undertaken. Radiographs are mandatory.

Classification of preaxial polydactyly is radiographic and is based on the presence of complete or incomplete duplication of each phalanx (Wassell classification) (Figure 9.3):

Type I:	Bifid distal phalanx,
Type II:	Duplicate distal phalanx,
Type III:	Bifid proximal phalanx,
Type IV:	Duplicate proximal phalanx; this is the most common,
Type V:	Bifid metacarpal,
Type VI:	Duplicate metacarpal,
Type VII:	Triphalangism.

Type IV is the most common (>40%) and Type I the least common. Type VII is the most complex; many consider it a separate entity.

Management

Surgical management is usually delayed until after 12 months, as this reduces the overall anaesthetic risk, allows for full and thorough pre-operative assessment and eases surgery, thanks to a larger hand size. Only an unclassified 'pouce flottant' (floating thumb) on a narrow skin only stalk is managed earlier, with simple excision (as for postaxial Type 1 duplications).

The surgical principles are to produce a well-aligned, normally sized stable thumb before the age of 2 while preserving the epiphyseal plates where feasible. Despite this, the reconstructed thumb is nearly always smaller than the normal, contralateral thumb.

Overall, nail appearance and joint motion are less important to a successful outcome, as stiffness at one thumb joint is functionally well tolerated.

Surgical treatment ranges from total ablation of one thumb to reconstruction using half of the components from each duplicate. In general, the ulnar-sided digit is preserved in favour of the radial duplicate, to save the ulnar collateral and provide MCPJ (metacarpophalangeal joint) stability.

Types I and II: Symmetrical duplication

Consider excision of the central composite tissue segment from both thumbs and approximation of the outer halves: this is called the Bilhaut–Cloquet procedure (Figure 9.4).

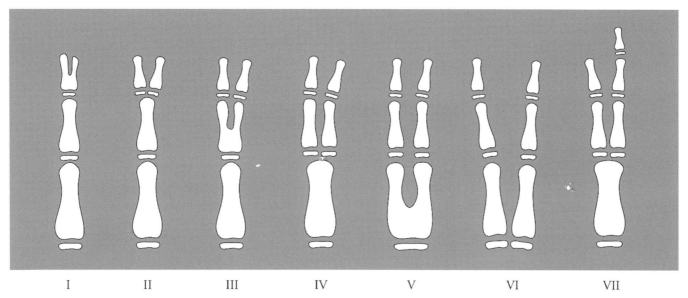

Figure 9.3 Wassell classification.

I II III IV V VI VII

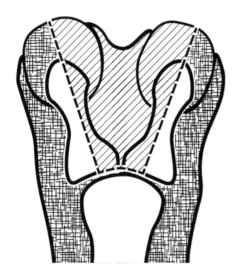

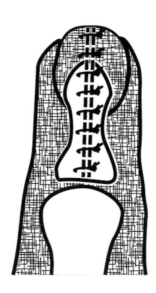

Figure 9.4 Bilhaut–Cloquet procedure.

Significant limitations include joint stiffness, a wide distal phalanx, angular deformities, nail ridging and poor cosmesis.

The modified Bilhaut–Cloquet procedure alleviates some of the limitations with the nail bed by using the nail bed of only one thumb.

Types III–VI: Asymmetrical duplication

Consider deletion or excision of the smaller duplicate. The deleted thumb is usually (and preferably) the radial digit, so as to preserve the more functionally important ulnar collateral ligament.

Deletion of the radial duplicate usually involves (Figure 9.5):

- Racquet shaped incision with or without proximal and distal z-plasty extensions,
- Abductor pollicis insertion preservation,

- Radial collateral ligaments preservation from the deleted thumb for later reconstruction,
- Assessment and centralization of extrinsic tendons,
- Reduction of radial condyle; preservation of growth plate and ulnar collateral ligament (UCL),
- Excision or fillet of duplicate ulnar digit, with or without wedge osteotomy of retained digit if angulation present,
- Check for pollex abductus (an abnormal connection between the extensor and flexor structures),
- Removed digit soft-tissue components can be used to augment extrinsic tendons and soft tissue as required.

Types III–VII

For Types III to VII, deletion is performed, as described. For Type VII, a complex reconstruction is required.

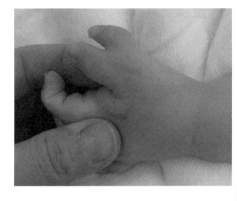
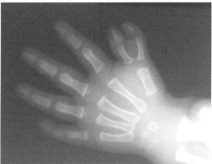
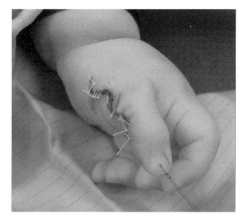
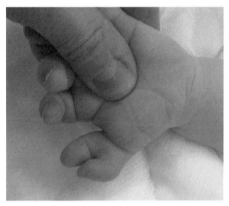
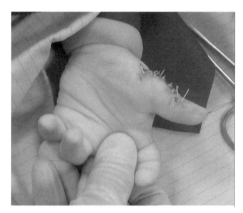

Figure 9.5 Wassell IV Thumb Polydactyly; deletion of radial duplicate.

Syndactyly

Syndactyly translates literally as together (*syn*) finger (*dactyl*) and is one of the most common congenital hand deformities, with an incidence of 1 per 2000 live births. It carries an autosomal dominant inheritance pattern with variable penetrance, although up to 40% have a positive family history.

The pathological process is not precisely understood; it is thought to arise from a failure of apoptosis (programmed cell death) in interdigital tissue.

In 50% of cases, syndactyly is bilateral, with a 2:1 male-to-female ratio; whites have the highest racial predilection. Although often non-syndromic, it may be associated with such syndromes as Poland, Down's, Carpenter, Holt–Oram, Pfeiffer and Apert (although the Apert hand is more properly termed acrosyndactyly) (Figure 9.6).

The most commonly involved web is the third (50% of cases), with the first, second and fourth webs accounting for 5%, 15% and 30% of cases, respectively.

Syndactyly is classified, based on the extent of web involvement into complete, with fusion at least up to the distal interphalangeal joint, or incomplete. It is further classified into simple (skin only) or complex (bone and skin involved). A final category of 'complicated' is reserved for cases where both syndactyly and polydactyly are present (Figure 9.7).

Diagnosis and investigations

Clinical examination should assess the number of rays involved, the completeness of the syndactyly, identification of syndromic features and a basic assessment of upper-limb function. Examination should include evaluation of passive range of motion, to assess associated symphalangism (stiff digits) and compare the digit lengths with the contralateral hand for brachysyndactyly. The pectoralis major should be examined: this will be hypoplastic in brachysyndactyly associated with Poland syndrome (Figure 9.8).

An X-ray is mandatory, to evaluate bony involvement and assess for the presence of transverse bars or more complicated hidden duplications. Both false positives and false negatives may result, owing to incomplete ossification. Arteriography is rarely indicated.

Syndactyly may also affect the toes. Surgical release is not advocated because of the risk of painful hypertrophic scars. An exception, however, is the first web (Figure 9.9).

Management

Syndactyly release is advised between 12 and 18 months, as most hand function is learnt between 12 and 24 months.

The exception to this is syndactyly involving the border digits (i.e. the first and fourth webs) and the complex Apert

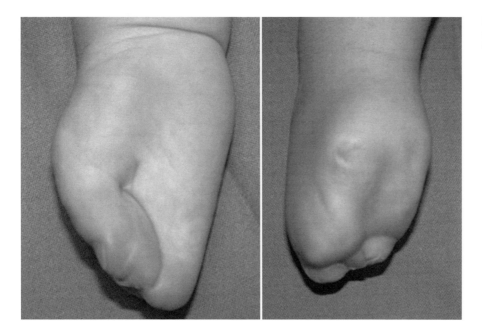

Figure 9.6 The rosebud hand. This is the most severe acrosyndactyly associated with Apert syndrome.

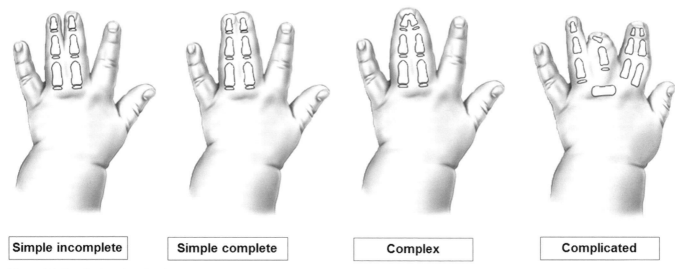

| Simple incomplete | Simple complete | Complex | Complicated |

Figure 9.7 Classification of syndactyly.

hand. The rationale for early surgical release (younger than 1 year) in these cases is that with continued growth any complex bony involvement is expected to cause tethering, impede development and adversely affect future digital growth.

Relative contraindications to surgery include:

- A minor degree of webbing (which is not cosmetically or functionally significant),
- Hypoplastic digits (where one digit functions better than two would),
- Feet (little functional benefit is offered but painful hypertrophic scarring may result).

Surgical release involves the following principles:

- Release only one side of a digit at a time, to prevent vascular compromise,
- Avoid straight-line incisions or incisions in the web,
- Use dorsal skin flap for web space reconstruction,
- Use large simple ulnar and radially based interdigitating flaps.

Many cases can be completed without using grafts if properly planned, but always reserve the option of full-thickness grafts with the preservation of paratenon (Figure 9.10):

- Identify neurovascular bundle proximally and volar; dissecting from the level of bifurcation.
- Joints and tendon slips must be preserved and exposed bone and joint covered with flaps as opposed to graft.
- Plan tip and lateral nail fold reconstruction with pulp-plasty and Buck–Gramcko flaps (Figure 9.11).

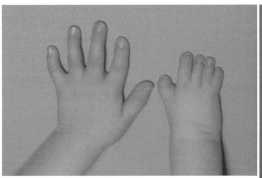
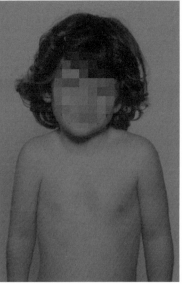

Figure 9.8 Brachysyndactyly and pectoralis major hypoplasia associated with Poland syndrome.

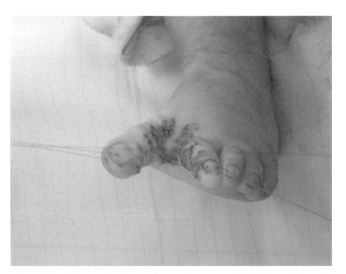

Figure 9.9 Release of the first and second toes using full-thickness skin grafts.

Camptodactyly

Camptodactyly is a congenital flexion deformity of the digit involving the proximal interphalangeal joint (PIPJ). It can be found in approximately 1% of the population but may be as high as 20% in adolescent girls. Camptodactyly is alternatively known as campylodactyly. This name is derived from the Greek *kampylos* (arched) and *dactyl* (finger).

Camptodactyly has an autosomal dominant inheritance and a variable penetrance pattern and tends to have a bimodal distribution. It is commonly bilateral and is classically defined as involving the little finger (although all digits may be involved, in order of frequency, little finger, ring, middle, index).

It is classified by its distribution into:

Infantile: At or soon after birth,

Pre-adolescent: Can be more severe and progressive,

Syndromic: Often severe with multiple digits.

In infancy, the male:female ratio is 1:1, whereas the adolescent variant has a female predominance. This has led some to believe they represent separate entities.

The aetiology is poorly understood with almost all structures crossing the volar aspect of the PIPJ being implicated. Abnormalities found on exploration include abnormal lumbrical insertion, a short or tethered superficialis tendon, anomalous fibrous tissue and abnormalities in the retinacular or extensor system. The distal interphalangeal joint is not pathological but may develop late compensatory changes.

Diagnosis and examination

Presentation of an abnormal posture involving the PIPJ requires a careful history to help rule out non-congenital or traumatic aetiologies. The time of onset of symptoms and progression of deformity allow for the classification of camptodactyly, if appropriate.

Clinical assessment is focused on the digits affected and assessment with measurement of both passive and active range of motion, classifying the PIPJ into reducible or irreducible.

To aid in localizing the abnormality, examination should include assessment for intrinsic tightness, which may indicate lumbrical pathology. Furthermore, increased extension on MCPJ flexion may indicate deforming or tight volar structures. Careful examination must include a study of overall finger morphology and examination for the presence of flexion creases, as associated brachydactyly with very stiff PIPJ and absent creases may represent a diagnosis of symphalangism.

When the PIPJ flexion deformity is irreducible, the suggestion is of significant joint pathology, which is not likely to be correctable by surgery. Distal interphalangeal joint involvement is not diagnostic of camptodactyly and may represent other aetiologies, including trauma.

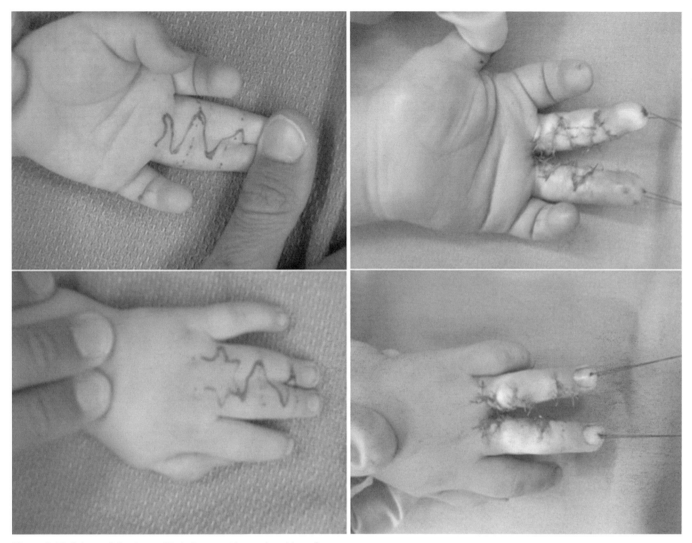

Figure 9.10 Release of the ring and little fingers without using skin grafts.

Radiographic examination is mandatory, as pathological changes involving the PIPJ are a poor prognostic sign, i.e. flattening out of base of middle phalanx and hypoplasia of proximal phalangeal head with volar notching of the neck and loss of joint space (Figure 9.12). Lateral radiographs will further rule out congenital synostosis.

Management

Camptodactyly rarely affects function and can be managed conservatively, particularly when contracture is less than 40°. Serial splintage and physiotherapy are the mainstays of treatment. If early correction is achieved, further splinting may be necessary in adolescence to prevent recurrence with growth.

In general, surgery should be avoided if the deformity is mild and not progressive. Relative indications for surgery are:

- Functional problems (with PIPJ flexion deformity >40°),
- Progressive disease,
- Failed conservative therapies.

In the absence of skeletal abnormalities, surgery involves a Brunner-type or midline incision with secondary z-plasty and the release of all abnormal or anomalous tissue on the volar aspect of the proximal interphalangeal joint, including any capsular contracture, with stepwise release of the flexor sheath and accessory collateral until satisfactory correction is achieved. The flexor digitorum superficialis and intrinsic should also be examined.

Other described procedures include tendon transfers, i.e. flexor digitorum superficialis (FDS), lumbrical to lateral band and central slip. If passive MCPJ stability during examination allows active extension at the PIPJ, a 'lasso' procedure using a superficialis slip may be indicated.

If skeletal abnormalities are present, opening or closing wedge osteotomies may be required in addition to soft-tissue procedures. This compromises extension without increasing the arc of motion, and is thus rarely performed. Arthrodesis is reserved for the most severe cases, when no useful function at the PIPJ can be attained.

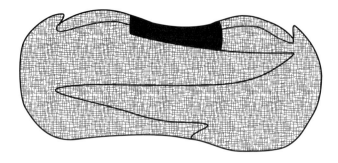

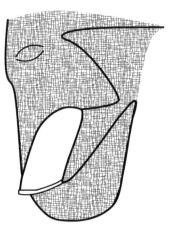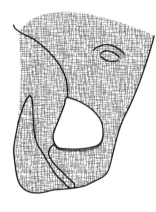

Figure 9.11 Buck–Gramcko pulp flaps.

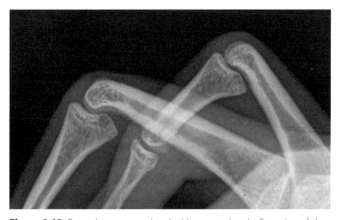

Figure 9.12 Bony changes associated with camptodactyly: flattening of the base of the middle phalanx, hypoplasia of the head and notching of the neck of the proximal phalangeal.

Clinodactyly

Clinodactyly is characterized by radioulnar curvature of a digit distal to MCPJ and has a reported incidence of between 1% and 19% of live births. It translates literally as sloped (*clino*) and finger (*dactyl*). It usually follows an autosomal dominant pattern with variable penetrance, although it may be associated with such syndromes as Poland, Treacher Collins, Kleinfelter and Down's (up to 80% of patients with Down's syndrome

have clinodactyly). It is often bilateral and most commonly affects the little finger and involves the middle phalanx.

The aetiology of clinodactyly is unclear. However, clinical deformity results from abnormalities in growth plate morphology. Abnormalities include a C-shaped physeal plate, previously termed a bracketed epiphysis but more correctly termed a longitudinal epiphyseal or diaphyseal bracket. Growth in the longitudinal portion of the epiphysis leads to asymmetrical growth and progressive abnormal phalangeal morphology. The triangular shaped bone that results from this abnormal growth pattern is called a delta phalanx.

Classification is based on the degree of angulation and physeal and phalangeal morphology:

I. Minor angulation, normal length (very common),
II. Minor angulation, short phalanx, associated with Down's syndrome,
III. Marked deformity, associated delta phalanx (wedge-shaped) with C-shaped physis.

History and examination

The assessment of a patient with clinodactyly should start with a general review and identification of syndromic features. The involved digit should be assessed for degree of deformity, based on degree of angulation and the presence of shortening. Limited range of motion is common with a bracketed epiphysis. Clinodactyly is generally painless. A painful deformity suggests trauma.

Radiographic assessment is mandatory to assess the skeletal maturity, degree of bony involvement, presence of abnormal epiphysis and morphology of the phalanges.

Management

Reassurance is all that is required in the majority of patients who have a mild deformity and no functional deficit. Surgery for cosmesis only should be avoided.

The indication for surgery is severe angulation with shortening or thumb involvement.

In the skeletally immature, resection of the abnormal bracket epiphysis and interposition fat grafting (Vickers' procedure) allows for longitudinal growth catch up over a 2-year period (Figure 9.13).

In the skeletally mature, corrective osteotomies are advised. Opening and reverse wedges are preferred over closing wedge osteotomies, which compromise phalangeal length. K-wires are required to stabilize the osteotomies and z-plasty may be required in the presence of skin deficiency.

Trigger thumb

Trigger thumb is described as a congenital deformity, even though there is no evidence that it is present at birth. Around 25% of trigger thumbs are bilateral and the estimated incidence is 3:1000.

Diagnosis and examination

The typical presentation is with the thumb held fixed and flexed at the interphalangeal joint, although some cases are intermittent. There is usually a palpable nodule (Notta's node) at the level of the metacarpophalangeal joint. Clinical catching or triggering is more difficult to elicit than in adult patients.

Management

The initial management is non-operative, as 30% of cases resolve before the age of 1 year. Flexion contractures do occur but correct spontaneously if the triggering resolves or if surgical release is performed during childhood. There is no place for steroid injection in the child.

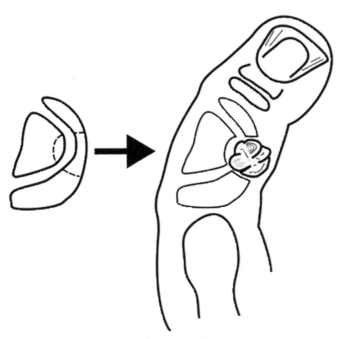

Figure 9.13 Vickers' procedure for clinodactyly.

Surgery is indicated if the deformity does not resolve by 2 years of age; this involves release of the A1 pulley through a volar approach with a short small transverse incision between the MCPJ flexion creases (Figure 9.14). Release is generally undertaken on the radial side to avoid injury to the oblique pulley and should be performed only enough to allow full extension at the interphalangeal joint.

Congenital clasped thumb

Clasped thumb is a deformity associated with a heterogeneous group of congenital anomalies and is characterized by a persistent flexed and adducted thumb. It is caused by a weakness or deficiency of the extensor pollicis brevis or longus, or both, and is usually accompanied with a degree of first web space contracture.

It is associated with anomalies such as arthrogryposis, digitotalar dysmorphism and Freeman–Sheldon syndrome.

The male:female ratio is quoted as between 1 and 2.5:1. Although one-third of cases are sporadic, a genetic defect is the likely causative factor and inheritance follows an autosomal dominant pattern with variable penetrance.

History and examination

The diagnosis of clasped thumb is often delayed with infants frequently holding the thumb in the palm for the first 3 to 4 months of life. However, assessment of the patient with clasped thumb should start with a general review of limb posture and function, with identification of syndromic features. Clinical examination should focus on assessment of the thumb posture, passive range of motion and assessment of the first web space. The clasped thumb is usually held in the palm with an extension lag (most commonly at the MCPJ, which is suggestive of extensor pollicis brevis deficiencies). A simultaneous lag at the interphalangeal joint indicates deficiency of the extensor pollicis longus with adduction of the metacarpal implying abductor insufficiency. An important differential diagnosis is trigger

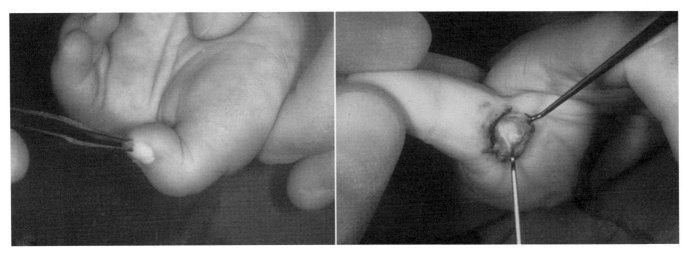

Figure 9.14 Trigger thumb release.

thumb, where the abnormality is localized to the interphalangeal joint and associated with Notta's node.

Radiographic assessment is not mandatory but commonly undertaken to assess joint morphology.

Tsuyuguchi classified clasped thumb into:

Type I: Supple clasped thumb: the thumb can be passively abducted and extended against the resistance of thumb flexors; with or without other digital anomalies.

Type II: Clasped thumb with hand contractures: the thumb cannot be passively extended and abducted; with or without other digital anomalies.

Type III: Clasped thumb associated with arthrogryposis.

Management

If the extensor tendons are present and the joint is supple (Type I), non-operative treatment is the mainstay and consists of thumb splintage in extension for at least 6 months, followed by night splinting for a further 6 months once active extension of the thumb is achieved.

Surgery is indicated:

- If conservative treatment fails or there is functional impairment,
- For significant adduction contracture,
- In severe deformity (Types II and III).

Surgery should be individualized according to the degree of narrowing of the first web, the stability of the metacarpophalangeal joint (MCPJ) and muscle deficiency.

The main aims of surgery are improvement in thumb span with release of the first web and tendon transfers to overcome tendon deficiencies.

Soft-tissue augmentation is achieved with simple z-plasty, four-flap plasty, rotation or transposition flaps, depending on the degree of deficit. If full passive extension and abduction cannot be achieved after adequate skin release, release of adductor pollicis insertion, the first dorsal interosseous and the carpometacarpal joint (CMCJ) capsule plus K-wire stabilization and metacarpophalangeal joint chondrodesis for MCPJ instability may be required.

Tendon transfers may be required to restore active extension of the stable or stabilized MCPJ, with the extensor indicis as the preferred tendon for transfer. If this is absent, one slip of the flexor digitorum superficialis muscle can be transferred to the vestigial remnant of the deficient thumb extensors.

Joint fusion remains an option in severe cases with fixed deformities.

Thumb hypoplasia

Thumb hypoplasia represents a spectrum of deformity from mild deficiency to complete thumb adactyly. Although classified as a 'Class V: Undergrowth', it is best considered a part of radial deficiencies, in terms of both its genetic cause and associated syndromes.

The overall incidence is approximately 1 per 100 000 live births, with an equal male:female ratio. It is bilateral in 60% of patients. Associated syndromes include Holt–Oram, TAR, VACTERL and Fanconi's anaemia. Inheritance varies with associated syndromes; it is dominant with Holt–Oram but recessive with TAR and Fanconi's.

History and examination

The diagnosis is clinical and although more severe adactylies or 'floating thumbs' are diagnosed early, mild thumb hypoplasia may go unnoticed until fine motor skills begin to develop and it is noticed that the thumb is ignored or smaller than the contralateral side. All patients with thumb hypoplasia should be managed in a multidisciplinary team including paediatricians, owing to the associations with blood dyscrasias and cardiac abnormalities.

Clinical examination involves bilateral inspection and palpation, comparing thumb size, consistency, thenar muscle bulk and the first web space. The ipsilateral elbow and wrist should be examined for associated radial longitudinal deficiencies and the index finger assessed, to allow consideration of future pollicization. Good function in an index finger makes for good function after pollicization.

Gentle lateral stress is applied for the assessment of MCPJ and CMCJ stability. This is vital in determining surgical options, i.e. thumb reconstruction versus ablation and pollicization.

Pollex abductus, an abnormal insertion or communication between the flexor pollicis longus and the extensor mechanism, should be actively assessed and is suggested when there is abduction on thumb flexion.

Radiography is mandatory and should include both hands, wrists and forearms.

Classification (Blauth)

This is based on the degree of thumb hypoplasia, intrinsic and extrinsic hypoplasia, skeletal hypoplasia and joint stability:

1. Minor generalized hypoplasia,
2. Absence of or hypoplasia of intrinsic muscles, first web space contracture and MCPJ instability,
3. Type 2 plus hypoplastic extrinsic muscles or tendons and greater skeletal deficiency; subdivided into:
   3a. stable CMCJ,
   3b. unstable CMCJ.
4. 'Pouce flottant' or floating thumb: rudimentary appendage with small skin bridge,
5. Thumb adactyly.

Management

Treatment is aimed at improving function and not cosmesis. A normal-sized thumb with a normal range of movement should not be promised. Surgical treatment is largely governed by Blauth classification:

- Type 1 hypoplasia usually has good function and requires no treatment.
- If the CMCJ is present and stable (Types 2 and 3a), reconstruction of the thumb is advocated.
- Reconstructive options include:
  - MCPJ stabilization with UCL reconstruction.
  - Exploration and release of pollex abductus abnormalities (if present), deepening of the web space (usually with four-flap plasty) and augmentation of the intrinsic musculature with opponensplasty (most commonly ring finger flexor digitorum superficialis (FDS) or abductor digiti minimi (ADM) (Huber) transfer).
- In Type 3a thumbs, extrinsic extensor hypoplasia can be augmented with extensor indicis transfer.
- If the CMCJ is absent or unstable (Type 3b) and in Types 4 and 5 thumbs, pollicization is preferred to reconstruction. It may be difficult to explain this to parents, as often the surgeon will need to discard a very reasonable looking thumb (Figure 9.15).

Pollicization techniques have been refined over the last century but this remains a complicated procedure requiring attention to detail. The basic principles are as follows:

- Raising of dorsal skin flap from the radial side of the index finger with transposition to create the first web.
- Intrafascicular dissection of the index finger common digital nerves to the second web level, with preservation of accompanying digital vessels.
- Excision of the index finger metacarpal with resection of the metacarpal epiphysis (preserving the metacarpal head to act as a neotrapezium).
- Extension of the index MCPJ (as it can hyperextend), then rotation of the metacarpal head in 120° pronation and securing in 45° palmar abduction.
- Shortening of extensor and reposition of:
  - Extensor indicis → extensor pollicis longus,
  - Extensor digitorum communis index → abductor pollicis longus,
  - First palmar interosseous → adductor pollicis,
  - First dorsal interosseous → abductor pollicis brevis (Figure 9.16).

Pollicization often provides improved cosmesis, as well as an opposable digit.

Macrodactyly

The term macrodactyly is derived from *macros* (large) and *dactyl* (finger). It is characterized by enlargement of both soft tissue and osseous elements and belongs to a group of heterogeneous disorders referred to as 'Class IV overgrowth'.

Figure 9.15 Pollicization of the index finger.

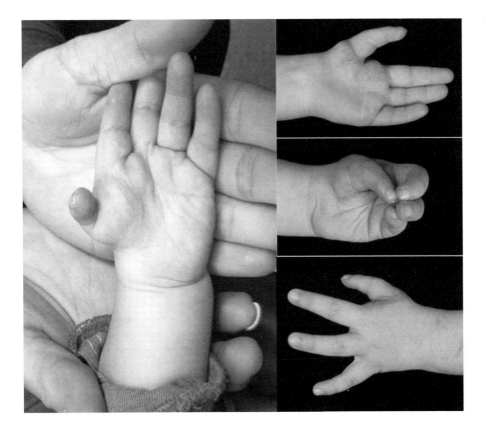

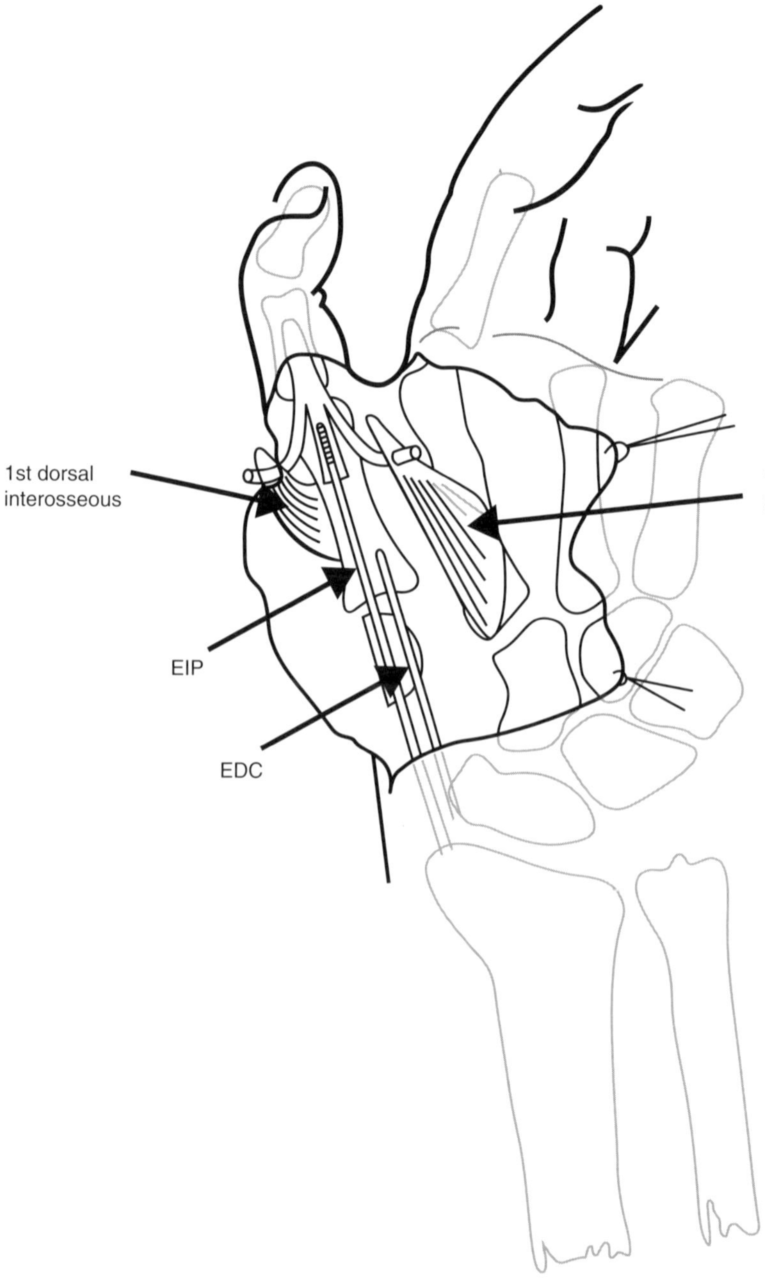

Figure 9.16 Pollicization of the index finger; surgical technique. EDC, extensor digitorum communis; EIP, extensor indicis proprius.

The aetiology is unknown but the most common theory relates to a nerve-stimulated overgrowth mediated by abnormal neural control or a localized form of neurofibromatosis.

Macrodactyly is rare with no clear inheritance pattern (Figure 9.17); it most commonly involves the index finger. There is a male predilection. The upper and lower limbs may be involved with multidigit involvement present in about 50% of cases.

History and examination

Not all overgrowths are macrodactyly and the condition should be distinguished from other conditions, such as haemangiomas, vascular malformations and Ollier disease.

History is therefore based on the chronology of the overgrowth (static versus progressive), the localization of the abnormality to anatomical area and nerve territory, the presence of features suggesting vascular abnormality (compressibility, warmth, thrill) the degree of osseous involvement or overgrowth, and systemic features, including those of neurofibromatosis.

Comparison radiographs are mandatory to document growth and assess for osseous involvement. Arteriography or MRI may be required to rule out vascular abnormality.

Macrodactyly has been classified by its evolution into either static or progressive types, with Upton further classifying it into:

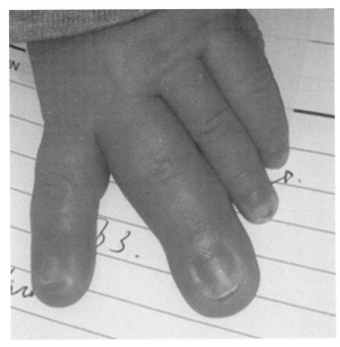

Figure 9.17 Macrodactyly.

1. Macrodactyly with lipofibromatosis:
   - Static subtype: born with large digit, enlarges proportionally with age,
   - Progressive subtype: near-normal at birth, progressive growth until epiphyseal closure.
2. Macrodactyly with neurofibromatosis,
3. Macrodactyly with hyperostosis,
4. Macrodactyly with hemihypertrophy.

Management

Surgery for macrodactyly is often complex and often unsatisfactory, yet psychological consequences can be severe. Social counselling and family involvement are imperative. The goals of surgery are control or reduction in deformity with maintenance of sensibility and function.

The surgical options vary, depending on the aetiology, anatomical location, severity and subtype, and include soft-tissue reduction, epiphysiodesis, neurolysis, nerve excision and grafting, corrective osteotomies, arthrodesis and, in severe cases, amputation.

Epiphysiodesis should be performed when the digit approaches adult size. In general, it is best to perform few definitive procedures, rather than multiple ones.

Arthrogryposis

The term arthrogryposis is derived from *arthro* (joint) and *gryposis* (curved or hooked). Arthrogryposis is a congenital disorder affecting the muscles and is thought to be secondary to abnormality in the motor nerves. It is properly termed 'arthrogryposis multiplex congenita', literally meaning a congenital anomaly in the newborn involving multiple curved joints.

The overall incidence is approximately 1 per 10 000 live births. It is important to note that arthrogryposis is essentially a descriptive term and not an exact diagnosis. It has numerous underlying pathologies which broadly fall into three groups:

Type 1: Classical arthrogryposis multiplex congenita, primarily involving the limbs with deficient or absent muscles,

Type 2: Arthrogryposis associated with major neurogenic or myopathic dysfunction,

Type 3: Arthrogryposis associated with other major anomalies and syndromes.

Pathologically, there is always a defect in the motor unit as a whole or at some point between the anterior horn cells and the muscle itself. It can therefore also be classified as neurogenic or myogenic. The aetiology is unclear, with theories postulating inflammatory or infective causes or maldevelopment secondary to increased immobility *in utero*. Some of these include: structural abnormality of the uterus, oligohydramnios, increased intra-uterine pressure or mechanical compression of the fetus and breech presentation or prematurity.

Examination and management

Clinical examination remains the best modality for establishing the diagnosis. The classical presentation involves all four limbs, with multiple rigid joint deformities and defective, fibrosed or absent muscle groups but normal sensation. Muscle and joint contractures result with cylindrically appearing limbs lacking skin creases. Adducted and internally rotated shoulders, extended knees or elbows and club-like hand and wrists are typical, although isolated distal variants may occur (Figure 9.18). Clasped thumb and thin waxy skin are often present.

In arthrogryposis, unlike paralytic disorders, joint deformities are stiff or rigid from birth and there is a tendency for symmetrical involvement with increasingly severe contractures moving more distally along the affected limb.

Radiographs of the limbs are mandatory and may demonstrate osseous abnormality with loss of subcutaneous fat and muscle. Muscle biopsies and CT or MRI are rarely indicated unless CNS involvement or myopathic disorder is suspected.

Management

Arthrogryposis should be managed in a multidisciplinary team involving surgeon, therapist, paediatrician and geneticist. Early use of splints and serial casting is the mainstay of treatment to encourage elbow flexion and wrist extension, with prevention of contracture being preferred over surgery.

Surgery may be reserved for cases of failed splintage or late presentation and aims to address posture and limb function, achieving improved position of the shoulder, elbow, wrist and hand posture. Historically, one limb was aimed at perineal

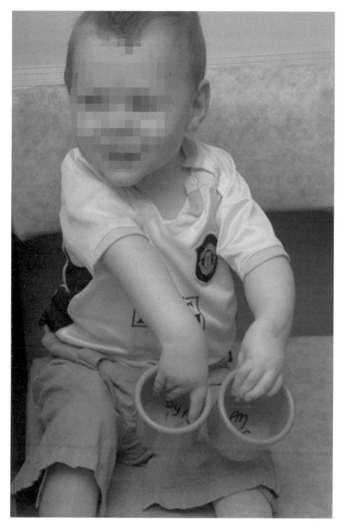

Figure 9.18 Arthrogryposis multiplex congenita.

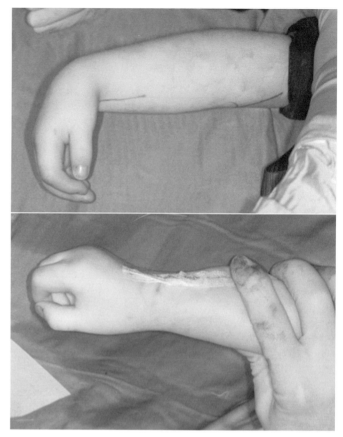

Figure 9.19 Surgery for arthrogryposis multiplex congenita. Position of the wrist before and after dorsal wedge osteotomy of carpus and transfer of flexor carpi ulnaris and flexor carpi radialis.

hygiene, and the other for 'hand-to-mouth' use. However, this destroys the very useful bimanual function, as demonstrated in Figure 9.18. In principle, whatever is done to one upper limb should also be done to the other. Hand-to-mouth function and bimanual hand use are the key goals.

Surgery, where indicated, can be staged, with initial soft-tissue release followed by bony surgery to achieve elbow flexion. The aim of wrist surgery is to put the wrists in a good position for keyboard use and is usually achieved by carpal wedge osteotomy and tendon transfer (Figure 9.19). Recurrence is common and ongoing splintage is required to maintain the correction until skeletal maturity.

Transverse arrest

Transverse arrest is classified as a failure of formation (Type 1). It is characterized by either the complete absence of the upper limb distal to a point, producing an amputation stump (complete type), or the absence of a part of the limb (intercalated type).

Complete arrests (also known as congenital amputation, failure of development, terminal absence and transverse amelia) may occur at any level but are most common in the forearm at the junction of proximal and middle thirds. The incidence is unknown and it appears not to be inherited.

Intercalated variants (most commonly related to maternal thalidomide ingestion → phocomelia) may present as:

Complete: Hand attached directly to torso,

Proximal: Normal hand and forearm attached to torso,

Distal: Hand attached to normal upper arm at elbow.

The prevalence of the intercalated variant is 0.6 per 100 000 births, with the majority of cases being isolated, although syndromic associations include musculoskeletal, cardiac and intestinal abnormalities.

Complete arrests and intercalated arrests are therefore postulated to be separate entities with differing aetiologies, despite being grouped together as 'transverse failures of formation'.

History and examination

Maternal drug history and clinical examination help classify the deformity.

In complete transverse arrest, examination should entail palpation of the distal portions assessing for any range of motion of the distal portion, which may represent buried vestigial metacarpals or digits with the potential for independent function.

Management

Prosthetics is the mainstay of treatment, with limited possibilities for surgical intervention.

In complete transverse arrest, surgery may occasionally be indicated where some functional distal remnant exists that could be expected to allow pincer function after release or improve prosthetic fitting or function. In these rare cases, distraction manoplasty or free phalangeal transfers may be indicated.

In intercalated arrest, prosthetic fitting is required for most phocomelic patients, who may activate the device using digits. Surgery is only indicated to achieve prosthetic fitting or to improve function of the terminal digits. Many patients choose to do without prosthetics.

Brachydactyly

Brachydactyly (*brachos*, short; *dactyl*, finger) refers to disproportionately short fingers or toes and may occur either as an isolated malformation or as a part of a complex malformation syndrome. In the majority of isolated brachydactylies (and some syndromic forms,) genetic abnormalities have been isolated.

In isolated brachydactyly, the inheritance is mostly autosomal dominant with variable penetrance.

Brachydactyly encompasses a number of pathological entities including:

1. A distal form of true transverse arrest with the more proximal part being relatively well developed (note: fingernail absent).
2. Amputations as part of constriction ring syndrome with proximal structures being entirely normal (note: fingernail absent).
3. Symbrachydactyly with significant reduction in bone and soft-tissue elements and severely hypoplastic digits or nubbin-like remnants. There is hypoplasia of more proximal parts, i.e. hand, wrist and forearm (note: fingernails or remnants are present on hypoplastic digits or nubbins).

Symbrachydactyly

Blauth has further subdivided symbrachydactyly into four descriptive types (Figure 9.20):

Figure 9.20 Symbrachydactyly classification.

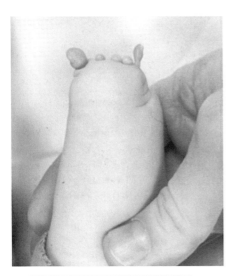

Peromelic type

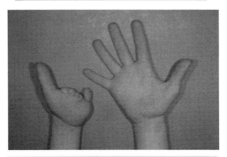

Short finger type

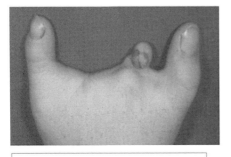

Atypical cleft type

Monodactylous type

Peromelic type:	Absence of all digits and metacarpals,
Short finger type	
Cleft hand type:	Absence of one or more central digits,
Monodactylous type:	Absence of all digits other than the thumb.

History and examination

The severity of digital shortening is variable with mild shortening only apparent due to the loss of normal cascade. Careful examination, including examination of the length and function of brachydactylous digits and the presence of remnant nail plates is mandatory for diagnosis. Associated abnormalities may include syndactyly, clinodactyly and symphalangism.

Examination of the shoulder, chest wall and contralateral limb is required to exclude such conditions as Poland syndrome.

Management

The functional and aesthetic aspects of symbrachydactyly vary depending on the degree of shortening, status of digital remnant and number of digits involved. Hence surgical intervention also varies.

For an isolated deformity, the indication for surgery is function. Options include:

- Lengthening of the brachydactylous digit, either as a single stage, with step-cut osteotomy, or as a multistaged procedure with distraction osteogenesis, can be fraught with problems (particularly in the digit as opposed to the metacarpal). Soft-tissue release, lengthening or ligamentous reconstruction may be required and result in an aesthetically unpleasing, stiff and contracted digit with reduced function.
- In general, with regard to lengthening of the brachydactylous digit, the preferred treatment for short phalanges is to avoid surgery, whereas for short metacarpals, lengthening, particularly with distraction osteogenesis, produces a more favourable response.
- Functional improvements are more predictable, with soft-tissue procedures including widening of web space, z-plasty lengthening of constriction bands and ablation of short useless nubbins, especially from the first web.
- Segments of one digit may be used to augment another digit and a microvascular toe transfer is often the best option to restore a degree of pinch in a digitless or monodactylous hand.
- Free phalangeal transfer (taking a non-vascularized toe middle phalanx and transferring it to the digit) yields disappointing long-term results, often with a significant deformity in the donor toe.

Radial longitudinal deficiency

Radial longitudinal deficiencies consist of a spectrum of abnormalities that are characterized by deficiency of the radius and radiocarpal structures and are classed under 'Class 1: failure of formation'. Although skeletal hypoplasia can occur in the whole arm, including the humeral and ulnar elements, a characteristic radial deviation of the wrist secondary to reduced radial support for the carpus is observed (Figure 9.21).

The prevalence is approximately 1:30 000 live births with radial deficiencies; it is frequently bilateral and asymmetric.

Both environmental causes (including maternal use of thalidomide), and syndromic associations are well documented. Associated syndromes include VACTERL, Holt–Oram, TAR, Fanconi's anaemia and Trisomy 13 and 18. Inheritance patterns follow their syndromic causes when present, being recessive in Fanconi's and TAR, dominant in Holt–Oram and sporadic in VACTERL, Trisomy 13 and 18.

History and examination

Owing to the associated syndromes, children with radial longitudinal deficiencies should be managed by a multidisciplinary team involving paediatricians and therapists. Haematological testing, echocardiography, renal ultrasound and genetic screening are also mandatory.

In addition to examination to assess shoulder, elbow and hand function, a full examination is required to assess for syndromic associations.

Careful examination of the elbow is required, as severe forms of radial deficiencies are associated with poor elbow function. In theory, hand-to-mouth function may be worsened by correcting the radial deviation in a child with a stiff elbow.

Stiffness or flexion contractures of the index and middle fingers is observed in association with thumb hypoplasia or aplasia in up to 60% of patients with total radial absence. Careful examination of index finger movement and function is required, as a stiff and ignored index finger will not make a good pollicized thumb.

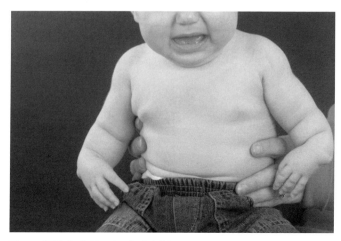

Figure 9.21 Radial longitudinal deficiency.

Radiography is mandatory and should be bilateral, including the digits, hands, wrists and forearms (including the elbows).

Classification is based on radiographic severity, as outlined by Bayne:

Type 1: Short distal radius (>2 mm shorter than ulna with normal proximal radius),

Type 2: Hypoplastic distal and proximal radius,

Type 3: Partial absence of radius,

Type 4: Complete absence of radius.

A fibrocartilaginous radial ruminant or anlage may be identified at surgery.

Management

Treatment is based on the severity of deformity, although functional impairment, secondary to forearm length, wrist instability and thumb hypoplasia, is the main indication for treatment. Physiotherapy is required in all but the most minor of cases and helps prevent progression of stiffness.

In Types 1 and 2, management is primarily with stretching and splintage. Severe Type 2 deficiencies occasionally require soft-tissue release or tendon transfers. Centralization of the carpus on the ulna is rarely warranted.

In Types 3 and 4 with wrist instability and more severe radial deviation, soft-tissue distraction and surgical realignment of the carpus on the ulna is usually required.

Contraindications include major organ defects making anaesthetic risk unacceptable, inadequate elbow flexion and firmly established functional patterns in adults.

Pre-operative stretching through the use of serial casting has now been largely superseded by soft-tissue distraction using external fixators. Distraction offers both osseous realignment, making wrist stabilization easier, and soft-tissue lengthening, thus reducing the requirement for local skin flaps to cover radial shortages and reducing the need for tendon lengthening procedures. Tendon transfer and rebalancing is still required to help maintain the carpus in its new position.

Once adequately distracted, the realignment procedure may be by:

Centralization: With the carpus repositioned over the ulna (usually by making a notch in the carpus) and stabilized with pin fixation through the third metacarpal,

Radialization: With the scaphoid placed over the ulnar head and secured through the second metacarpal.

The decision is usually based on expected outcomes and the presence of an adequate radial carpus stock for a carpal slot to fit the scaphoid. Radialization is preferred as the risk of physeal injury is low, thus maximizing potential longitudinal growth.

Pollicization to reconstruct an absent or hypoplastic thumb is then undertaken.

Ulnar longitudinal deficiency

Ulnar deficiencies are far less common than their radial counterparts and occur in approximately 1:100 000 live births. The occurrence is sporadic, more commonly unilateral and is not associated with systemic conditions.

History and examination

Ulnar deficiencies differ from radial-sided deficiencies, with marked elbow pathology but a stable wrist. Despite this, the hand and carpus are always abnormal; most are associated with adactly, one-third have syndactyly and over two-thirds have thumb hypoplasias.

Examination is based on assessing bilateral upper limbs, with a focus on elbow and wrist function and identification of associated abnormalities. Radiographs of both upper limbs are mandatory for comparison and diagnosis.

Classification is into four types, depending on the degree of ulna hypoplasia:

Type 1: Hypoplastic ulna,

Type 2: Partial absence of ulna,

Type 3: Total absence of ulna with normal radiohumeral joint,

Type 4: Total absence of ulna with synostosis of radiohumeral joint.

Management

Patients with the more common unilateral ulna deficiency usually function well, preferring the normal limb for one-handed tasks and adapting well for bimanual function.

Surgical treatment depends on severity, with better outcomes in Types 1 and 2. In such cases, surgery for associated thumb hypoplasia or syndactyly is all that is usually required.

Indications for surgery in the progressive or unstable Types 2 and 3 deficiencies remain controversial. Options include:

- Excision of the ulna anlage (fibrocartilaginous ruminant); this is advocated by some for progressive deformity.
- Realignment and formation of a one-bone forearm: this is described but there are risks in sacrificing forearm rotation for forearm stability.

Type 4 deficiencies result in marked internal rotation of the limb, which severely limits limb function. If functional compensation is not achieved through conservative measures, an osteotomy may be required to facilitate external rotation.

Central longitudinal deficiency

Central ray deficiencies typically involve aplasia of the central digits, forming what is also known as a typical cleft hand

Table 9.1 Differentiation between the typical and the atypical cleft hand

Typical	Atypical
Autosomal dominant	Sporadic
Bilateral	Unilateral
V-shaped	U-shaped
Feet involved	
No finger nubbins	Nubbins or nails present
Little finger present if monodactylous	Thumb present if monodactylous

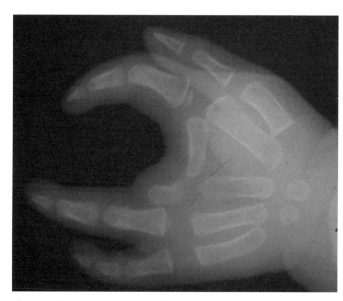

Figure 9.23 Transverse bar in a cleft hand.

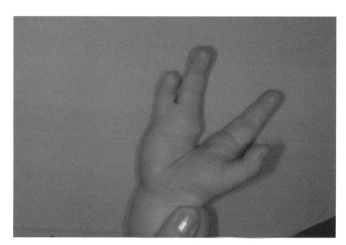

Figure 9.22 'Typical' cleft hand.

(Figure 9.22). It is characterized by partial or complete absence of a central ray, forming a deep V-shaped cleft. It is often bilateral and may involve both hands and feet; a family history is common. The incidence is estimated at 1:10 000 live births. Bones are either absent or malpositioned, but never hypoplastic.

Central ray deficiencies may present as part of a syndrome or as an isolated abnormality. They are thought to result from abnormalities of the apical epidermal ridge (AER) *in utero*, with multiple genetic loci identified for non-syndromic variants. Associated conditions include ectrodactyly–ectodermal dysplasia–clefting (EEC), acrorenal, Cornelia de Lange and ectrodactyly and craniofacial syndromes.

Examination

The characteristic appearance is a deep V-shaped cleft associated with absence or deficiency of a central ray. Associated first web syndactyly may be observed.

A number of significant characteristics differentiate true from atypical cleft hands (Table 9.1). Radiographs are mandatory and may demonstrate transverse bony elements within the cleft, which will require excision (Figure 9.23).

Management

In the absence of first web space contractures, hand function is often remarkably good. This has led it to be labelled a 'functional triumph but a social disaster'.

Indications for early surgical intervention include border syndactyly and the presence of transverse bones within the cleft. If left untreated, marked length discrepancies may develop between the syndactylized digits that can severely affect growth potential, while transverse bone growth within the cleft will result in progressive cleft widening.

Closure of the cleft is the mainstay of surgical management and may involve transfer of the second metacarpal to the third metacarpal base and reconstruction of the transverse metacarpal ligament with skin adjustment to provide a good first web.

Bibliography

1. Swanson AB (1983) A classification for congenital limb malformation. *J Hand Surg* **8**:693–702.

2. Siegert JJ, Cooney WP and Dobyns JH (1990) Management of simple camptodactyly. *J Hand Surg Br* **15**:181–9.

3. Eaton CJ and Lister GD (1990) Syndactyly. *Hand Clin* **6**:555–75.

4. Blauth W (1967) The hypoplastic thumb. *Arch Orthop Unfallchir* **62**:225–46.

5. Marks TW and Bayne LG (1978) Polydactyly of the thumb: abnormal anatomy and treatment. *J Hand Surg* **3**:107–16.

6. Tsuge K (1985) Treatment of macrodactyly. *J Hand Surg Am* **10**:968–9.

Neuromuscular diseases

Simon L. Barker

Recognizing 'normal'

In any paediatric orthopaedic examination, it is vital that progress in achieving developmental milestones is evaluated. Familiarity with the normal will alert the examiner to the abnormal.

Mobility and ambulation

Approximately 90% of normally developing infants are able to:

- Roll themselves by 6 months,
- Sit without support by 8 months,
- Pull themselves up to stand by 10 months,
- Walk by 15 months,
- Hop on one foot by 4 years.

Note, however, that 10% of children will normally achieve these milestones later, but failure to walk by 2 years of age should be investigated.

A normal toddler gait is wide-based and stiff-kneed. A mature 'adult' gait, with its characteristic reciprocal arm swing, develops from 3.5 years onward.

Upper-limb development

- Transfer of objects between hands: normally from 8 months,
- Opposition and release of objects: from 1 year,
- Proper grasp and release: 18 months,
- Finger-grip to hold a crayon: 2 years,
- Writing: from 4 to 5 years.

The following red flags should prompt further evaluation:

- Not rolling over by 6 months,
- Not sitting by 8 months,
- Handedness before 12 months,
- No words by 14 months,
- Not walking by 18 months.

Developmental reflexes normal for this stage of development?

Early assessment of a particular pathology is difficult; the picture usually 'evolves'. Some early indicators are abnormalities in developmental reflexes. As the neurological system matures, the developing brain cortex inhibits these reflexes. The absence or presence of these reflexes can indicate an underlying neurological abnormality. Developmental reflexes include the palmar grasp, walking and stepping, startle, Moro, tonic neck, Babinski and abdominal reflexes.

Gait analysis

Gait analysis represents a dynamic complement to static clinical examination. There are several commonly used descriptors in any form of gait analysis.

The five prerequisites of normal gait (Perry, modified by Gage) are:

1. Stability in stance,
2. Foot clearance in swing,
3. Prepositioning of foot in swing,
4. Adequate step length,
5. Energy conservation.

Energy is conserved by:

1. Minimizing excursion of the centre of gravity,
2. Control of momentum (eccentric contraction),
3. Transfer of energy between limb and body segments.

Three foot rockers are described:

1. Initial contact (heel is fulcrum) – deceleration through eccentric contraction,
2. Mid-stance (ankle is fulcrum),
3. Terminal stance (metatarsal heads are fulcrum) – acceleration through concentric contraction.

Gait cycle

This describes distinct stages from the point when one foot strikes the floor to the point when that same foot next strikes the floor. It is usually described in ordinary walking but can be described in a modified fashion for running. There are two phases:

| Stance phase: | The foot is in contact with the floor (60% of the cycle). It starts with initial contact. |

Postgraduate Paediatric Orthopaedics, ed. Sattar Alshryda, Stan Jones and Paul A. Banaszkiewicz. Published by Cambridge University Press. © Cambridge University Press 2014.

Swing phase: The foot is not in contact with the floor (40% of the cycle). Starts from toe-off and ends with the next initial contact.

Confusion often arises when considering the other foot, which has the same cycle of stance and swing but offset so that its swing starts 10% into the first leg's cycle and initial contact at 50%. Two periods of double support are described when both feet are in contact with the floor, each representing 10% of the cycle. Running is defined when double support gives way to double float, when both feet are off the floor at the same time.

The gait cycle is divided by seven events into seven periods. Four of these occur in the stance phase and three in the swing phase (Figure 10.1 and Table 10.1).

Table 10.1 Gait cycle events, periods and phases

Phases	Events	Periods
Stance phase	Initial contact	Loading response
	Opposite toe-off	Mid-stance
	Heel rise	Terminal stance
	Opposite initial contact	Preswing
Swing phase	Toe-off	Initial swing
	Feet adjacent	Mid-swing
	Tibia vertical	Terminal swing

Gait by observation

It is possible to utilize the descriptors of the gait cycle to describe the gait of any individual qualitatively by simple observation. It is good practice to assess posture and balance while the patients is standing at rest and then gait while as the patient walks up and down a corridor (most clinic rooms are not large enough to establish a normal gait pattern). Assess gait both shod (with orthoses fitted where appropriate) and unshod.

3D instrumented gait analysis

This involves the addition of technology to support gait by observation. There are several proprietary systems. A compliant patient is essential; usually this means a child 5 years or older and over 1 m tall.

Essentially, the 'laboratory' is a predefined space through which the patient moves. Landmarks on the patient (such as the anterior superior iliac spine) are identified to the cameras around the room by means of markers attached to the skin. A computer program recreates an electronic 3D image of the patient's movements, usually synchronously with orthogonal video image capture. The movement (kinematic) data are supplemented by data from force plates embedded in the floor of the laboratory to generate moments, powers and ground reaction forces (kinetic data). Kinetic data can only be reliably

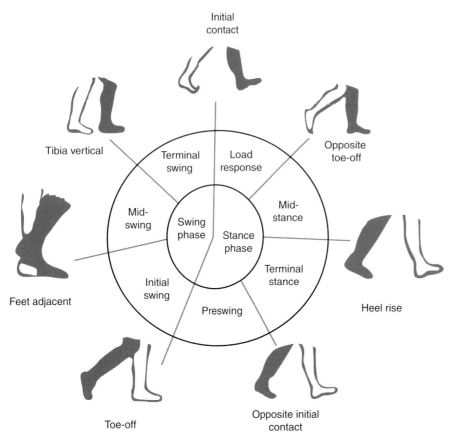

Figure 10.1 Gait cycle. Initial contact: the first point of contact of a given foot with the floor. This was traditionally known as 'heel strike', but in an equinus foot the contact might be flat-footed or first contact might even be the metatarsal heads or toes. Loading response: deceleration, energy absorption. The ankle plantarflexes to a position where the foot is flat. This is coincident with double support. Mid-stance: a period of single limb support, as the centre of mass decelerates and approaches centre of the base of support (with terminal stance this is equal in time to the opposite leg in swing). Terminal stance: period of single limb support as the centre of mass accelerates forward, regaining absorbed energy. Preswing: second period of double support. Toe-off: last point of contact (usually great toe) before swing commences. Initial swing: acceleration of the swinging leg (like a pendulum). Mid-swing: transition. Terminal swing: deceleration of the swinging leg as it is positioned for stance.

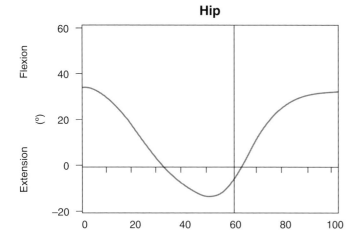

Hip

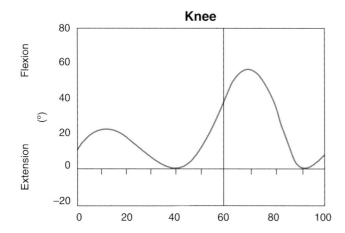

Knee

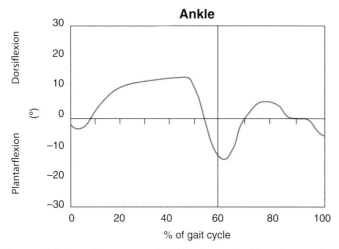

Ankle

% of gait cycle

Figure 10.2 Normal kinematic graphs of hip, knee and ankle in the sagittal plane. Each rectangle represents one gait cycle (100%), divided into stance phase (60%) and swing phase (40%). Hip joint motion: the hip extends and flexes once in each gait cycle. At initial contact, the hip is flexed to 35°; it starts extending to about −15° just before the swing phase starts, then flexes back to 35° as it approaches the next initial contact. Knee motion: this involves two flexion and two extension peaks during each gait cycle. The knee is extended at initial contact, flexes during loading response, reaching a peak at the mid-stance phase, extends fully again at the end of the mid-stance, and then starts flexing again, reaching a peak during the initial swing phase. It extends

captured in those who are able to walk unaided. Once crutches or frames are used, the load distributed through the force plate becomes meaningless.

The technique can be further supplemented with electromyograms, to evaluate whether given muscles are firing in a predicted fashion (the rectus femoris, for example, frequently exhibits inappropriate activity or 'cospasticity' in cerebral palsy and is thought to be responsible for a 'stiff-kneed gait' in such individuals).

The data generated from 3D instrumented gait analysis are superficially bewildering but generally follow a conformed layout, often displayed in specially designed viewing software (e.g. Polygon®). Data include:

1. Patient demographics.
2. Temporal data:
   a. Velocity,
   b. Step length (distance between two feet),
   c. Stride length (the distance between two initial contacts of the same foot, which equals the sum of both step lengths).

3. Video footage – an orthogonal video of the walking pattern that can be slowed down. This is a very useful way to see more than the eye can comprehend at normal walking speeds.
4. Kinematics – individual graphs that represent the linear or angular deviation of different limb segments (Figure 10.2). The x axis is time, with a vertical line identifying the point of toe-off (transition from stance to swing). The y axis is the deviation (linear or angular) of a given segment when compared with the more proximal segment. Traditionally, the pelvis, hip, knee, foot and ankle are used. On each graph, there are two lines (one for each limb) and a normal range. Sometimes there are additional lines to represent the use of orthoses or comparator data from previous gait lab sessions. Figure 10.3 shows some abnormal kinematic graphs.
5. Kinetic graphs are usually displayed on a second screen. The x axis still represents time, but the y axis demonstrates power generated and absorbed, e.g. at the ankle.

There remains significant scepticism in the orthopaedic community over the value of instrumented gait analysis. Much like a radiograph or CT scan, it is not self-interpretive and is dependent on observers to analyze it. Interpretation is hampered by:

again prior to the next initial contact. Ankle joint movement: this is a bit more complex than the other joints. It is neutral at initial contact, followed by plantarflexion to bring the foot flat on the ground (first rocker). During mid-stance, the tibia moves forward over the foot and the ankle joint becomes dorsiflexed (second rocker). Before opposite initial contact, the ankle joint plantarflexes to propel the body forward using the forefoot as a fulcrum (third rocker). During the swing phase, the ankle dorsiflexes again to clear the ground, after which it plantarflexes to neutral position preparing the foot for the next initial contact.

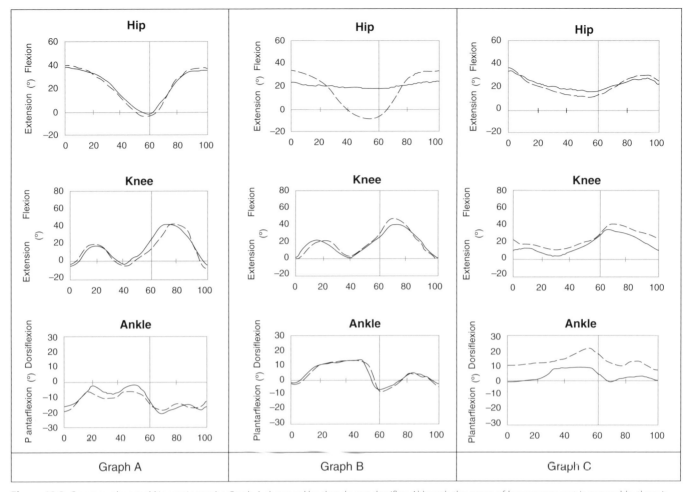

Figure 10.3 Common abnormal kinematic graphs. Graph A shows ankles that do not dorsiflex. Although the range of knee movement is reasonable, there is hyperextension of the knee at initial contact and at the end of mid-stance. The hip movement is normal. These features are of a toe walker. Graph B shows a left hip movement that remains constant around 25°, giving the impression that the hip is fused. Graph C shows all joints (hip, knee and ankle) flexed throughout the gait cycle and a reduced range of movement; these are features of a crouch gait. These findings have to be correlated with history, examination, video analysis, moment and power graphs, and electromyography.

Patient: The variability of a given individual's gait pattern.

Equipment: The reliability of marker placement (some output data are very vulnerable to magnified error due to misplaced markers, e.g. when orthoses are worn, landmarks are covered and marker placement error increases).

Interpreter: There is an evolving understanding of 'normal' and 'deviation from normal'.

Nevertheless, this represents an attempt to gather objective data where otherwise none exists. A data gathering and analysis session provides a useful introduction to the technique. Studying a set of normal walking data alongside the gait cycle will give a deeper appreciation of the data.

Cerebral palsy
Definition
Cerebral palsy is a disorder of movement and posture that results from permanent and non-progressive damage to the immature brain in the antenatal period or the first 2 years of life. Although the brain damage is not progressive; secondary effects on the growth and function of the musculoskeletal system may progress until skeletal maturity.

Epilepsy is coincident in one-third, visual problems in one-half and mental retardation in one-half of cases. The risk of coincident pathology is increased with more severe motor problems.

Diagnosis is now usually supported by MRI of the brain, although the clinical picture is not always concordant with imaging, and on occasion profound disability can accompany a 'normal scan'.

Periventricular leucomalacia is associated with spastic diplegia.

Incidence
The incidence is 2 per 1000 live births. It is increased in resource-poor perinatal care environments but also increased in a resource-rich setting, where enhanced care leads to increased survival.

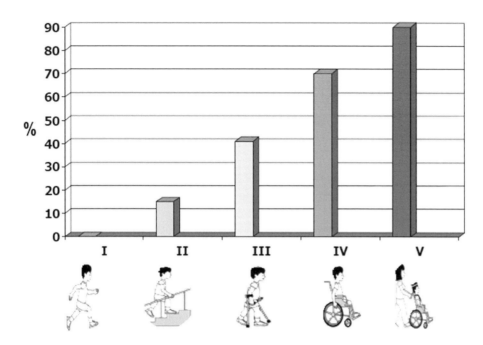

Figure 10.4 Hip migration associated with GMFC levels. The higher the GMFC levels, the greater the likelihood of hip dislocation. 90% of patients with GMFCS level V have hips with migration >30%.

Classification

Several systems are described, each considering a different aspect of the condition.

Physiological

- Spastic: Increased muscle tone due to motor cortex and pyramidal tract damage – by far the most common.
- Dyskinetic: Abnormal movements caused by damage to the extrapyramidal system and basal ganglia. A few types have been described:
    - Athetoid: Slow writhing movements of the fingers and hands, and the rest of the upper limb. The mouth and lower limbs may also be involved.
    - Ballismus and hemiballismus: Infrequent jerky, purposeless movement involving a single limb.
    - Chorea: Random movements of the limbs that increase during rest and may improve with movement.
    - Dystonia: Involuntary sustained muscle contraction that results in abnormal posture. The muscle tone fluctuates and often increases with effort and emotion.
- Ataxic: Problems with balance and coordination caused by damage to the cerebellum.
- Mixed.

Anatomical

Monoplegia:	Single limb,
Hemiplegia:	One side of body,
Diplegia:	Both lower limbs involved, mild upper-limb involvement,
Quadriplegia:	Total body involvement.

Functional

The 'Gross Motor Function Classification System' (GMFCS) describes the child's abilities based on self-initiated movement, with emphasis on mobility:

  I. Walks without limitation,
 II. Walks with limitations,
III. Walks with a hand-held mobility device (e.g. crutch),
 IV. Self-mobility limited, may use powered mobility,
  V. Transported in a manual wheelchair.

This system is widely used and has prognostic significance (it is linked to the risk of hip dislocation, Figure 10.4). It has been extended and revised to enable meaningful classification at differing stages of child development (http://motorgrowth. canchild.ca/en/GMFCS/resources/GMFCS-ER.pdf).

Hoffer described four grades with respect to potential for ambulation:

1. Community ambulator,
2. Household ambulator,
3. Therapeutic ambulator,
4. Non-ambulator.

The sensitivity of functional evaluation can be increased by the 'Functional Mobility Scale', which describes ambulatory ability at three distances; 5 m (e.g. around the house), 50 m (e.g. at school) and 500 m (e.g. in the community).

Aetiology

This is unknown in one-third of cases. Risk factors include:

I. Prenatal:
    1. Placental insufficiency,
    2. Toxaemia,

3. Tobacco,
4. Alcohol,
5. Drugs,
6. Infections (ToRCHeS infections: toxoplasmosis, rubella, cytomegalovirus, herpes II and syphilis),
7. Epilepsy,
8. Haemorrhage in the third trimester.

II. Perinatal:

1. Prematurity (commonest),
2. Anoxia,
3. Infection,
4. Erythroblastosis fetalis and kernicterus,
5. Birth trauma,
6. Placental abruption.

III. Postnatal:

1. Infection (encephalitis and meningitis),
2. Head trauma (accidental or non-accidental),
3. Low birth weight (often premature) is a strong factor but two-thirds are born at term,
4. Hypoxia is often overplayed; it is only evident in 10% of cases.

Specific areas of brain injury are associated with specific patterns of cerebral palsy. Kernicterus is associated with damage to the basal ganglia and presents as athetoid cerebral palsy. In contrast, subdural or intradural bleeding causes damage to one segment of the brain, resulting in a spastic hemiplegia. Hypoxia is a non-selective insult that usually gives rise to total body involvement cerebral palsy. Periventricular leucomalacia occurs in the corona radiate before motor efferents form the pyramidal tract in the internal capsule. Here, it selectively damages lower-limb motor neurons and is therefore associated with spastic diplegia. These relationships are far from absolute, but the advent of routine MRI may prove helpful in understanding and predicting the extent of the pathology.

Assessment of children with cerebral palsy

Assessment should include:

- Identification of patient-determined goals,
- Determination of GMFCS,
- Observation of posture, balance and gait,
- Upper-limb functional assessment (where appropriate),
- Attention to progressive spinal deformity,
- Determination of strength and selective control (or lack thereof) and joint contractures (hip, knee and ankle) (Table 2.3),
- Foot position, skin condition and footwear,
- Rotational profile of the lower limbs, to assess for any torsional deformity (see Chapter 2),
- Leg lengths (may disclose a true or apparent difference (consider hip dysplasia as well as unequal leg segment lengths),
- A check of orthoses and walking aids.

Gait analysis in cerebral palsy

Central nervous system (CNS) lesions manifest peripherally via secondary musculoskeletal changes:

1. Reduced selective muscle control,
2. Persistent primitive reflexes,
3. Abnormal tone,
4. Imbalanced muscle actions across joints,
5. Poor balance.

In cerebral palsy, the physiological 'cost' of walking is typically three or four times the norm.

Although controversy remains concerning the validity of instrumented gait analysis, it has been found to be helpful as an objective tool in serial assessment of the natural history and surgical impact in ambulant children with cerebral palsy.

Management of cerebral palsy
Principles

The management of cerebral palsy is an exemplar of the multi-disciplinary team model, facilitating coordinated care between surgeon, paediatrician, physiotherapist and occupational therapist. There is usually a requirement for close liaison with other services, such as wheelchair, orthotics and community paediatrics.

Orthopaedic considerations tend to focus on the spine, hips, knees and feet, with the upper limb becoming more topical in recent years.

Because of the tendency for problems to evolve in response to growth, affected children tend to be kept under regular (e.g. annual review) until they reach skeletal maturity.

Orthopaedic effort is directed to:

1. Facilitate independence,
2. Maintain activities of daily living,
3. Anticipate and mitigate future problems.

Initially, these goals are necessarily negotiated with parents and guardians, but the child's increasing autonomy will complicate the balance of priorities in any given case (for example, adolescents who struggle to walk with crutches may elect to keep up with their peers by using a wheelchair, to the frustration of their parents).

The opportunity to intervene effectively is very limited in the athetoid and ataxic cerebral palsy subtypes. Inconsistent gait and variable tone do not respond predictably to surgery. Efforts must focus on supportive measures and assistive devices.

In the more common spastic subgroup, several common features help to direct the therapeutic approach:

1. Increased limb, but decreased truncal and neck tone,
2. Lower threshold to stretch reflex with exaggerated contraction at joints,
3. Untreated, prolonged, dynamic tone matures into static contractures across joints,

4. Uncoordinated agonist or antagonist activity and reduced or abnormal mobilization causes abnormal forces on developing bones and joints (e.g. hip),
5. Persistent primitive reflexes, lack of voluntary control and voluntary weakness masked by spasticity.

Treatment principles

- Range of movement – physiotherapy-led stretching programme,
- Maintain position and accommodate weakness – appropriate splintage,
- Decrease spasticity:
  - General (baclofen),
  - Regional (selective dorsal rhizotomy),
  - Specific (botulinum toxin).
- Correct deformity – musculotendinous or bony surgery.

General interventions

Owing to the complex and varied presentations in cerebral palsy, it is not possible to give a formula for management. However, some interventions are frequently employed. In each case, it is vital that physiotherapy is coordinated to make the most of any intervention. This list cannot be exhaustive and there is no substitute for attending several combined cerebral palsy clinics to gain an appreciation of the decision-making process in the orthopaedic care of these children.

Treatment of spasticity

- Oral medications (baclofen, benzodiazepines, dantrolene and tizanidine),
- Intramuscular (botulinum toxin A, phenol and alcohol),
- Intrathecal baclofen,
- Selective dorsal rhizotomy.

Baclofen acts by binding to the gamma-aminobutyric acid receptors. The side effects include sedation, confusion, memory loss, dizziness, ataxia and weakness. Oral baclofen is usually used in children who are too small or too young for a more effective treatment. Intrathecal baclofen has fewer systemic side effects (although there is significant local risk) and the therapeutic dose is 1% of the oral dose. It is usually delivered through a programmable pump implanted under the skin. The dose is titrated based on clinical response. The pump must be refilled every 1–5 months.

Botulinum toxin A is a potent neurotoxin that presynaptically and irreversibly binds to the motor endplate, preventing acetyl choline release thereby reducing muscle activity (both involuntary spasm and voluntary contraction). Muscle function (and spasticity) gradually recovers over a 3-month period, as new motor endplates replace those that have been irreversibly blocked. Systemic side effects are rare with cerebral palsy; however, pain, generalized muscle weakness, blurred vision, ptosis, dysphagia, dysphonia, dysarthria, urinary incontinence and breathing difficulties have been described.

Botulinum toxin is used in cerebral palsy to reduce muscle spasm, typically in hip adductors, hamstrings and gastrocnemii. It is also employed in selective control of forearm muscles, and can be useful in reversibly establishing the likely impact of a more permanent surgical (tendon or muscle) procedure. Often, botulinum toxin therapy is used to postpone the date of formal surgery in the hope that fewer surgical procedures will be required overall.

Blind injections have a very poor accuracy of motor endplate localization in all but the gastrocnemii, therefore ultrasound or nerve stimulator guidance is usually employed.

Selective dorsal rhizotomy has shown promising results; however, it is irreversible and it is important to recognize that the selection of suitable patients is as important as selecting the dorsal sensory rootlets in the procedure.

The current technique involves stimulating the rootlets from each of the sensory nerve roots from L1 to S2 on both sides, to identify those that contribute most to the spasticity. These are then divided. There are several variations in the technique but the broad principle is the same in each case.

Considerable and evolving debate surrounds the correct circumstances for its use. Current criteria include children between 4 and 11 years of age with a diagnosis of spastic diplegia, usually following premature birth with adequate muscle strength in the legs and trunk and moderate to severe spasticity. The most recent NICE guidelines may be found at http://www.nice.org.uk/nicemedia/live/11220/52085/52085.doc.

Orthoses

Orthoses are frequently employed in children with cerebral palsy. They are often employed to:

- Maintain position (e.g. an ankle–foot orthosis in a planovalgus foot or dynamic equinus).
- Redirect forces (e.g. in a crouch gait a ground reaction ankle–foot orthosis or bivalved 'stonker' ankle–foot orthosis will redirect the ground reaction force from the plantigrade foot to the anterior tibia, forcing it into an extended position). This is a very successful way to maintain ambulation, as children with spastic diplegia tend to develop a crouch gait as they age.
- Improve function. For example, a wrist splint can re-establish a functional position for a hand. The muscles operating the hand may not improve but what selective strength there is may be more usefully directed and if, nothing else, the hand is more useful as a post with an extended wrist than a flexed one.
- Thoracolumbar orthoses are employed as temporizing measures in the scoliotic immature spine. While spinal braces do not improve the ultimate prognosis of a spinal curvature (in the same way that a brace against a collapsing wall would not make the wall stronger once the brace was removed), yet they can helpfully 'buy time' so that a child is larger and closer to maturity when surgery becomes necessary.

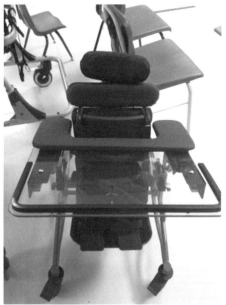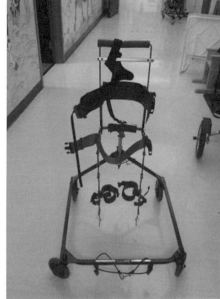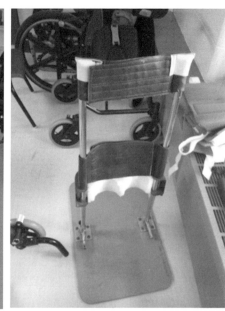

Figure 10.5 Different types of stander.

Assistive devices

A variety of assistive devices are used to improve and maintain the functional capabilities of children with cerebral palsy:

- Canes and crutches (standard, forearm crutches, tripod and quad cane),
- Walkers to help with balance: a rear walker is most often used as it promotes extension of the lower limbs and the back,
- Wheelchair (manual or motorized),
- Standers to maintain the child in an upright position to facilitate social interaction and some mechanical loading (Figure 10.5).

Surgical interventions

Traditional 'birthday surgery' (an operation every year determined by the child's annual review appointment) has been largely superseded by single event multilevel surgery, where necessary procedures are combined to restore more normal anatomy.

Soft-tissue surgery –– Muscles and tendons are lengthened or recessed (divided) to reduce joint tightness. Dividing muscles or tendons inevitably weakens them; therefore, bony procedures are preferred where possible. Soft-tissue procedures are, however, frequently considered for the hamstrings and gastrocnemii (but not the Achilles tendon, which should be preserved in the ambulant to avoid an iatrogenic crouch gait).

Tendon transfer is most commonly seen in flexor-to-extensor forearm rebalancing or in the thigh to redirect hamstring or rectus femoris function.

Bony surgery –– This involves osteotomies, temporary epiphysiodesis and arthrodesis. A key consideration in cerebral palsy is the rotational profile of the lower limb. This has often become compromised, with persistent femoral anteversion permitting internal rotation with compensatory external tibial torsion. Derotation osteotomy can be usefully employed to restore lever arms and maximize the impact of diminished strength in a limb affected by cerebral palsy. Hip surgery is considered when there is progressive subluxation, generally assessed as a migration percentage greater than 30%. Varus osteotomy of the proximal femur may be accompanied by pelvic surgery to deepen the acetabulum (e.g. Dega osteotomy). Temporary epiphysiodesis of the anterior aspect of the growth plate of the distal femur can be employed in the growing child to gradually correct fixed flexion at the knees. Extension osteotomy of the distal femur is also possible. Bony foot surgery is considered for planovalgus feet (e.g. subtalar arthrodesis, os calcis lengthening) where orthoses are no longer successful.

Salvage surgery –– This is done to reduce pain in a situation where other techniques have not been successful. In cases where hip surgery has failed to maintain reduction and the deformed hip is painful, few options are available. Local anaesthetic infiltration can give surprising longevity of pain control. The option of proximal femoral excision carries with it the risk of heterotopic ossification and intractable recurrent pain. Therefore, significant effort is employed in keeping hip joints reduced.

Surgical treatment of specific deformities
The hip

At the hip, particular attention is paid to abduction range, since limitation of abduction (<30°) is a herald of joint

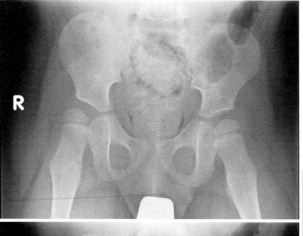

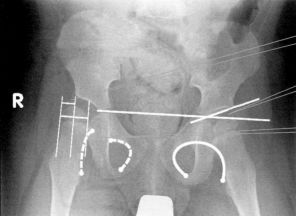

Figure 10.6 Pelvis X-ray of a child with cerebral palsy, demonstrating right hip significant subluxation (right RMI >45%, left RMI <30%), acetabular dysplasia (right AI = 28°), broken Shenton's line and extreme coxa valga. Some of the coxa valga may be apparent, as there is usually significant femoral anteversion.

Reimer's migration index = width of uncovered capital epiphysis / total capital epiphysis width × 100 (the measurements are taken perpendicularly to Hilgenreiner's line through the triradiate cartilages)

Left AI = 22°
Right AI = 28°

Broken Shenton's line

subluxation. Standardized AP pelvis radiographs are used where necessary and often in a surveillance protocol. There is strong evidence from Swedish studies in support of this approach to reduce the incidence of dislocation. Other radiographic parameters used to evaluate the hip in children with cerebral palsy are the femoral neck-shaft angle, Shenton's line, Reimer's migration index (RMI) and the acetabular index (AI) (Figure 10.6).

Reimer's migration index is the percentage of uncovered head. Normal RMI is less than 30%. Traditionally, an RMI between 30% and 50% is considered subluxation, >50% indicates a dislocation, and >90% a severe dislocation.

Surgery for neurogenic hip dysplasia could involve any of the following procedures, depending on the severity:

1. Adductor release through a small medial incision. The adductor longus, gracilis and adductor brevis can be released while protecting the anterior division of the obturator nerve. In a non-ambulatory child, the psoas tendon can be released by the same approach.

2. Flexion contracture is usually released by intramuscular lengthening of the iliopsoas tendon over the pelvic brim (Smith-Petersen approach). This preserves muscle power and prevents excessive weakness associated with dividing the tendon.

3. Femoral varus and derotation osteotomy through a lateral subvastus approach. The main purpose of the femoral osteotomy is to reduce the excessive femoral anteversion; however, it may be useful to add varus to better direct the femoral head. Excessive varus should be avoided in an ambulatory child (keep the neck–shaft angle above 110°).

4. Pelvic osteotomy is usually undertaken through an anterior hip approach. In contrast with DDH, the acetabular deficiency in a neurogenic hip is usually posterior and lateral or global, rendering Salter's osteotomy inappropriate, as it uncovers the hip further. A Dega osteotomy (or one of its modifications) is usually indicated for acetabular dysplasia. A curved osteotomy is made 1 cm above and parallel to the acetabular margin. It is then deepened toward the triradiate cartilage and the acetabulum is levered down to reduce the acetabular size and provide lateral and posterior cover (Figure 10.7).

5. Salvage procedures for non-reconstructable hip dislocation:

   • Proximal femoral resection at the subtrochanteric level,
   • Proximal valgus osteotomy,

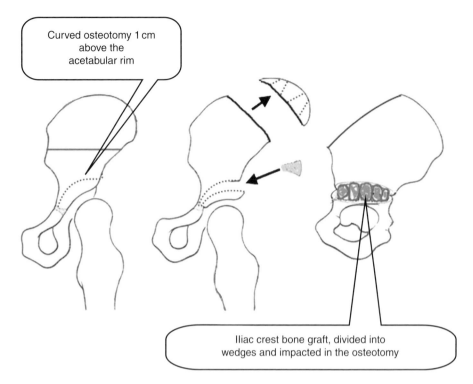

Curved osteotomy 1 cm above the acetabular rim

Figure 10.7 Dega osteotomy.

Iliac crest bone graft, divided into wedges and impacted in the osteotomy

- Hip fusion (unpopular),
- Prosthetic replacement (either total hip replacement or hemi-arthroplasty using a humeral prosthesis) in patients who can walk and have good muscle strength and no pelvic obliquity.

The knee

Two important deformities that require orthopaedic surgical intervention are:

1. Hamstring contracture, which is usually manifested by an increased popliteal angle and is common in patients with diplegia and quadriplegia. The medial hamstring (which includes the semitendinosus, semimembranosus and gracilis) is usually lengthened. In severe deformity, a recession of the biceps femoris (lateral hamstring) may also be indicated. Anterior hemiepiphysiodesis (in younger patients) or extension osteotomy of the distal femur may be added to provide more correction or to avoid weakening the hamstring. Complications of the procedure include damage to the sciatic or common peroneal nerve, genu recurvatum and increased anterior pelvic tilt.
2. Tight rectus femoris that results in a stiff knee gait. This impairs knee clearance in the swing phase. The rectus tendon is dissected from the rectus intermedius, passed under the vastus medialis and secured to the semitendinosus. This has been shown to increase knee flexion in the swing phase, aiding foot clearance.

The foot and ankle

Foot and ankle deformities associated with cerebral palsy include equinus, equinovarus, equinovalgus and hallux valgus.

Equinus –– This is usually caused by gastrocnemius tightness, with or without a contribution from the soleus. The Silfverskiöld test is used to differentiate between the two. Lengthening the gastrocnemius preserves the power of push-off (by the soleus) and is less likely to result in overcorrection. Several techniques have been described:

- The Silfverskiöld procedure involves proximal gastrocnemius tenotomy.
- Bauman describes deep gastrocsoleus recession through a medial approach in the interval between the gastrocnemius and soleus.
- Strayer lengthens the gastrocnemius selectively by dividing the tendon just proximal to where it blends with the soleus fascia. The tendon is usually resutured to the soleus fascia at a higher level.
- Superficial gastrocsoleus recession at the musculotendinous junction is described by Vulpius (chevron-type cut) and Baker (tongue-in-groove type cut).
- Achilles tendon lengthening by open z-plasty or by percutaneous techniques. White used two percutaneous cuts (distal medial and proximal lateral) while Hoke described a three-incision technique (proximal and distal medial and middle lateral).
- Overcorrection causes a calcaneus deformity and exacerbates a crouch gait, which is more problematic.

Equinovarus –– This is most often seen in hemiplegic cerebral palsy. Treatment options include:

- Tendo Achillis and tibialis posterior lengthening.
- Split tibialis posterior tendon transfer to the peroneus brevis or split tibialis anterior to the cuboid. The confusion

test is proposed to help determine which muscle to transfer; with active hip flexion, if the forefoot supinates, the tibialis anterior is probably involved and split tibialis anterior to the cuboid bone is indicated, while pure dorsiflexion suggests involvement of the tibialis posterior. However, this has been contended by gait analysis studies.

- A lateral calcaneal shift osteotomy may be required in severe and rigid deformity.

Equinovalgus –– This is more common in diplegics and quadriplegics. It is usually caused by tight Achilles tendon, spastic peronei and weak tibialis posterior.

The hindfoot valgus can occur at the subtalar and ankle joints. Radiographs are essential to establish the pathoanatomy. Surgical treatment involves lengthening the contracted muscles (Achilles tendon and peroneus brevis) and lateral column lengthening through the calcaneum. Other options include extra-articular subtalar fusion or triple fusion, depending on the severity of the deformity and the state of the surrounding joints.

Hallux valgus –– This is usually associated with equinovalgus foot and external tibial torsion. The most reliable procedure is arthrodesis of the MTPJ, as other procedures have a high recurrence rate.

The spine

This is discussed in Chapter 6.

The upper limb

Upper-limb deformities that may benefit from surgery are seen more frequently in the hemiplegic patient and include:

1. Internal rotation deformity at the shoulder,
2. Elbow flexion deformity, often with forearm fixed pronation,
3. Flexed ulnar-deviated wrist,
4. Swan neck deformities of the fingers,
5. Adduction of the thumb (thumb-in-palm deformity).

The goals of surgery are to improve function (grasp, release and pinch) and positioning for care and hygiene. These can be achieved by tendon lengthening, tendon transfer, osteotomy or arthrodesis. The effectiveness of these interventions is generally more cosmetic than functional.

Spina bifida

Neural tube defects comprise varying degrees of abnormalities, ranging from spina bifida occulta to the devastating rachischisis. The terminology used by different authors for different categories of spina bifida is overlapping and can be confusing.

Spina bifida occulta is a developmental failure of the arch to close at one or more vertebral levels. The cord and meninges are confined. It occurs in 10% of the population and is not a source of pathology.

Spina bifida cystica describes significant pathologies with various subcategories:

Meningocele:	Meninges protrude through defect in spine; children are usually neurologically intact.
Myelomeningocele:	Meninges and cord protrude through defect in spine.
Rachischisis:	Fissure in spine (Greek: *rachis*, spine; *schisis*, cleavage). A severe form with neural elements exposed (no coverings).

Anencephaly (absence of brain) and encephalocele (herniation of the brain through the skull) are technically also part of spina bifida. Lipomeningocele is a subcutaneous lipoma connected to an intraspinal lipoma through a fibrofatty stalk. Neurological deficits are common. Diastematomyelia is a split in the spinal cord with a bony or cartilaginous septum.

Embryology

The spinal cord develops in three phases:

Gastrulation (2–3 weeks *in utero*):	The embryonic disc forms three distinct layers of ectoderm, mesoderm and endoderm.
Primary neurulation (3–4 weeks *in utero*):	The notochord and overlying ectoderm form the neural plate, which then folds along its long axis to form the neural tube, which closes proximally and distally.
Secondary neurulation (5–6 weeks *in utero*):	A secondary neural tube is formed by the caudal cell mass. This cavitates, eventually forming the tip of the conus medullaris and filum terminale by a process called retrogressive differentiation.

To explain the pathoaetiology of spina bifida, two theories have been proposed: von Recklinghausen proposed a primary failure of neural tube closure while Morgagni proposed a rupture of a closed neural tube.

Aetiology

1. Failure of genes controlling neural tube closure: the risk of having a neural tube defect is 2–4% if one sibling is affected and 10–25% if more than one are affected.
2. Environmental factors:
   a. Maternal insulin-dependent diabetes mellitus,
   b. Maternal hyperthermia (attributed to saunas, etc.),
   c. Maternal intake of valproate (antiepileptic medication),
   d. Maternal folate deficiency. Grain product fortification with folic acid in the USA (begun in 1996) resulted in a 19–25% reduction in live births with spina bifida over 5 years.

Table 10.2 Spina bifida classification by level

Anatomical level[†]	Functional level[†]	Ambulation	Notes on orthoses
High thoracic	No control of any muscles of ambulation	Non-walker	Cumbersome orthoses are available but require strong motivation and support. Thoracic–hip–knee–ankle–foot orthoses and crutches or a swivel walker convert the side-to-side motion of the thorax into forward motion with a swivelling base.
Low thoracic, high lumbar	Lack or weakness of the hip muscles	Non-walker	Reciprocating gait orthoses are abandoned by 99% of patients. The rationale is that when one hip flexes actively (L1), the other is passively extended using cord and pulleys. Hip–knee–ankle–foot orthoses help position the legs under the trunk but most patients have flexion contracture, rendering them less functional.
Low lumbar	Lack or weakness of quadriceps	Walk using knee–ankle–foot orthosis or ankle–foot orthosis and crutch	The quadriceps is important for ambulation, to extend the knee in the swing phase and keep it straight in a stance phase. Patients with weak quadriceps (L3–4) benefit from a hinged knee–ankle–foot orthosis with drop locks to stabilize the knee. If the quadriceps is not significantly weak but the tibialis anterior is weak, causing foot drop and impaired foot clearance in the swing phase, a rigid ankle-foot orthosis alone will suffice.
High sacral	Lack or weakness of gastrocsoleus	Walk using ankle-foot orthosis, no crutches; 98% walkers with gluteal lurch	The ground reaction ankle-foot orthosis produces a posteriorly directed force on the tibia, helping to compensate for weak gastrocsoleus during stance. Other customized ankle–foot orthoses can be used to hold flexible deformities, such as heel varus, valgus, supination or pronation.
Low sacral	Good gastrocsoleus function	Normal walkers	

[†] The anatomical and functional levels may not correlate and there is often a grey area. It is important to assess the individual patient's capabilities.

Diagnosis

Maternal levels of α-fetoprotein, antenatal ultrasonography and amniotic levels of α-fetoprotein can diagnose this condition by 18 weeks of pregnancy.

Postnatal classification by neurosegmental level has prognostic implications; however, the level is seldom clear cut and it may take up to 3–4 years to finally declare itself (Table 10.2).

An annual assessment of muscle function should be undertaken, since deteriorating function may be caused by treatable conditions (tethered cord, syrinx, Arnold–Chiari malformation, malfunctioning shunt or worsening hydrocephaly) and an MRI scan is indicated.

Management

The standard treatment of spina bifida is still urgent closure after birth. Surgery *in utero* has a potential promise but carries significant risk for child and mother.

Orthopaedic issues

Spine

The incidence of scoliosis is related to the level of the lesion:

- <10% in sacral lesions,
- 40% in low lumbar lesions,
- >90% in high lesions.

Any developing curvature mandates an MRI scan to exclude cord tethering or syringomyelia.

Bracing or surgical correction is considered when curves progress beyond a Cobb angle of 30°.

Kyphosis is common in higher lesions. There is no bracing solution; however, surgery is fraught with significant complications.

Hip

The hip may present with contractures, subluxation or low tone dislocation.

Contractures are generally addressed by surgical release of the offending muscles.

Dislocation is more common with higher-level lesions (L2 and above). Surgery for dislocated hips may not be successful in relocating the hip and carries significant complication. Consideration is given to unilateral dislocation in lower lesions (i.e. in the ambulant); however, there is general agreement that bilateral dislocation is best untreated.

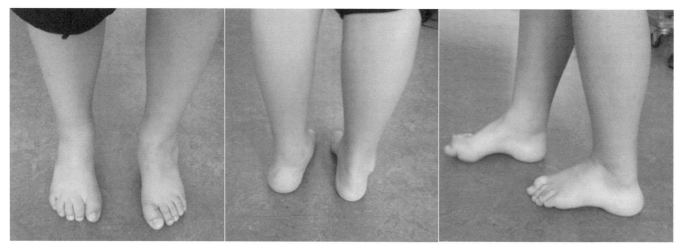

Figure 10.8 Foot deformity in spina bifida. A child with lumbar spina bifida (lipomeningocele) developed asymmetrical foot deformities; right cavovarus foot and left calcaneovalgus deformity.

Knee

Contractures are common; flexion, extension contracture (recurvatum) and valgus deformities are the commonest.

The former two can be treated by serial casting and surgical releases of the contracted muscles. Osteotomy is rarely necessary. Valgus deformity may accompany external tibial torsion. Knee–ankle–foot orthoses are used to protect the knee from valgus stress in patients with a low lumbar level. Derotation osteotomy can be considered when the torsion is significant (>20°).

Night extension splints are advised, to reduce the development of contractures.

Foot and ankle

More than three-quarters of children with myelomeningocele will develop a foot and ankle deformity. Several types of deformity have been associated with spina bifida (including club foot, calcaneus, calcaneovalgus, planovalgus and cavus deformities; see Figure 10.8). The aim is for a plantigrade braceable foot. Casting is certainly a good starting point for most deformities; however, division of tendons (e.g. Achilles tendon) can be contemplated in the non-ambulant to address resistant deformity. A more aggressive approach in ambulant children may be warranted. Insensate skin is vulnerable and extra care is needed with splintage. Careful consideration should be given to seating and wheelchairs, to reduce pressure sores.

Intercurrent issues

It is important to be mindful of the associated features of spina bifida:

Hydrocephalus

Some 90% of children with myelomeningocele require shunting. Shunting is associated with a worse cognition and motor prognosis and with complications (infection, shunt blockage).

Arnold–Chiari malformation

This describes herniation of the hindbrain through the foramen magnum:

Type I: Limited to cerebellar tonsils, causes adolescent headaches, lower-limb spasm and upper-limb pain.

Type II: Presents in infancy and is more common with herniation of the brain stem, cranial nerve dysfunction (feeding problems) and hydrocephalus (Figure 10.9).

Type III: An encephalocele.

Tethered cord

This is a feature of myelomeningocele at birth, in which a fibrous band connects the conus medullaris to the bony sacrum, preventing the normal cranial migration of the conus with growth. It frequently persists with scarring – demonstrable on MRI – but less than one-third of cases manifest clinically with reduced motor function, spasticity, scoliosis or bladder problems. Surgical release is only indicated when there is a confirmed neurological deterioration.

Syringomyelia

This is a fluid-filled cavity in the cord in up to one-half of patients. It may cause pressure problems with spasticity, weakness and scoliosis.

Urological problems

Significant renal dysfunction (due to postrenal obstruction) has been significantly reduced in this patient group by close monitoring and early intervention (e.g. self-catheterization). Urinary tract infection should be considered and antibiotic prophylaxis given when undertaking orthopaedic procedures.

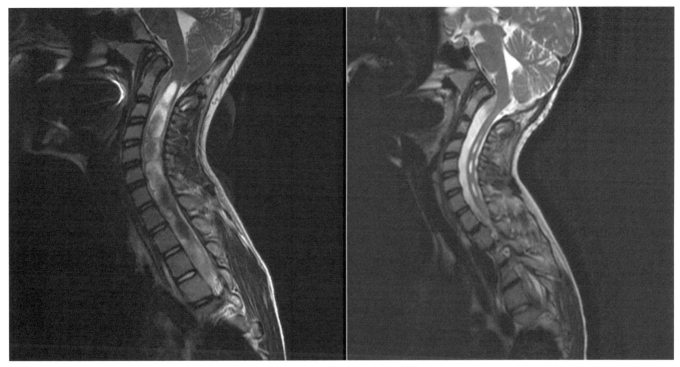

Figure 10.9 Arnold–Chiari malformation and syrinx. MRI scans of the neck. Left: cerebellar tonsil projects below the foramen magnum. There is an expansile syringohydromyelia, which extends from the inferior aspect of C1 with multiple internal septations. Right: significant improvement after surgical decompression. Notice the position of the cerebral tonsils, the cerebral spinal fluid around the cord and the resolution of the syrinx.

Latex

As many as 8 out of 10 children with spina bifida have latex allergy compared with 1% of the general population; this may be related to frequent catheterization or hospital contact.

Muscular dystrophies

These are a series of conditions due to gene mutations on X chromosomes or autosomes involved in muscle protein production.

Duchenne muscular dystrophy

The most common type (incidence 13–33 in 100 000); it is X-linked recessive, hence boys are affected and girls are carriers.

The muscle fibres are gradually replaced with fibrofatty infiltrate. This causes significant muscle weakness despite an incongruous increase in the size of the muscle (pseudohypertrophy). Steroid treatment has been shown to slow the progression of disease, including orthopaedic deformities.

Presenting history

- 'Floppy infant',
- Delayed milestones,
- Toe walking,
- Clumsy, fatigable, waddling gait from 4 years of age.

Clinical features

- Pseudohypertrophy of calf,
- Scapular winging (facioscapulohumeral dystrophy – autosomal dominant),
- Scoliosis due to paraspinal muscle weakness,
- Proximal weakness precedes distal weakness,
- Gower's sign – climbs up legs with hands to rise from sitting,
- Cardiorespiratory failure in late teens.

Diagnosis

- Clinical features,
- Significantly raised creatine phosphokinase levels,
- Genetic testing,
- The use of electromyography and muscle biopsy has diminished since the advent of genetic testing.

Orthopaedic aspects of management

- Physiotherapy to maintain strength.
- Orthotics to assist in maintaining ambulation and independence.
- Contracture release for wheelchair seating (release in ambulant patients is controversial).
- Scoliosis is progressive in 90%; hence, early consideration for surgery is necessary before respiratory compromise precludes it. Scoliosis is usually observed around the age of 2 years. Although scoliosis at the early stages gets worse

slowly, it can deteriorate quite dramatically over short period of time (30° per year; often referred to as spinal collapse). The indications for surgery are different from those for idiopathic scoliosis. Surgery should be performed once a curve reaches 30° and the patient is non-ambulatory. Pre-operative planning must include a cardiac evaluation and pulmonary function tests.

There is some controversy on including the pelvis in the scoliosis corrective surgery.

Becker

This is also X-linked recessive but less severe and slower to progress, with longer survivorship into adulthood. The onset is after 7 years. Symptomatic management is as for Duchenne.

Arthrogryposis multiplex congenita

This condition, also known as amyoplasia, includes a number of subtypes with the common feature of joint contracture due to failure to innervate the muscles across a given joint. Chromosome 5q, 9p, 11p and X linkage have all been implicated, together with possible environmental factors.

Although eight subtypes are described, Type I (upper limb) and Type III (lower limb) are the most common.

Management is focused around maintaining independence:

- Maintaining functional position of lower limbs,
- Bracing and splinting,
- Serial casting,
- Correct unilateral dislocated hips where possible,
- Osteotomies for functional positioning of upper limbs.

Bibliography

1. Perry J (1985) Normal and pathologic gait. In *Atlas of Orthotics*, 2nd edition, ed. Bunch WH. St Louis: Mosby, pp. 76–111.

2. Gage JR (1991) *Gait Analysis in Cerebral Palsy*. London: Mac Keith Press.

3. Samilson RL (1975) *Orthopaedic Aspects of Cerebral Palsy*. London: William Heinemann.

4. Graham HK Harvey A, Rodda J, Nattrass GR and Pirpiris M (2004) The functional mobility scale (FMS). *J Pediatr Orthop* **24**(5): 514–20.

5. Cramer KE and Scherl SA (2004) *Orthopaedic Surgery Essentials: Paediatrics*. Philadelphia: Lippincott Williams & Wilkins.

Musculoskeletal infections

Richard O.E. Gardner and Simon P. Kelley

Paediatric musculoskeletal infection manifests in several ways. The following will be discussed in this chapter:

- Septic arthritis and the differentiation from transient synovitis,
- Acute and chronic osteomyelitis.

Septic arthritis

Septic arthritis is an inflammation of synovial joints due to bacterial infection of the joint. It typically affects large joints, such as the hip (35%), knee (35%) and ankle (10%), though other joints may be affected. One joint is usually affected, though in severe infection multiple joints may be involved.

It is more common in the younger child (<2 years), though children of all ages may get septic arthritis. Premature and immunocompromised children are at greater risk.

Aetiology

Septic arthritis may be the result of:

1. Haematogenous spread from an infective focus elsewhere in the body by the bloodstream (commonest mechanism),
2. Local spread from adjacent bone or soft-tissue infection, i.e. osteomyelitis,
3. Direct seeding into a joint following surgery or penetrating trauma.

In early infancy, before the formation of the growth plate, the transphyseal blood vessels may act as a route for the transfer of bacteria into the joint, e.g. the hip.

In the hip, elbow and shoulder joints, septic arthritis may develop after metaphyseal osteomyelitis, as the metaphyses of these joint are intra-articular.

The organisms that cause septic arthritis are depicted in Table 11.1. *Staphylococcus aureus* is the commonest (56%) and Group A *Streptococcus* is usually observed after chicken pox.

Clinical features

- Constitutional upset (fever, malaise, anorexia),
- Limp or inability to bear weight,

Table 11.1 Causative organisms [1]

Group	Causative organism
Neonate	*Staphylococcus aureus**, Group B *Streptococcus, Escherichia coli, Haemophilus influenza* (now rare due to immunization)
Early childhood (to 3 years)	*Staphylococcus aureus**, *Kingella kingae***, *Streptococcus pneumonia, Neisseria meningitidis*
Childhood (3–12 years)	*Staphylococcus**, Group A β-haemolytic *Streptococcus*
Adolescent (12–18 years)	*Staphylococcus aureus**, Group A β-haemolytic *Streptococcus, Neisseria gonorrhoea*

Other risk factors:
- Sickle cell   *Salmonella* species, *Staphylococcus aureus, Streptococcus pneumonia*
- Foot puncture   *Pseudomonas aeruginosa, Staphylococcus aureus*

* There is an increasing incidence of MRSA across all age ranges.
** *Kingella kingae* is a fastidious Gram-negative bacillus that is increasingly noted to be a major cause of osteomyelitis and septic arthritis in children under 4 years. It can be cultured in aerobic blood culture bottles and PCR techniques have been described to aid diagnosis [2].

- Joint effusion, overlying erythema, warmth and tenderness,
- Restricted range of movement,
- If the hip joint is involved, the child may be observed to hold the lower limb with the hip in external rotation, abduction and a degree of flexion. In the infant, the only positive sign may be 'pseudoparalysis' – a lack of active movement of the affected joint.

Investigations

Clinical suspicion should be combined with blood tests and imaging to confirm the diagnosis.

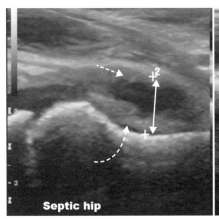
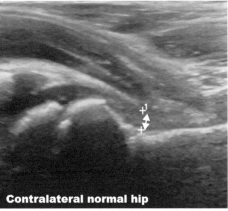

Septic hip

Contralateral normal hip

Figure 11.1 Ultrasound images of the right hip in a 3-year-old girl. A large effusion is evident (solid arrow) with layering suggestive of debris (curved dashed arrow). Capsular thickening (dashed arrow) is also evident.

Blood tests

Tests for full blood count with differential, erythrocyte sedimentation rate (ESR) and C-reactive protein (CRP) should be taken, and blood cultures obtained. The white blood cell count may be raised in only 30–60% of cases. The level of CRP is elevated early on in the disease process and normalizes within a week of effective treatment; hence, this marker is effective in monitoring response to treatment. In contrast, ESR may take 24–48 hours to elevate and 3 weeks to normalize [3].

Radiography

In septic arthritis, X-rays help exclude other diagnoses but may also show evidence of an effusion, e.g. joint space widening of the hip. Soft-tissue swelling may be seen early on but bone changes often take 2 or more weeks to become evident [4].

Ultrasonography

This is the first-line imaging modality for septic arthritis. It is useful in determining the presence of a joint effusion (Figure 11.1). Findings of synovial thickening and capsular thickening can help to differentiate septic arthritis from transient synovitis [5], though not reliably [6].

MRI

MRI should be considered if the clinical picture is not convincing or ultrasonography fails to reveal a joint effusion, as it may reveal features of osteomyelitis or other abnormalities, such as a tumour.

Aspiration

Joint aspiration should be performed when joint sepsis is suspected, and ideally prior to administration of antibiotics. Aspiration of the hip is ideally done under sterile precautions in the operating room, using an image intensifier and an arthrogram. A Gram stain may confirm the presence of organisms. A white cell count >50 000 /ml with >75% polymorphonuclear cells is suggestive of sepsis. A positive Gram stain is noted in only 30% of cases of confirmed joint sepsis (Figure 11.2).

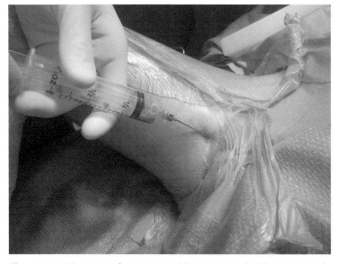

Figure 11.2 Hip aspirate from a 3-year-old boy using a subadductor approach. Purulent fluid was obtained and culture confirmed *Staphylococcus aureus*.

Differential diagnosis

- Transient synovitis,
- Osteomyelitis,
- Juvenile rheumatoid arthritis.

Transient synovitis (aseptic inflammation of the synovium) has a similar presentation to septic arthritis, but typically runs a benign course and does not require treatment. It is therefore essential to differentiate it from septic arthritis.

In a study of 282 patients, Kocher *et al.* [7] identified four independent predictors to differentiate between transient synovitis and septic arthritis:

- Fever (>38.5°C),
- Inability to bear weight,
- Erythrocyte sedimentation rate >40 mm/h,
- White blood cells >12 000 /mm^3.

A diagnosis of true septic arthritis (38 patients) was assigned when a patient had a positive finding on culture of joint fluid or a white blood cell count (WCC) in the joint fluid of at least 50 000 cells/mm^3, with positive findings on blood culture.

A diagnosis of presumed septic arthritis (44 patients) was assigned when a patient had a WCC in the joint fluid of at least 50 000 cells/mm^3, with negative findings on culture of joint aspirate and blood.

A diagnosis of transient synovitis (86 patients) was assigned when the patient had a WCC in the joint fluid of less than 50 000 cells/mm^3, with negative findings on culture, resolution of symptoms without antimicrobial therapy, and no further development of a disease process as documented in the medical record.

The group with septic arthritis (88 patients) included both the group with true and the group with presumed septic arthritis. The predicted probability of septic arthritis with one predictor was 3%, two predictors 40%, three predictors 93% and four predictors 99.6%.

Kocher validated his criteria prospectively in a later study [8].

Caird *et al.* noted that the level of C-reactive protein (>20 mg/l) was a further independent predictor for septic arthritis of the hip [9]. Table 11.2 summarizes the three studies' findings. Other authors have used these criteria and found the predictive value to be less reliable [10].

A rare but important differential diagnosis is juvenile rheumatoid arthritis, which is an autoimmune disease with an incidence of about 5/100 000. It is not unusual for patients to present with a single joint involvement (at least at first). The white cell count and inflammatory markers are usually raised. Synovial fluid is usually turbid but sterile. The WCC in the synovial fluid is usually high but often less than 50 000. Uveitis is a serious associated problem and may ultimately affect the child's vision; hence, a high degree of suspicion and early referral to a rheumatologist (or ophthalmologist) is regarded as good practice.

Treatment

The management of septic arthritis is considered an orthopaedic emergency. Joint destruction is closely associated with time to treatment. Bacteria and leucocytes release proteolytic enzymes, resulting in rapid proteolytic breakdown, an inflammatory effusion and joint destruction.

Table 11.2 Predictors for septic arthritis

Number of predictors	Predicted probability of septic arthritis (%)		
	Kocher *et al.* 1999 [7]	Kocher *et al.* 2004 [8]	Caird *et al.* 2005 [9]
0	0.2	2	16.9
1	3	9.5	36.7
2	40	35	62.4
3	93.1	72.8	82.6
4	99.6	93	93.1
5			97.5

Once the diagnosis is confirmed, prompt surgical drainage and administration of intravenous antibiotics are required to prevent avascular necrosis and permanent chondral destruction to the joint (Figure 11.3). A delay in acquiring an ultrasound should not delay surgical drainage. Open surgical lavage remains the gold standard; however, this may be done arthroscopically in joints such as the knee and ankle.

Some authors have reported good results in undertaking multiple joint aspirations. This is done under ultrasound guidance or in the operating theatre with an arthrogram.

The initial antibiotic coverage is with a broad-spectrum cephalosporin and in line with local microbiology guidelines. This is administered once joint fluid has been acquired for an urgent Gram stain. A positive Gram stain is observed in only 30% of cases of septic arthritis.

The initial antibiotic regimen is altered based on the sensitivities of the Gram stain. Drains and immobilization of the joint are not advisable. Antibiotics are administered for a period of 3–6 weeks. As with acute osteomyelitis, the decision to convert from intravenous to oral therapy is taken when clinical signs resolve, the patient has been afebrile for 48 hours and CRP/ESR levels return to close to baseline. It should be noted that repeat washouts are sometimes required, especially in *Streptococcus* infection.

Sequelae include chondral damage, avascular necrosis, growth arrest, angular deformity, leg length discrepancy and Tom Smith arthritis.

Osteomyelitis

Osteomyelitis usually occurs in the first decade of life and predominantly involves the lower extremity: 27% of cases occur in the femur, 26% in the tibia, 9% in the pelvis and 8% in the humerus [4]. It may be acute, subacute (>3 weeks) or chronic (Figure 11.4).

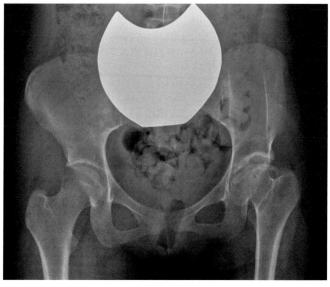

Figure 11.3 Long-term outcome following delayed management of septic arthritis of left hip as a neonate.

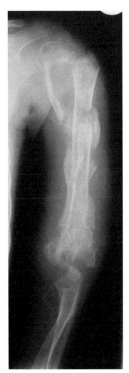
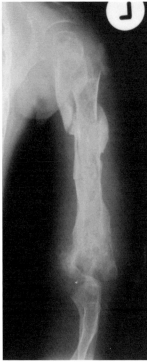
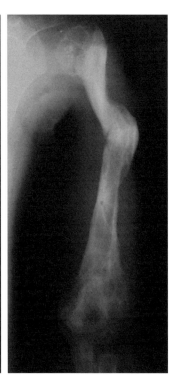

Figure 11.4 Chronic osteomyelitis of the humerus in a 4-year-old boy. The entire diaphysis was sequestrated. The involucrum can be seen to develop in the first two images. The sequestrum was removed when the involucrum was deemed to offer structural support.

Pathogenesis

Children have a predisposition to developing osteomyelitis. The reasons include:

1. Turbulent, sluggish blood flow in the vascular loops in the metaphysis,
2. Relative paucity of reticulo-endothelial cells adjacent to the physis,
3. Increased blood flow.

Acute haematogenous osteomyelitis has a predilection for the metaphysis of long bones, where the sluggish blood flow causes blood-borne organisms to be deposited. A collection may form in the metaphysis, resulting in thrombosis of the endosteal blood supply. Localized bone is resorbed through a combination of osteoblast death and osteoclast activation. The release of prostaglandin E_2 stimulates further resorption [11].

The metaphyseal cortex is thin and pus may penetrate it, resulting in a subperiosteal abscess. This in turn deprives the cortex of periosteal blood supply. If effective management is not instituted, the segment of cortex becomes necrotic and forms a sequestrum. The periosteum, however, retains osteogenic properties and new bone is laid down, the involucrum. The sequestrum and involucrum are the hallmarks of chronic osteomyelitis.

In the neonate, vascular channels from the metaphysis link into the epiphysis. Osteomyelitis in the metaphysis can result in thrombosis of these vessels, leading to severe osteonecrosis of the epiphysis. With development of the femoral ossific nucleus, the epiphyseal and metaphyseal blood supply become independent, with the physis providing a barrier to spread [12, 13].

Clinical features

A cute osteomyelitis can have a similar presentation to septic arthritis but with typically more motion in the adjacent joint.

Investigations

Radiography

This is the primary imaging investigation for osteomyelitis. Soft-tissue swelling may be seen early on but bone changes often take 2 or more weeks to become evident [4].

Ultrasonography

In osteomyelitis, ultrasound can detect subperiosteal abscesses.

Bone scan (technetium 99m)

This is a good investigation for localizing osteomyelitis; it is especially useful in neonates and in children with multifocal osteomyelitis. Results may be negative in the first 24 hours [13].

MRI

This is the gold standard for osteomyelitis but it should be reserved for the more complicated case (Figure 11.5). It can help to differentiate infection from tumours; the latter are shown as a reduced signal on a T1 sequence image and a high signal on a T2-weighted image. Careful correlation with the clinical picture is needed, as fractures, bone bruising and bone

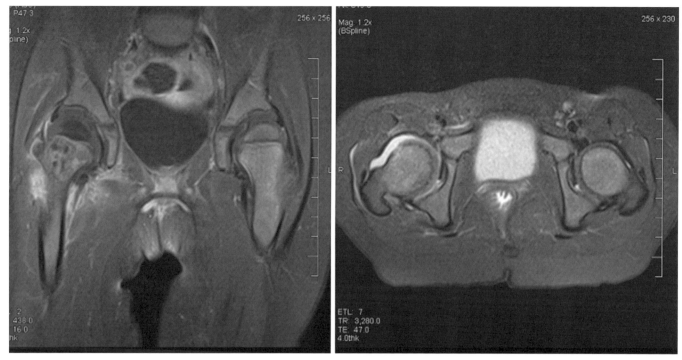

Figure 11.5 MRI of infected hip. Left: Coronal MRI demonstrating osteomyelitis in the proximal femoral metaphysis. Reduced signal in the right epiphysis suggestive of avascular necrosis. Right: Axial view demonstrating right hip effusion.

infarcts can have a similar appearance. Fat-suppression sequences obtained with gadolinium as a contrast agent highlight marrow changes, while abscesses demonstrate rim enhancement [14].

Aspiration

Aspiration may be performed in suspected osteomyelitis. Fluid may be aspirated from a subperiosteal abscess and a large-bore spinal needle can be used to perforate the thin metaphyseal cortex and aspirate a purulent intramedullary collection.

Differential diagnosis of osteomyelitis

Osteomyelitis may be mistaken for neoplasia. Leukaemia has similar radiological findings, as well as a frequent presentation of fever, raised ESR and CRP levels and leucocytes. A blood film is helpful, if leukaemia is suspected. Eosinophilic granuloma, Ewing's sarcoma and osteosarcoma should also be considered.

Treatment

Acute haematogenous osteomyelitis

Most hospitals follow a local protocol for bone and joint infections and this should be followed or considered.

In general, in the absence of an abscess, the mainstay of treatment is with antibiotics, initially administered intravenously followed by a period of oral antibiotics, usually for up to 4 weeks [15]. The conversion to oral antibiotics should depend upon the resolution of clinical signs: temperature, overlying erythema and tenderness and a level of C-reactive protein that is returning to baseline [4, 16].

Failure to show signs of improvement with antibiotics suggests either inappropriate antibiotics or the presence of an abscess. Attempts should initially be made to confirm that the microorganism is sensitive to the selected antibiotic, especially in this era of increasing MRSA (methicillin-resistant *Staphylococcus aureus*). Bone aspiration may be considered for a sample to culture.

An abscess requires drainage. Pelvic abscesses (>2 cm) should also be considered for drainage [4, 17].

Chronic osteomyelitis

As discussed, the hallmark of chronic osteomyelitis is the presence of a sequestrum and adjacent involucrum. The infection will not resolve until a sequestrectomy is performed, but in the severe case, when the sequestrum is large, this may be delayed until the involucrum provides some structural integrity (Figure 11.4). The management of extensive bone defects is complex and may require reconstructive surgery, including bone transport or the Masquelet technique [18]. Prolonged use of antibiotics remains controversial – complete sequestrectomy is the most effective means of resolving the infection [19].

Complications of osteomyelitis include pathological fractures, angular deformities and leg length discrepancy.

References

1. Herring JA (2008) *Tachdjian's Pediatric Orthopaedics*, 4th edition, volume 1. Philadelphia: Saunders Elsevier.

2. Ceroni D, Cherkaoui A, Ferey S, Kaelin A and Schrenzel J (2010) *Kingella kingae* osteoarticular infections in young children: clinical features and contribution of a new specific real-time PCR assay to the diagnosis. *J Pediatr Orthop* 30(3):301–4.

3. Stans AA (2005) Osteomyelitis and septic arthritis. In *Lovell and Winter's Pediatric Orthopaedics*, 6th edition, volume 1, ed. Morrissy RT and Weinstein SL. Philadelphia: Lippincott Williams & Wilkins, pp. 440–80.

4. Dartnell J, Ramachandran M and Katchburian M (2012) Haematogenous acute and subacute paediatric osteomyelitis: a systematic review of the literature. *J Bone Joint Surg Br* 94(5): 584–95.

5. Dorr U, Zieger M and Hauke H (1988) Ultrasonography of the painful hip. Prospective studies in 204 patients. *Pediatr Radiol* 19(1):36–40.

6. Zamzam MM (2006) The role of ultrasound in differentiating septic arthritis from transient synovitis of the hip in children. *J Pediatr Orthop B* 15(6):418–22.

7. Kocher MS, Zurakowski D and Kasser JR (1999) Differentiating between septic arthritis and transient synovitis of the hip in children: an evidence-based clinical prediction algorithm. *J Bone Joint Surg Am* 81(12): 1662–70.

8. Kocher MS, Mandiga R, Zurakowski D, Barnewolt C and Kasser JR (2004) Validation of a clinical prediction rule for the differentiation between septic arthritis and transient synovitis of the hip in children. *J Bone Joint Surg Am* 86-A(8):1629–35.

9. Caird MS, Flynn JM, Leung YL *et al.* (2006) Factors distinguishing septic arthritis from transient synovitis of the hip in children. A prospective study. *J Bone Joint Surg Am* 88(6): 1251–7.

10. Luhmann SJ, Jones A, Schootman M *et al.* (2004) Differentiation between septic arthritis and transient synovitis of the hip in children with clinical prediction algorithms. *J Bone Joint Surg Am* 86-A(5):956–62.

11. Speers DJ and Nade SM (1985) Ultrastructural studies of adherence of *Staphylococcus aureus* in experimental acute hematogenous osteomyelitis. *Infect Immun* 49(2): 443–6.

12. Trueta J (1957) The normal vascular anatomy of the human femoral head during growth. *J Bone Joint Surg Br* 39-B(2):358–94.

13. Pennington WT, Mott MP, Thometz JG, Sty JR and Metz D (1999) Photopenic bone scan osteomyelitis: a clinical perspective. *J Pediatr Orthop* 19(6):695–8.

14. Lawson AB and Copley MD (2008) Bone and joint infection. In *Tachdjian's Pediatric Orthopaedics*, 4th edition, volume 1, ed. Herring JA. Philadelphia: Saunders Elsevier, Chapter 35.

15. Jagodzinski NA, Kanwar R, Graham K and Bache CE (2009) Prospective evaluation of a shortened regimen of treatment for acute osteomyelitis and septic arthritis in children. *J Pediatr Orthop* 29(5):518–25.

16. Peltola H, Pääkkönen M, Kallio P, Kallio MJ and the Osteomyelitis-Septic Arthritis Study Group (2010) Short-versus long-term antimicrobial treatment for acute hematogenous osteomyelitis of childhood: prospective, randomized trial on 131 culture-positive cases. *Pediatr Infect Dis J* 29(12):1123–8.

17. Connolly SA, Connolly LP, Drubach LA, Zurakowski D and Jaramillo D (2007) MRI for detection of abscess in acute osteomyelitis of the pelvis in children. *Am J Roentgenol* 189(4):867–72.

18. Donegan DJ, Scolaro J, Matuszewski PE and Mehta S (2011) Staged bone grafting following placement of an antibiotic spacer block for the management of segmental long bone defects. *Orthopedics* 34(11):e730–5.

19. Jones HW, Beckles VL, Akinola B, Stevenson AJ and Harrison WJ (2011) Chronic haematogenous osteomyelitis in children: an unsolved problem. *J Bone Joint Surg Br* 93(8):1005–10.

Chapter

12

Musculoskeletal tumours

Richard O.E. Gardner, Gino R. Somers and Sevan Hopyan

Background

This chapter aims to cover the commonest benign and malignant bone tumours in paediatric orthopaedics. Table 12.1 summarizes the bone tumours and their cells of origin and Table 12.2 summarizes bone-tumour-like conditions. The tumours selected in this chapter are those that are most frequently addressed in the FRCS examination. Current evidence is discussed and identifiable radiological and histological features are illustrated. With this aim, we have also included the soft-tissue tumour rhabdomyosarcoma.

Benign tumours

- Unicameral bone cyst,
- Aneurysmal bone cyst,
- Fibrous dysplasia,
- Osteochondroma or multiple hereditary exostosis,
- Osteoid osteoma,
- Chondroblastoma.

Malignant tumours

- Ewing's sarcoma,
- Rhabdomyosarcoma,
- Osteosarcoma.

Grading system

The Enneking classification (Table 12.3) is used to stage malignant tumours of bone and soft-tissue. It is used to guide prognosis and evaluate the results of treatment. Tumours are categorized according to their histological grade, their containment within the compartment and whether metastases are present.

A low-grade tumour (e.g. chondrosarcoma) is well-differentiated with minimal atypia and few mitotic figures. A high-grade tumour (e.g. osteosarcoma, Ewing's sarcoma) is poorly differentiated with cellular atypia, mitotic figures and a higher rate of metastasis. Grading is described as G1 (low grade) or G2 (high grade). Low-grade bone tumours

Table 12.1 Bone tumours and their cells of origin

Cells of origin	Benign	Malignant
Haematopoietic		Myeloma, Lymphoma
Chondrogenic	Osteochondroma, Chondroma, Chondroblastoma, Chondromyxoid fibroma	Primary chondrosarcoma (LG), Secondary chondrosarcoma (LG), Dedifferentiated chondrosarcoma (mixed), Mesenchymal chondrosarcoma, Clear cell chondrosarcoma
Osteogenic	Osteoid osteoma, Osteoblastoma	Osteosarcoma (HG), Parosteal osteosarcoma (LG), Periosteal osteosarcoma (IG)
Unknown origin	Giant cell tumour (fibrous), Histiocytoma	Ewing's sarcoma (HG), Malignant giant cell tumour (HG), Adamantinoma (LG)
Fibrogenic	Fibroma (metaphyseal fibrous defect, non-ossifying fibroma), Desmoplastic fibroma (LG)	Fibrosarcoma (HG), Malignant fibrous histiocytoma (HG)
Notochordal		Chordoma
Vascular	Hemangioma	Hemangioendothelioma (LG), Hemangiopericytoma
Lipogenic	Lipoma	
Neurogenic	Neurilemoma	

LG, low grade; IG, intermediate grade; HG, high grade; mixed, mixture of high and low grades.

Table 12.2 Bone-tumour-like conditions

Condition	Description
Eosinophilic granuloma	Highly destructive lesion with well-defined margins; cortex may be destroyed and there is soft-tissue swelling. Treatment: self-limiting, steroids, radiotherapy, curettage and bone grafting.
Osteomyelitis	
Avulsion fractures	
Aneurysmal bone cyst	75% in <20 years, eccentric, lytic, expansile in the metaphysis. Treated with curettage and bone grafting or radiotherapy.
Fibrous dysplasia	Lytic lesion with ground glass appearance. There is often a fine sclerotic rim. The classical feature in the proximal femur is the 'shepherd's crook' appearance. Treated with observation, corrective osteotomy with open reduction and internal fixation, bisphosphonate.
Osteofibrous dysplasia	<10 years, tibia, no biopsy or radiography is necessary. Biopsy shows fibrous tissue stroma and a background of bone trabeculae with osteoblastic rimming.
Heterotopic ossification	
Unicameral bone cyst	Central lytic and symmetrical; thinning of the cortex; active when touching the physis. Commonly affects the humerus. Treated with aspirate and methylprednisolone injection, curettage and bone grafting with or without internal fixation.
Giant cell reparative granuloma	
Exuberant callus	

Table 12.3 Enneking classification of malignant tumours of bone and soft tissue

Stage	Subgroup	GTM (grade, tumour site, metastases)	Description
I	IA	G1T1M0	Low grade, intracompartmental, no metastases
	IB	G1T2M0	Low grade, extracompartmental, no metastases
II	IIA	G2T1M0	High grade, intracompartmental, no metastases
	IIB	G2T2M0	High grade, extracompartmental, no metastases
III	IIIA	G1/2T1M1	Any grade, intracompartmental, with metastases
	IIIB	G1/2T2M1	Any grade, extracompartmental, with metastases

Table 12.4 Classification of benign tumours of bone

Stage	Group	Characteristics
Stage 1	Inactive (latent)	Refers to lesions that are not causing pain and show no evidence of active growth. Stage 1 lesions are generally treated with observation only.
Stage 2	Active	Refers to lesions that are causing pain or some form of disability. A lesion that has weakened the structure of the bone such that fracture may occur would also be considered Stage 2.
Stage 3	Aggressive	Refers to lesions that are large, have extended into the soft tissues, or have caused a pathologic fracture. These lesions are prone to local recurrence despite treatment.

metastasize in 10% of cases, intermediate-grade tumours in 10–30% of cases and high-grade tumours in more than 50% of cases.

The anatomical site of the tumour is confirmed by further imaging, typically MRI. The lesion is considered intracompartmental (T1) if it is contained within the bone or, if it is a soft-tissue mass, within the fascial compartment. If these boundaries are breached, the tumour is extracompartmental (T2). If metastases are present, the annotation M1 is used; when no metastases are present, M0 is recorded.

The system for benign lesions is divided into three groups – inactive (latent), active and aggressive (Table 12.4).

Unicameral bone cyst

This may be described as a unicameral (single chamber) or simple bone cyst. It is a common benign lesion of bone; the true incidence is unknown, as many are asymptomatic. Following a fracture, multiple septations may be evident on plain radiographs. There is a male:female preponderance of 3:1. Diagnosis is typically made in the first decade.

The aetiology is unknown, but clonal chromosomal rearrangements have been identified [1, 2]. It is predominantly

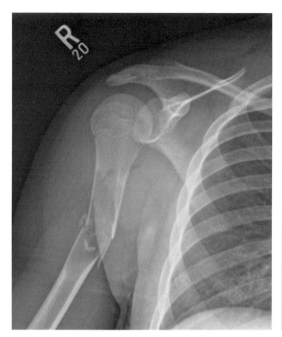
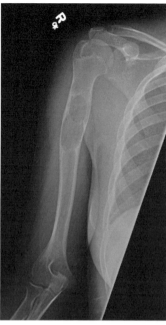

Figure 12.1 Pathological fracture through simple bone cyst in humeral diaphysis ('fallen fragment' sign is evident) and 2 months later following fracture union, demonstrating persistence of cyst.

located centrally in the metaphysis of bones, most commonly in the proximal humerus and proximal femur (94%).

The cyst contains straw-coloured serous fluid. High levels of prostaglandin have been found [3]. The lesions are frequently an incidental finding on X-ray or discovered secondary to a pathological fracture. Occasionally, patients present with a dull ache (possibly secondary to a microfracture).

Cysts can be considered to be active or latent. The cyst is active when it is located immediately adjacent to the physis, often with a thin, partially expanded cortical shell. Cysts are considered latent when the cyst grows away from the physis with intervening normal bone. The cortex becomes more substantial, there are no signs of progression and there is evidence of metaphyseal remodelling.

The natural history is for simple bone cysts to improve or resolve in late adolescence, though the incidence is unclear. This is why most treatments are minimally invasive.

Do the cysts tend to heal spontaneously post fracture?

No: while abundant callous may initially form, it tends to resorb after 6 months and there is a low likelihood of the cyst healing after a fracture. The true incidence is unknown, but it is likely to be less than 5% [4]. However, while the cyst often persists, the bone usually heals rapidly.

Imaging

Imaging reveals a central, well-defined, lucent metaphyseal lesion. Cortical thinning may be present with ballooning or expansion of the metaphysis. In the absence of a pathological fracture, no soft-tissue swelling or periosteal reaction is evident. The 'fallen fragment sign' may be present (Figure 12.1). This represents a pathological fracture (a small flake of bone that settles in the base or dependent region of the lesion), indicating the cystic rather than solid nature of the lesion [5].

When to stabilize

Consider stabilization in a symptomatic young patient with evidence of an enlarging cyst with or without a history of previous fracture or a probable impending fracture. When 85% or more of the transverse diameter of the bone is involved, the risk of fracture increases [6]. A lower threshold for stabilization should be considered in an adolescent with a large cyst in a weight-bearing bone. Pathological fracture through the femoral neck can be treated in 90/90 traction followed by a spica cast.

Management

If the bone is fractured, allow it to unite and therefore contain the cyst before treating the cyst. There is a relatively high recurrence rate with all treatment modalities, commonly involving recurrence by around one year after evidence of initial healing. Higher rates of recurrence following surgical intervention have been noted in cysts immediately adjacent to the physis, in large cysts and in cysts that are multiloculated. There are a number of treatment options (Figure 12.2).

Observation

This is indicated when symptoms are minimal and the risk of pathological fracture is low, especially in the proximal humerus.

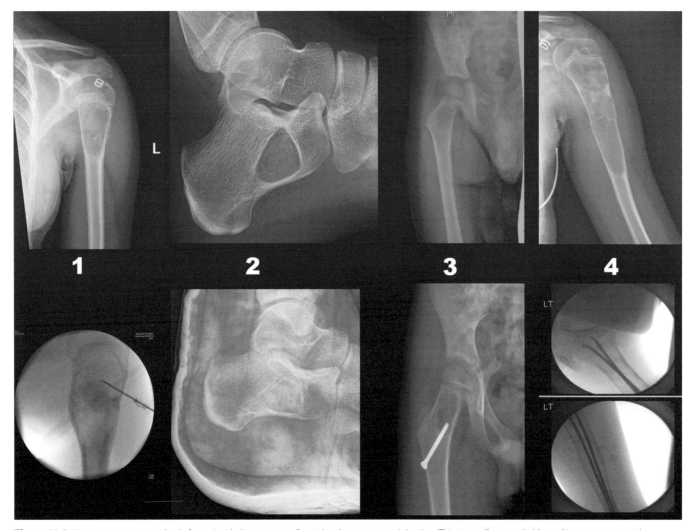

Figure 12.2 Various treatment methods for a simple bone cyst. 1: Steroid or bone marrow injection. This is usually preceded by radio-opaque material injection to ensure accuracy. 2: Curettage and bone graft. 3: Drainage using a cannulated screw. 4: Intramedullary stabilization.

Steroids

Aspiration and injection with methylprednisolone has an unpredictable outcome with reported rates of healing of up to 60% [7]. The rationale for steroid use is the high level of prostaglandin noted in cyst fluid [3]. However, successful healing may require multiple injections of methylprednisolone.

Aspiration followed by autologous bone marrow injection

A study reported healing in 76% of cases following a single injection [8].

In a level I study, Wright *et al.* [9] reported a randomized clinical trial comparing intralesional bone marrow ($n = 39$) and methylprednisolone ($n = 38$) injections. This trial involved 24 centres and 47 surgeons across North America and India with a follow-up period of 2.2 years. The results of the trial indicated that steroid injection (42% healed) was significantly better than bone marrow (23% healed) for healing bone cysts ($P = 0.01$). The authors also found that both

subsequent fracture ($P = 0.04$) and increased cyst area ($P = 0.03$) were significantly associated with non-healing of the cyst. Complications included nine subsequent fractures and two infections in the bone marrow injection group, and eleven fractures and no infections in the steroid group ($P = 0.12$).

Curettage-mechanical disruption of the cyst

This has been shown to be an effective treatment. In a retrospective study of 46 patients with bone cysts treated by isolated curettage (10), methylprednisolone injection (17) or autologous bone marrow injection (19), the healing rates were 70%, 41% and 21% respectively ($P = 0.08$) [10].

In another study [11], 40 patients were treated by one of four methods: serial percutaneous steroid and autogenous bone marrow injection (group 1; 9 patients); open curettage and grafting with a calcium sulfate bone substitute either without instrumentation (group 2; 12 patients) or with internal instrumentation (group 3; 7 patients); or minimally invasive

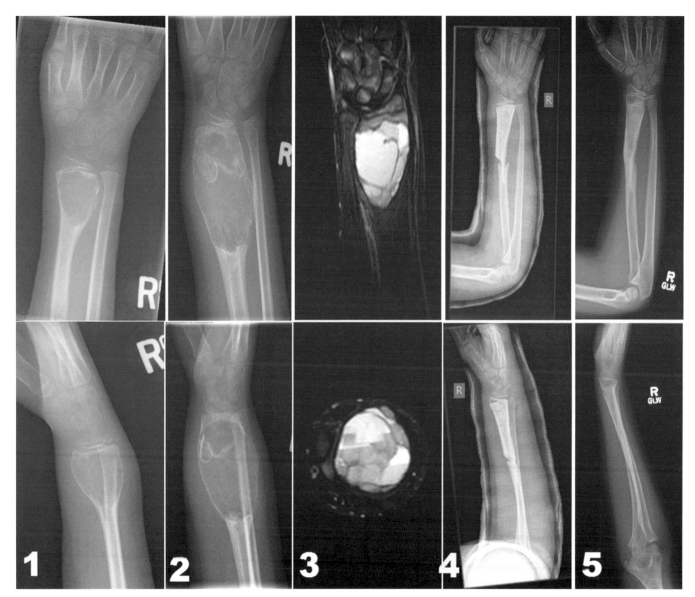

Figure 12.3 Aneurysmal bone cyst in the distal radius. 1: This 9-year-old boy presented with pain and swelling distal radius due to ABCs. 2: He underwent unsuccessful curettage with subsequent expansion of ABC after one year. 3: MRI demonstrated fluid–fluid level and no other pathologies. 4: The cyst was saucerized, the membrane was resected with curette and high-speed burr and a distal radius allograft was inserted. 5: Incorporation of allograft 6 months post-operation.

curettage, ethanol cauterization, disruption of the cystic boundary, insertion of a synthetic calcium sulfate bone graft substitute, and placement of a cannulated screw to provide drainage (group 4; 12 patients). Group 4 patients had the highest healing rate (11/12) compared with 3/9 in group 1, 8/12 in group 2 and 6/7 in group 3.

Intramedullary stabilization using elastic nails

This should be considered in a young patient who is symptomatic and has evidence of an enlarging cyst, a history of previous fracture or an impending fracture.

The threshold for stabilization should be low in an adolescent with a large cyst in a weight-bearing bone. The risk of fracture increases if 85% or more of the transverse diameter is involved. There is a relatively high recurrence rate with all treatment modalities. Higher rates of recurrence following surgery have been noted in cysts immediately adjacent to the physis, large cysts and cysts that are multiloculated.

Aneurysmal bone cyst

These are benign, expansile, vascular lesions that usually involve the metaphyses of long bones but have been identified throughout the skeleton. Aneurysmal bone cysts (ABCs) represent the most common benign aggressive tumour in the paediatric population. They predominantly occur in the first

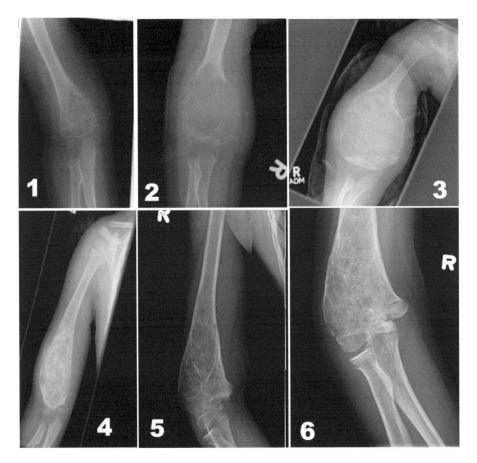

Figure 12.4 Aneurysmal bone cyst in the distal humerus. 1: Initial presentation with pain and restriction in movement at 2 years 9 months of age. 2: Continued expansion with pathological fracture despite intralesional sclerotherapy aged 3 years. 3: Curettage attempted but further expansion evident at 3 years 3 months. 4: Combination therapy with repeat curettage and embolization, demonstrating cortication of ABC and early remodelling (3 years 8 months). 5, 6: Final remodelling and healing of cyst with genu varum at 9 and 11 years of age. Later corrective osteotomy restored carrying angle.

two decades of life [12], most commonly in the humerus, femur and tibia. The spine is involved in 20% of cases and can cause neurological compromise that may even be acute due to vertebral collapse [4]. Approximately 70% present as a primary tumour while 30% are secondary [13], forming a cystic part of an osteosarcoma, giant cell tumour, osteoblastoma or chondroblastoma.

Aetiology

A chromosomal translocation t(16;17) is thought to be the cause of ABCs. This fuses the *CDH11* (osteoblast cadherin 11) gene to *USP6*, an oncogenic promoter [14]. High levels of insulin-like growth factor have been found in ABCs, suggesting a role in their pathogenesis [15]. Theories of historical interest include the presence of a localized vascular disturbance, resulting in increased intra-osseous pressure [13].

Clinical presentation

While the clinical course is heterogenous in children, aneurysmal bone cysts usually present with pain, swelling, discomfort and, occasionally, a pathological fracture. They can grow rapidly with extensive expansion and osteolysis of the host bone. Spinal lesions may be complicated by neurological compromise.

Imaging

Plain radiographs demonstrate an expansile, often eccentric, metaphyseal lesion. Depending on the active nature of the cyst, the cortex is thinned or the cyst is lined by a thin shell of subperiosteal new bone formation. Aneurysmal bone cysts may be described as:

Inactive:	The periosteal 'shell' is intact and has sclerotic margins,
Active:	Incomplete periosteal shell with defined border,
Aggressive:	Absent periosteal shell or evidence of bone formation [15] (Figures 12.3 and 12.4).

MRI demonstrates 'fluid–fluid' levels and contrast-enhancing walls of the cyst. The fluid–fluid level is not a pathognomonic feature as it is also seen in telangiectatic osteosarcoma, giant cell tumours and simple bone cysts following fractures [12].

Histology

There is a cavitary lesion with fibrous septa, filled with haemorrhagic tissue. There may be evidence of osteoid formation [12].

Treatment

Active treatment is recommended, owing to the risk of further bone destruction, fracture and infrequent rate of spontaneous healing [4].

The options include:

- Curettage and bone grafting. This is the traditional choice but there is a high rate of recurrence. Combining curettage with high-speed burring of the surrounding bone has been reported to result in healing rates of 90% [1] but higher rates of recurrence are noted in the skeletally immature.
- Cryotherapy and sclerotherapy.
- Arterial embolization may be used as an adjunct to surgery or in areas where surgical management is challenging, e.g. the pelvis and spine [16, 17].
- En-bloc resection may be considered where the bone is expendable, e.g. the rib and fibula [4].

Fibrous dysplasia

This is a benign condition that is characterized by expansile fibro-osseous tissue in one or more bones. The bone has a disordered woven appearance, as opposed to adult lamellar bone. There is not thought to be a hereditary component.

Classification

Monostotic:	Only one bone involved.
Polyostotic:	Several areas of the skeleton may be affected. Commonly, the metaphyseal and diaphyseal regions of the long bones, skull and mandible are involved.
McCune–Albright syndrome:	Polyostotic fibrous dysplasia with endocrine abnormalities, e.g. precocious puberty.

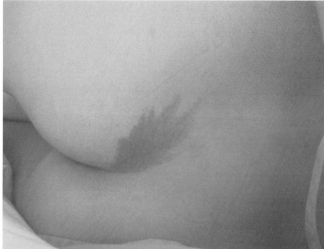
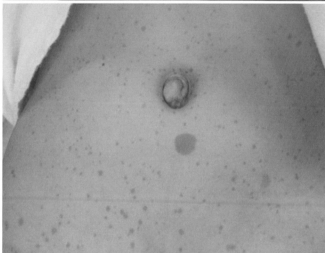

Figure 12.5 Café au lait spots. Top: Ragged border 'Coast of Maine' pattern café au lait spots in a patient with fibrous dysplasia. Bottom: Smooth border 'Coast of California' pattern seen in neurofibromatosis.

Aetiology

The exact cause of fibrous dysplasia is not known [18], though there is an association with a mutation in the α subunit of the $G_s\alpha$ binding protein. GTPase is inhibited, increasing cAMP production. It is postulated that mutation early in embryogenesis results in the mosaicism that accounts for the variable skeletal and cutaneous manifestations [19]. The increased production of cAMP has been shown to increase IL-6 production, which increases the number of osteoclast and resultant bone resorption. There is thus a failure of maturation of immature woven bone to lamellar bone [20].

The woven bone fails to adapt to mechanical stress (the trabeculae are inappropriately orientated and encased in fibrous tissue) and does not mineralize appropriately.

Clinical presentation

The incidental finding of an asymptomatic lesion is not unusual but patients usually present with pain, deformity or a pathological fracture. Bone pain is caused by fatigue fractures in the pathological bone. Deformity is particularly seen in the polyostotic form, commonly involving the proximal femur ('shepherd's crook sign'), tibia and humerus. Deformity may progress after skeletal maturity in polyostotic fibrous dysplasia but not in the monostotic form [18]. Café au lait spots with a ragged border (Coast of Maine) pattern are observed rather than the smooth border (Coast of California) seen in neurofibromatosis (Figure 12.5).

Radiographs

Radiographic findings may demonstrate an expansile lesion with cortical thinning or endosteal scalloping with a 'spreading flame' appearance. The involved bone is described as having a 'ground-glass' quality, owing to the homogenous appearance and absence of trabeculae. The classic deformity in the proximal femur is termed a 'shepherd's crook'

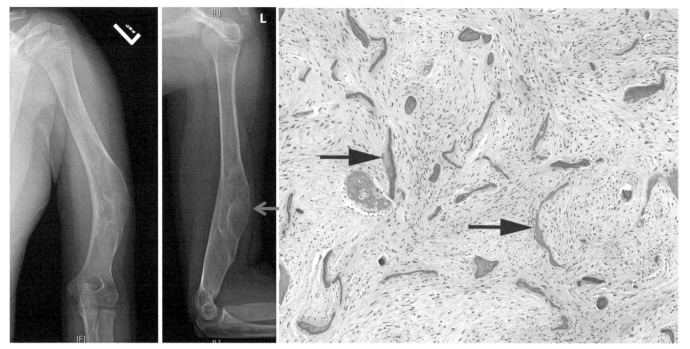

Figure 12.6 Fibrous dysplasia of the humerus in an 11-year-old girl. Left: Deformity is evident in the left humerus secondary to polyostotic fibrous dysplasia, with localized cortical expansion and endosteal scalloping. The bone has a homogenous 'ground-glass' appearance. The 'spreading flame' is marked by the arrow. Right: Photomicrograph of fibrous dysplasia, showing a variably cellular fibrous stroma, throughout which are scattered irregular trabeculae of unmineralized osteoid of variable shape and size (arrows). The appearance has been termed 'alphabet soup'. The trabeculae are not lined by osteoblasts and there is no significant atypia. Haematoxylin and eosin staining, original magnification ×100. The gross macroscopic appearance has a yellowish colour and gritty texture.

deformity; it is caused by repeated microfractures through pathological bone, resulting in a progressive varus deformity (Figure 12.6).

Treatment

Observation

This is the mainstay of treatment in asymptomatic lesions. Asymptomatic lesions may be monitored for progression. An endocrinology work-up should be performed when polyostotic fibrous dysplasia is diagnosed.

Bisphosphonates

These have been used successfully to treat bone pain and have been reported to improve cortical thickness in pathological bone.

Operative management

This is considered when progressive deformity or fracture occurs or is anticipated, typically with the more severe polyostotic involvement.

Curettage

This has a relatively high rate of failure due to recurrence. The choice of bone graft is an essential part of the decision-making process in the surgical management of fibrous dysplasia.

Autogenous cancellous graft resorbs in time; hence, cortical allograft is the preferred choice of graft, demonstrating the slowest rate of resorption [1, 4, 21].

Stabilization

If the deformity is diaphyseal, intramedullary stabilization using rods (e.g. Fassier–Duval growing rod insertion in the femur) is advised (Figure 12.7), though external fixators may be an alternative. If the deformity is localized to the proximal femur, corrective osteotomies are required with internal fixation.

Osteochondroma or exostosis

This is the commonest benign bone tumour; it is thought to be due to an aberrant growth of the physis at the perichondral ring. The lesion grows by endochondral ossification of the cartilaginous cap with the cortex and medulla continuous with the normal bone. It typically assumes a sessile or pedunculated appearance, with the latter directed away from the physis toward the diaphysis. Predominant locations are the metaphyses of the distal femur, proximal tibia and proximal humerus (Figure 12.8).

Pain may be due to mechanical trauma, muscle irritation or sarcomatous change.

Sarcomatous change to well-differentiated chondrosarcoma is rare (<1%). Signs include irregularity of the margin,

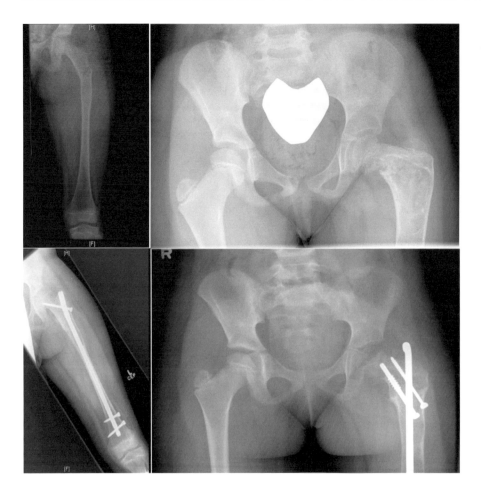

Figure 12.7 Two patients with fibrous dysplasia treated with intramedullary stabilization. The implant choice depends on the bone size, age of the patient (remaining growth and weight) and objectives of the operation (fracture treatment or corrective osteotomy).

heterogeneous mineralization, increase in size after skeletal maturity and a soft-tissue mass. A cartilage cap >20 mm in depth is also suggestive. Following wide excision, disease-free survival can be achieved [22].

Treatment

Symptomatic osteochondromas can be excised. Delaying surgery where possible until late adolescence minimizes the risk of recurrence and physeal injury.

Multiple hereditary exostoses

This is an autosomal dominant condition with a high penetrance (approximately 96%) caused by mutations in *EXT1*, *EXT2* and *EXT3* (chromosomes 8, 11 and 19 respectively). The exostosin (*EXT*) family of genes encodes glycosyltransferases, which are responsible for heparan sulfate biosynthesis. The reduction or absence of heparin sulfate results in disturbed chondrocyte signalling and abnormal endochondral ossification. The majority of mutations involve EXT1 and are associated with a greater burden of exostoses, deformity and risk of malignant transformation to chondrosarcoma [23].

Prevalence is around 1:100 000 with 10% of individuals having no family history [24]. Most patients have evidence of multiple exostoses in the first decade of life.

Clinical presentation

The most commonly involved sites are the metaphyses adjacent to the knee (>90%), proximal humerus, forearm, ribs and scapula. Short stature is common and 10% have a leg length discrepancy with genu valgum being the most common limb abnormality. Forearm asymmetry with increased radial inclination and ulnar negative variance is common (Madelung's appearance). Subluxation of the radial head occurs. The spinal canal may be involved, with occasional neurological symptoms. Pain due to mechanical symptoms from prominent exostosis is a common feature, with significant impact on the quality of life (Figure 12.9).

Malignant transformation

Variable rates are quoted in the literature (from 0.9 to 10%) but the rate is likely to be approximately 1%. Features of concern are identical to those for an isolated osteochondroma.

Treatment

During childhood it is advisable to assess the child regularly for leg length discrepancy or angular malalignment. At skeletal maturity an X-ray of the pelvis is advised to identify any axial exostosis.

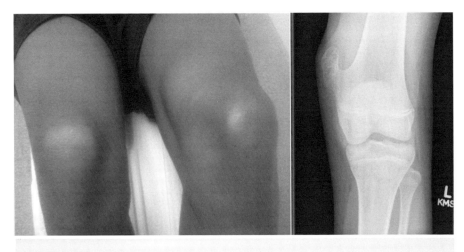

Figure 12.8 Top: Pedunculated distal femoral osteochondroma. Notice that the lesion is growing away from the physis and has cortical and medullary continuity with the femoral diaphysis. Bottom: photomicrograph of osteochondroma, showing cartilage cap with orderly chondrocyte growth (C), lined on its surface by pink periosteum (arrowhead). Also seen is evidence of enchondral ossification, with cartilage within the underlying bony trabeculae (arrow), and underlying bone marrow (BM). The cartilage cap is typically 1–3 mm thick (can be 10 mm thick in the younger patient). Haematoxylin and eosin stain, original magnification ×40.

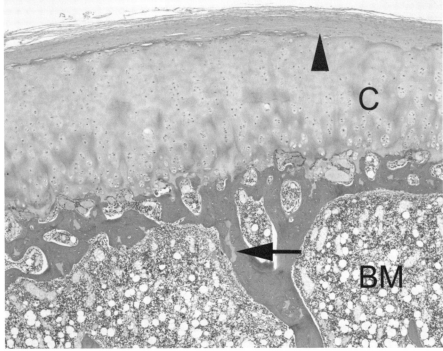

Figure 12.9 Patient with multiple hereditary exostoses affecting the metaphyses adjacent to the knee and the distal ulna. The large osteochondroma of the distal ulna has resulted in negative ulna variance and incongruity of the distal radioulnar joint and a resultant restriction in forearm rotation.

195

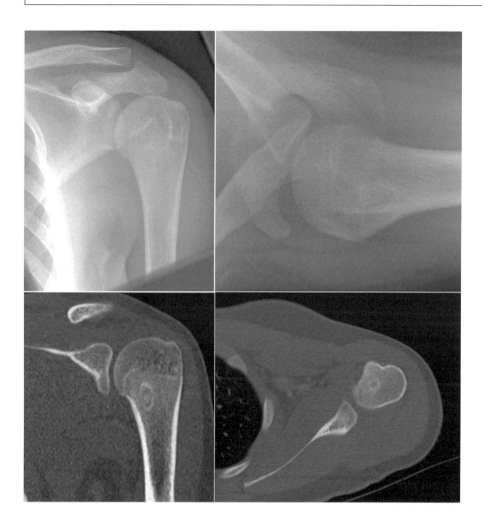

Figure 12.10 Osteoid osteoma of the proximal humerus. The lesion is subtle on the plain radiographs but the sclerotic margin and central nidus are clearly evident in the CT.

The options and indications for surgery are:

- Excision of symptomatic lesions (overlying irritation, pressure on neurological structures).
- Correction of angular limb deformity and leg length discrepancy may be required.
- Forearm involvement may be addressed by excision of the exostosis combined with ulna lengthening or radial shortening, although significant recurrence rates are reported [5].

Osteoid osteoma

Osteoid osteoma is a common benign osteoblastic lesion of uncertain aetiology. It has a 2:1 male:female predilection and is characterized by several features.

Symptoms

There is a chronic, dull, aching pain, which is typically worse at night and is responsive to NSAIDs. The pain has been attributed to the presence of high levels of prostaglandins within the nidus (hence the efficacy of NSAIDs), as well as histological evidence of unmyelinated axons.

Location

Osteoid osteomas are typically present in the diaphyses and metaphyses of the long bones and frequently, but not always, intracortical. They also occur in the posterior elements of the spine, where they are associated with a painful scoliosis (lesion on the concavity, possibly secondary to local muscle spasm). Occasionally, they are found in an intra-articular (with less reactive bone) or subperiosteal location.

Radiography

Plain radiographs often demonstrate a radiolucent nidus, surrounded by dense sclerotic bone. The nidus is typically <1.5 cm and may only be seen on axial CT images. Bone scans are also reliable in localizing the tumour, as technetium 99m is preferentially taken up by the nidus. The differential diagnosis includes: stress fracture, Brodie abscess and osteoblastoma (Figure 12.10).

Histologically, osteoblastomas are identical to osteoid osteomas, but they are usually much larger (2–10 cm). They usually occur in patients of 10 to 25 years of age. Unlike osteoid osteoma, 30–40% of osteoblastomas are found in the

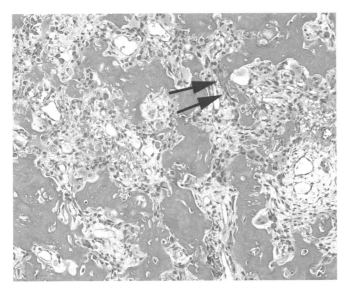

Figure 12.11 Nidus of osteoid osteoma. There are bland, pink bony trabeculae and osteoid matrix intermixed with a cellular fibrovascular stroma. Osteoblasts line up along some of the osteoid (arrows). No atypia is seen. Haematoxylin and eosin, original magnification ×200.

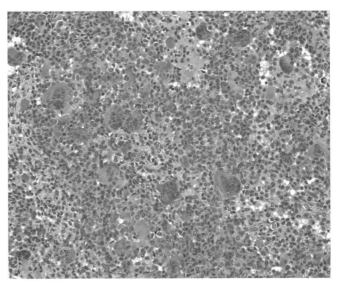

Figure 12.12 Chondroblastoma, showing a cellular tumour composed of sheets of polygonal cells with slightly irregular nuclei. Numerous osteoclast-like giant cells are present and a small amount of pale pink stroma is seen. Haematoxylin and eosin, original magnification ×200.

spine, where they most often affect the posterior elements, including the spinous transverse processes, laminae and pedicles. Treatment consists of curettage or local excision. The risk of recurrence after such treatment is approximately 10–20% (Figure 12.11).

Treatment

Osteoid osteomas are self-limiting but spontaneous improvement may take several years.

- CT-guided radiofrequency ablation is the treatment of choice. Under CT guidance, a radiofrequency probe is inserted into the lesion and the nidus heated to 80°C for 4 minutes with the skin protected. This reliably induces a 1 cm zone of necrosis. Treatment is successful in 95% of cases [1] but no histological analysis is possible.
- Non-steroidal anti-inflammatory drugs (NSAIDs) relieve symptoms in 50% of cases.
- Open surgical resection is generally not recommended but may occasionally be preferred when adjacent neurovascular structures are at risk. It has the advantage of histological confirmation of the lesion. Disadvantages include resection of normal bone potentially requiring grafting or stabilization and the risk of fracture.

Chondroblastoma

This is an uncommon benign cellular cartilage tumour that is most often located in the epiphyses of the long bones. The most common locations are the proximal humerus, distal femur and proximal tibia. The male:female ratio is 2:1. The majority of patients present before 30 years of age and the aetiology is still debated.

The symptoms are usually mild and consist of pain and localized tenderness. Pain may be present for many years before a diagnosis is made. Because the lesion is epiphyseal, the adjacent joint may be swollen and have a limited range of motion.

Histologically, chondroblastoma is characterized by polygonal cells (chondroblasts), giant cells, islands of chondroid or hyaline cartilage, 'chicken-wire' calcification and nodules of calcification in the stroma [4]. The chicken-wire calcification results when lace-like deposits of calcium are intermixed on the intercellular chondroid matrix (Figure 12.12).

Radiological features are often diagnostic (Figure 12.13). The differential diagnosis includes giant cell tumours (mature skeleton), clear cell chondrosarcoma, enchondromas, synovial lesions (e.g. pigmented villonodular synovitis, rheumatoid arthritis) and atypically located eosinophilic granuloma. Fine-needle aspiration yields satisfactory material for interpretation and confirmation of the diagnosis.

Complete curettage and excision of the lesion (using a high-speed burr) is often successful, with 80% local control. Preservation of the joint surface and physis is important for functional outcome. The defect is filled with either autogenous or allograft bone. About 2% of chondroblastomas may metastasize to the lung.

Osteosarcoma

This is the commonest malignant tumour of bone. The aetiology is unknown but genetic predispositions have been established. Patients with Li–Fraumeni syndrome (p53 tumour-suppressor gene mutation) and hereditary retinoblastoma (mutation of the *RB* gene) have a high incidence of developing osteosarcomas.

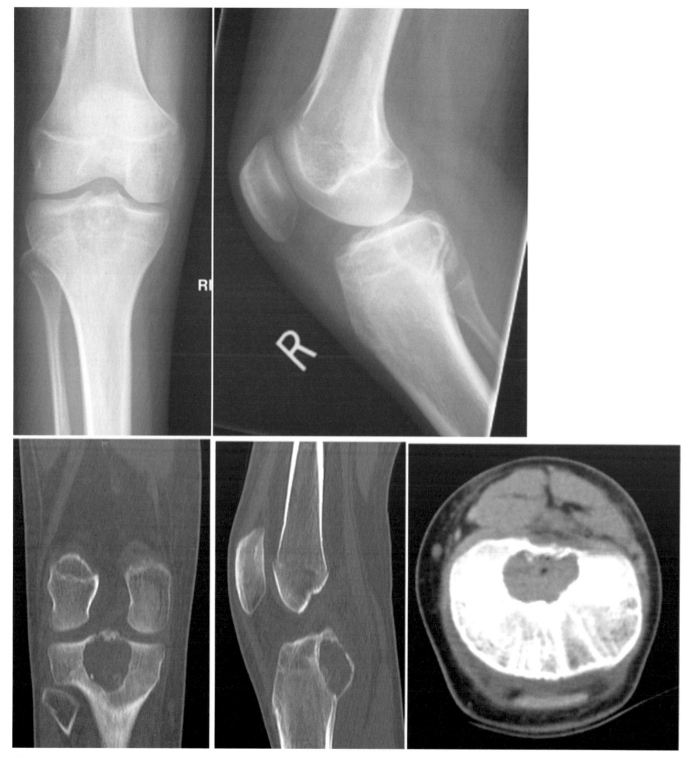

Figure 12.13 Chondroblastoma. Chondroblastomas are usually located in the epiphyses, but as in this case, they may extend into the metaphyseal region. They are usually eccentric, involving less than one-half of the entire epiphysis. The lesion is rimmed by a sclerotic margin, and small punctate calcifications are present in the tumour. Commonly, the physis adjacent to the lesion is present at the time of diagnosis.

There is a bimodal age distribution, with the majority of cases in the second decade and a second peak in the elderly, usually secondary to Paget's disease (Paget's sarcoma). The histological hallmark is the presence of malignant osteoblasts with osteoid production.

Subtypes

Intramedullary osteosarcoma

This is the classical form. It is typically high grade and arising from the metaphysis on either side of the knee joint.

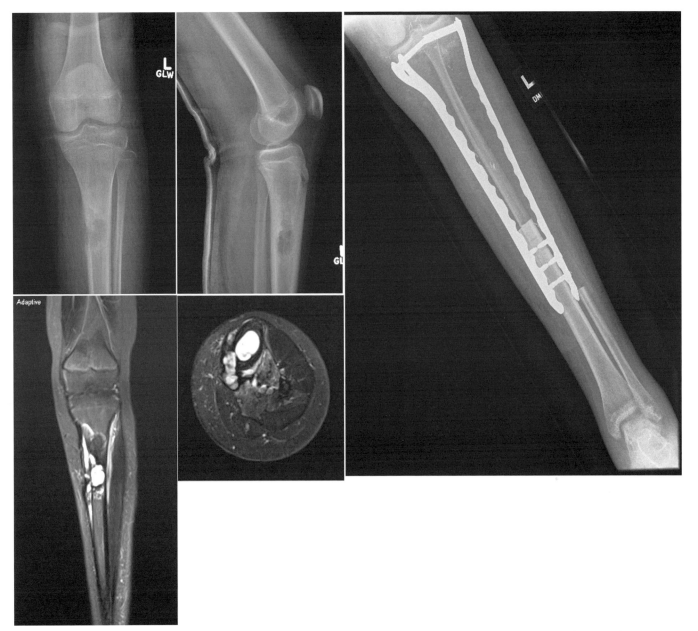

Figure 12.14 Osteosarcoma of the proximal tibia diaphysis in a 13-year-old girl. There is a permeative lesion, eccentrically located in the proximal diaphysis with cortical destruction and a wide zone of transition. The post-operation radiograph followed wide excision and reconstruction with ipsilateral vascularized fibula graft.

Parosteal osteosarcoma

This arises from the periosseous tissues, commonly the posterior aspect of the femur, sometimes with a linear separation from the bone (string sign). It is usually well-differentiated, slow growing and metastasizes late.

Periosteal osteosarcoma

This is a common variant. It presents as a poorly mineralized mass, extending from the surface of the diaphysis of the femur or tibia. Usually it is of intermediate grade (and prognosis). Radiographs demonstrate cortical erosion (periosteal surface) with 'sunray spicules', owing to the periosteal reaction.

Telangiectatic osteosarcoma

This is a high-grade, aggressive variant. The prognosis and management are similar to the classic intramedullary form. It usually presents as a rapidly growing painful mass. Radiographs reveal a destructive and expansile mass in the metaphysis of long bones.

Clinical presentation

There is localized pain; later a defined swelling may be palpable. An episode of trauma is often cited as the precipitating event by the patient.

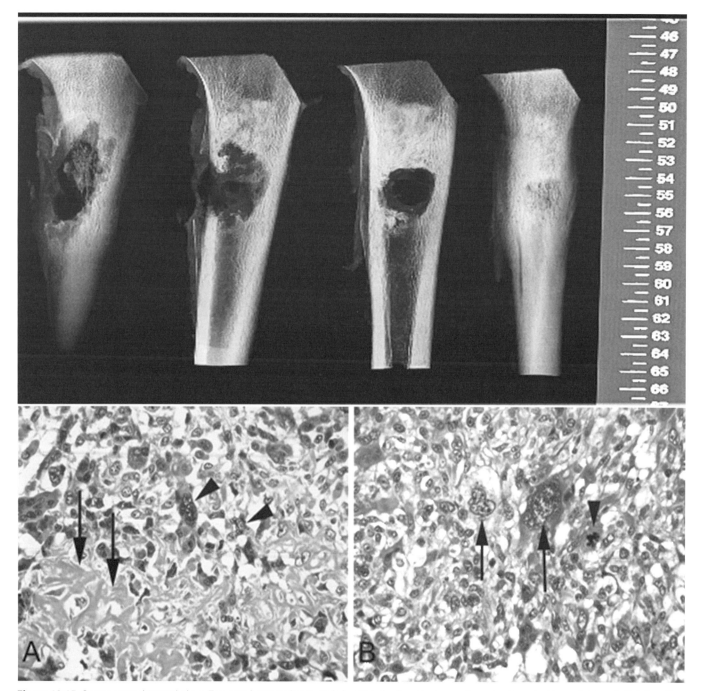

Figure 12.15 Osteosarcoma histopathology. Top: Lytic lesion and periosteal elevation clearly evident on radiograph of resected bone. Bottom: A. Pink, lace-like osteoid matrix (arrows) and significant atypia with numerous bizarre cells (arrowheads). B. Bizarre cells (arrows) and a mitotic figure (arrowhead). Haematoxylin and eosin, original magnification ×400.

Investigations

The common radiological features are demonstrated in Figure 12.14.

- On radiographs, the lesion is typically eccentrically placed in the metaphysis.
- MRI is invaluable in identifying the extent of intramedullary involvement, as well as the soft-tissue extension and the proximity to neurovascular structures.

The latter information will determine whether the tumour may be resected and limb salvage achieved.

- A spiral chest CT is performed once the diagnosis is made. Pulmonary metastases greater than 2 mm in diameter are identified in up to 20% of cases. In the absence of metastases, the 5-year disease-free survival is 60–80%. With pulmonary metastases, this falls to 0–40%, depending on the number of lesions. Bone metastases are generally not survivable.

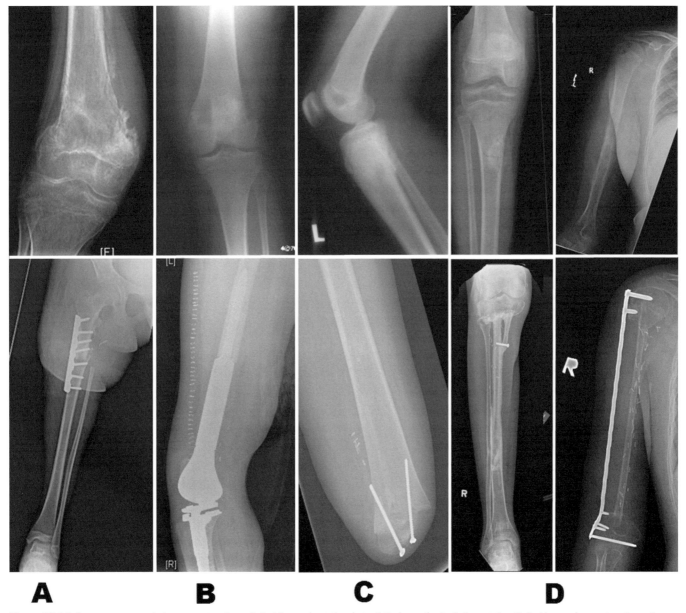

Figure 12.16 Osteosarcoma surgical treatment options. A: Excision and rotationplasty. B: Endoprosthesis. C: Amputation. D: Excision and reconstruction using vascularized fibular graft.

- A technetium 99m bone scan may be used to identify skip metastases and involvement elsewhere.
- Blood tests do not help with the diagnosis, but elevated levels of alkaline phosphatase and lactate dehydrogenase have been associated with poorer prognosis. The levels normalize with successful treatment and rise in the event of recurrence.

Biopsy

A carefully planned biopsy (core needle or open) should be undertaken by the treating surgeon. This confirms the diagnosis (Figure 12.15). The histological hallmark is the presence of malignant osteoblasts with osteoid production. The standard principles are employed:

- The surgeon performing the definitive procedure should perform the biopsy following careful evaluation of the MRI scan.
- The biopsy tract should be fully excised at the time of the definitive surgery; thus, the tract should be in line with the planned extensile approach.
- Longitudinal incisions are mandatory in limbs. Fascial planes must not be developed.
- Meticulous haemostasis is undertaken. If a drain is used, it should be in line with the incision so that the tract is also excised.

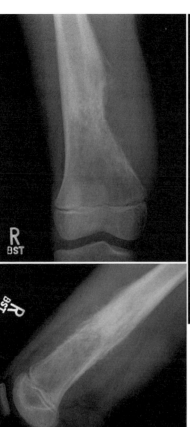

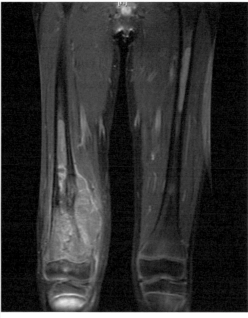

Figure 12.17 A 10-year-old boy with Ewing's sarcoma. Plain radiographs demonstrate a permeative lesion at the diaphyseal–metaphyseal junction with cortical erosion, periosteal elevation and 'sunray spicules'. A wide zone of transition is present with a substantial soft-tissue component. MRI confirms soft-tissue involvement and tumour spread to the proximal third of the medullary canal. The distal femoral epiphysis may be involved.

- Uninvolved compartments should be avoided if possible.
- A frozen section can be used to confirm that an adequate, viable sample has been taken.

Staging

Once the diagnosis is established, the tumour should be locally and systemically staged. The most useful local imaging modality is MRI. This is useful in identifying the extent of intramedullary and extracompartmental involvement, as well as skip metastases along the bone. The proximity or involvement of neurovascular structures is seen, as well as proximity to the physis or articular surface, to allow for surgical planning. Systemic staging is undertaken with chest CT and a whole-body bone scan.

Principles of management

Management involves a multidisciplinary team, including paediatric oncology, radiology and pathology.

Prior to definitive surgical treatment, neoadjuvant chemotherapy is undertaken. Chemotherapy has been shown to improve disease-free survival markedly (survival was 10–15% despite amputation prior to the use of chemotherapy in the late 1970s). The commonly used regimen combines cisplatin, Adriamycin and methotrexate. This is typically given for an 11-week period prior to surgery. Near the end of chemotherapy treatment, interval MRI is undertaken. With successful treatment, the soft-tissue component and reactive oedema diminishes in size.

Histological analysis following tumour excision with >90% tumour necrosis is associated with a better prognosis.

Surgical treatment is tailored to the individual case. The primary consideration is resection with a safe, negative margin. The treatment options can be divided into limb-sparing and amputation.

Amputation is generally reserved for cases:

- With neurovascular invasion or encasement,
- Where a safe margin cannot be achieved,
- When circumferential tumour necessitates resection of numerous important tissues (Figure 12.16).

Where possible the adjacent joint is preserved. This is based on whether the tumour extends beyond the physis or not. If not, a portion of the epiphysis with the articular surface is preserved, and intercalary reconstructive options include the use of:

- Autograft (e.g. vascularized fibula),
- Allograft,
- Endoprosthesis to restore the gap in the bone.

When the joint must be resected, reconstructive options include an endoprosthesis, osteoarticular allograft or rotation-plasty in carefully selected and informed patients. An endoprosthesis preserves limb length and may be extendable during growth, but will require revision and limits activities. Rotationplasty radically alters the appearance and necessitates an external prosthetic, but is durable with any activity and usually does not require revision.

Ewing's sarcoma

This is the second-most common primary malignant tumour of bone in children. It is part of a family of small, round, blue cell tumours including primitive neuroectodermal tumours. The cell of origin is unknown but these tumours share a translocation between chromosomes 11 and 22, t(11;22), combining the *ETS* gene (chromosome 11) to the *EWS* gene (on chromosome 22).

The tumour is rare in children under 5 years of age and peaks in the teenage years.

Location

It commonly presents in the pelvis, femur, tibia and proximal humerus (metaphyseal or diaphyseal).

Presentation

There is localized pain and swelling; the swelling may be tender. Patients may be febrile with raised inflammatory markers. Lactate dehydrogenase levels may be raised and can be monitored to assess response to treatment.

Radiology

This is more commonly diaphyseal than osteosarcoma. A substantial soft-tissue mass is often seen. There may be a permeative lesion with laminated periosteal reaction – described as an 'onion skin' appearance – but this is not always present. MRI is essential to quantify the level of medullary involvement and the presence of skip lesions. Systemic staging is undertaken with chest CT, a whole-body bone scan and bone marrow aspiration in children (Figures 12.17 and 12.18).

Treatment

Systemic chemotherapy is essential, and is given prior to (neoadjuvant) and after surgery for local control. Cycles of chemotherapy are given at 2–3 week intervals lasting for 6–9 months. Vincristine, doxorubicin and cyclophosphamide are used. The addition of ifosfamide and etoposide has been shown to improve the outcome in non-metastatic disease.

Surgery is preferred over radiotherapy for local control of resectable tumours because of a lower local recurrence rate. It is uncertain whether this alters survival. Occasionally,

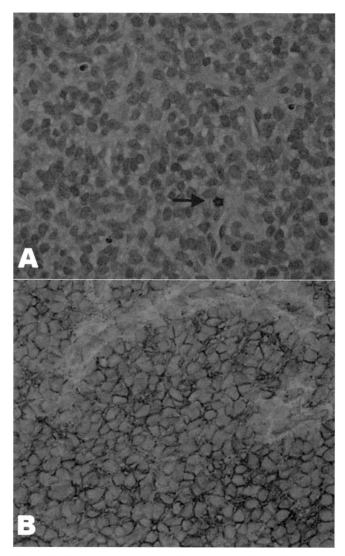

Figure 12.18 Ewing's sarcoma histopathology. A: Sheet-like proliferation of small round blue cells. The cells have vacuolar ('bubbly') cytoplasm and finely dispersed chromatin. No evidence of differentiation is seen. A mitotic figure is seen (arrow). Haematoxylin and eosin, original magnification ×600. B: Immunohistochemical stain of CD99 with membranous pattern of positivity characteristic of Ewing's sarcoma. CD99 immunostain (Dako®), haematoxylin counterstain, original magnification ×600.

radiotherapy and surgery are combined for massive pelvic tumours [25].

Radiotherapy alone may be considered in areas where reconstructive options are limited (e.g. acetabulum, bilateral sacrum) [26], but there is an associated risk of secondary malignancies [27, 28] and tumour recurrence.

Prognosis

This is influenced by the presence or absence of metastatic disease. Following successful local control, a 5-year survival of 70% can be achieved. This reduces to 30% with metastases at presentation.

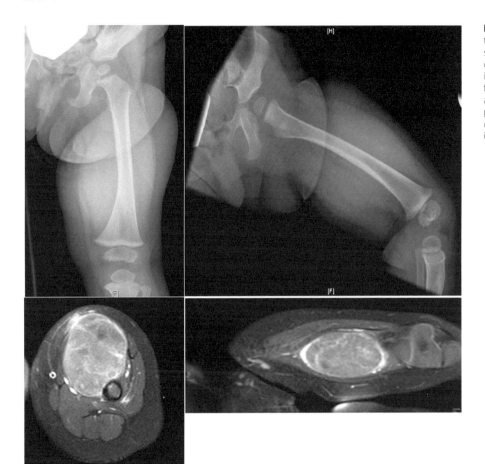

Figure 12.19 Alveolar rhabdomyosarcoma of the thigh in a 13-month-old girl. The soft-tissue swelling is notable on the plain radiograph. MRI demonstrates a large encapsulated soft-tissue mass in the anteromedial thigh, abutting the proximal femur. Wide surgical excision was combined with adjuvant chemotherapy. A biopsy of the lesion was performed using standard principles. Fluorescent *in-situ* hybridization (FISH) or RTPCR can be used to identify the translocation.

Rhabdomyosarcoma

This is the most common soft-tissue sarcoma in children. It can present anywhere in the body. There are two distinct forms that involve the extremities:

Embryonal rhabdomyosarcoma:	Usually occurs in infants and young children; has a more favourable outcome (80% 5 year survival).
Alveolar rhabdomyosarcoma:	Usually has a poorer prognosis and presents with a higher incidence of lymph node metastases; associated with a translocation of chromosomes 2 and 13, t(2;13).

Clinical presentation

Rhabdomyosarcoma usually presents with a painless firm deep soft-tissue swelling. It may grow quite rapidly.

There is an increased prevalence of rhabdomyosarcoma with the following conditions: neurofibromatosis, Li–Fraumeni syndrome (mutation in the p53 tumour-suppressor gene) and Beckwith–Wiedemann syndrome.

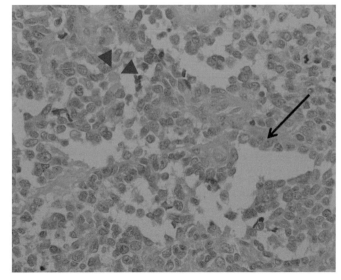

Figure 12.20 Photomicrograph of alveolar rhabdomyosarcoma. Cells are separated into vague nests by pink collagen, and are discohesive ('falling apart') within the centre of the nests. Tumour cells line up along the collagen (arrow) and some show striated muscle differentiation in the form of pink cytoplasm (arrowheads). Haematoxylin and eosin, original magnification ×400.

Radiological features

Plain radiographs are not usually helpful. MRI is the investigation of choice for diagnosis and surgical planning (Figure 12.19). Chest CT is required to identify metastases. A bone scan maybe performed to identify bone marrow involvement, and may be supplemented by a bone marrow biopsy. Some authors recommend sentinel-node biopsy, given the propensity for lymph node metastases in the alveolar variant (Figure 12.20).

Treatment

A multidisciplinary team is required for combination treatment, with chemotherapy, wide surgical excision (where possible) and possibly local radiotherapy. The chemotherapy regimen includes vincristine, cyclophosphamide and actinomycin D. Treatment is stratified according to stage, node involvement and histological type.

Prognosis

This varies according to stage of disease, presence of metastases at diagnosis and whether complete resection has been achieved. The overall survival rate is 74% without metastases, falling to 20–30% with metastases at presentation [29].

References

1. Campanacci M, Capanna R and Picci P (1986) Unicameral and aneurysmal bone cysts. *Clin Orthop Relat Res* **204**:25–36.

2. Vayego SA, De Conti OJ and Varella-Garcia M (1996) Complex cytogenetic rearrangement in a case of unicameral bone cyst. *Cancer Genet Cytogenet* **86**(1):46–9.

3. Shindell R, Connolly JF and Lippiello L (1987) Prostaglandin levels in a unicameral bone cyst treated by corticosteroid injection. *J Pediatr Orthop* **7**(2):210–12.

4. Herring JA (2008) *Tachdjian's Pediatric Orthopaedics*, 4th edition, volume 1. Philadelphia: Saunders Elsevier.

5. McGlynn FJ, Mickelson MR and El-Khoury GY (1981) The fallen fragment sign in unicameral bone cyst. *Clin Orthop Relat Res* **156**: 157–9.

6. Ahn JI and Park JS (1994) Pathological fractures secondary to unicameral bone cysts. *Int Orthop* **18**(1):20–2.

7. Scaglietti O, Marchetti PG and Bartolozzi P (1982) Final results obtained in the treatment of bone cysts with methylprednisolone acetate (depo-medrol) and a discussion of results achieved in other bone lesions. *Clin Orthop Relat Res* **165**:33–42.

8. Docquier PL and Delloye C (2003) Treatment of simple bone cysts with aspiration and a single bone marrow injection. *J Pediatr Orthop* **23**(6):766–73.

9. Wright JG, Yandow S, Donaldson S, Marley L and the Simple Bone Cyst Trial Group (2008) A randomized clinical trial comparing intralesional bone marrow and steroid injections for simple bone cysts. *J Bone Joint Surg Am* **90**(4):722–30.

10. Canavese F, Wright JG, Cole WG and Hopyan S (2010) Unicameral bone cysts: comparison of percutaneous curettage, steroid, and autologous bone marrow injections. *J Pediatr Orthop* **31**(1):50–5.

11. Hou HY, Wu K, Wang CT et al. (2010) Treatment of unicameral bone cyst: a comparative study of selected techniques. *J Bone Joint Surg Am* **92**(4):855–62.

12. Rapp TB, Ward JP and Alaia MJ (2012) Aneurysmal bone cyst. *J Am Acad Orthop Surg* **20**(4):233–41.

13. Cottalorda J, Kohler R, Sales de Gauzy J et al. (2004) Epidemiology of aneurysmal bone cyst in children: a multicenter study and literature review. *J Pediatr Orthop B* **13**(6):389–94.

14. Oliveira AM, Hsi BL, Weremowicz S et al. (2004) *USP6 (Tre2)* fusion oncogenes in aneurysmal bone cyst. *Cancer Res* **64**(6):1920–3.

15. Leithner A, Lang S, Windhager R et al. (2001) Expression of insulin-like growth factor-I (IGF-I) in aneurysmal bone cyst. *Mod Pathol* **14**(11):1100–4.

16. Zenonos G, Jamil O, Governale LS et al. (2012) Surgical treatment for primary spinal aneurysmal bone cysts: experience from Children's Hospital Boston. *J Neurosurg Pediatr* **9**(3): 305–15.

17. Gibbs CP Jr, Hefele MC, Peabody TD et al. (1999) Aneurysmal bone cyst of the extremities. Factors related to local recurrence after curettage with a high-speed burr. *J Bone Joint Surg Am* **81**(12):1671–8.

18. DiCaprio MR and Enneking WF (2005) Fibrous dysplasia. Pathophysiology, evaluation, and treatment. *J Bone Joint Surg Am* **87**(8):1848–64.

19. Weinstein LS, Shenker A, Gejman PV et al. (1991) Activating mutations of the stimulatory G protein in the McCune–Albright syndrome. *N Engl J Med* **325**(24):1688–95.

20. Yamamoto T, Ozono K, Kasayama S et al. (1996) Increased IL-6-production by cells isolated from the fibrous bone dysplasia tissues in patients with McCune-Albright syndrome. *J Clin Invest* **98**(1):30–5.

21. Enneking WF and Gearen PF (1986) Fibrous dysplasia of the femoral neck. Treatment by cortical bone-grafting. *J Bone Joint Surg Am* **68**(9):1415–22.

22. Ahmed AR, Tan TS, Unni KK et al. (2003) Secondary chondrosarcoma in osteochondroma: report of 107 patients. *Clin Orthop Relat Res* **411**:193–206.

23. Busse M, Feta A, Presto J et al. (2007) Contribution of *EXT1*, *EXT2*, and *EXTL3* to heparan sulfate chain elongation. *J Biol Chem* **282**(45):32802–10.

24. Schmale GA, Conrad EU 3rd and Raskind WH (1994) The natural history of hereditary multiple exostoses. *J Bone Joint Surg Am* **76**(7):986–92.

25. Dunst J and Schuck A (2004) Role of radiotherapy in Ewing tumors. *Pediatr Blood Cancer* **42**(5):465–70.

26. Yock TI, Krailo M, Fryer CJ et al. (2006) Local control in pelvic Ewing

sarcoma: analysis from INT-0091 – a report from the Children's Oncology Group. *J Clin Oncol* **24**(24):3838–43.

27. Bacci G, Longhi A, Barbieri E *et al.* (2005) Second malignancy in 597 patients with Ewing sarcoma of bone treated at a single institution

with adjuvant and neoadjuvant chemotherapy between 1972 and 1999. *J Pediatr Hematol Oncol* **27**(10): 517–20.

28. Henderson TO, Whitton J, Stovall M *et al.* (2007) Secondary sarcomas in childhood cancer survivors: a report

from the Childhood Cancer Survivor Study. *J Natl Cancer Inst* **99**(4):300–8.

29. Andrassy RJ, Corpron CA, Hays D *et al.* (1996) Extremity sarcomas: an analysis of prognostic factors from the Intergroup Rhabdomyosarcoma Study III. *J Pediatr Surg* **31**(1):191–6.

Chapter 13

Skeletal dysplasia

Anish P. Sanghrajka and James A. Fernandes

Introduction

A skeletal dysplasia can be defined as a congenital structural abnormality of bone, resulting in disturbances of normal growth or development of the trunk or extremities.

Making the diagnosis

This begins with a full history and examination, which is often enough to establish a differential diagnosis.

History

- Antenatal or postnatal complications including abortions and stillbirths,
- Developmental history,
- Past medical history and:
  - Problems with eyes,
  - Problems with hearing,
  - Respiratory problems.
- Family history.

Examination

- Standing height – most bone dysplasias cause short stature (defined as a height that is less than the third percentile for the chronologic age).
- Sitting height – compare with standing height on growth charts to determine whether shortening is proportionate (short trunk and limbs) or disproportionate (short limbs or trunk only).
- Determine pattern of limb shortening based upon the segment that is most affected (Table 13.1).
- Spinal examination – sagittal or coronal plane deformity.
- Lower-limb alignment.
- Examination for flexion contractures of hip, knee and elbow.

- Facies:
  - Forehead (e.g. frontal bossing of achondroplasia),
  - Trefoil (triangular) facies of osteogenesis imperfecta,
  - Dentition (abnormalities may indicate a collagenopathy).

Table 13.1 Patterns of limbs and trunk shortening

Pattern descriptor	Segment affected	Examples
Rhizomelic	Proximal (femur, humerus)	Achondroplasia (and hypochondroplasia, the rhizomelic type of chondrodysplasia punctata) Jansen's type of metaphyseal dysplasia Spondyloepiphyseal dysplasia (SED) congenita Thanatophoric dysplasia Diastrophic dysplasia Congenital short femur
Mesomelic	Middle (forearm, leg)	Langer and Nievergelt types of mesomelic dysplasia Robinow syndrome Reinhardt syndrome
Acromelic	Distal	Acrodysostosis Peripheral dysostosis
Micromelic	Entire limb	Achondrogenesis Fibrochondrogenesis Kniest dysplasia Dyssegmental dysplasia Roberts syndrome
Short trunk		Morquio syndrome Kniest syndrome Metatrophic dysplasia Spondyloepiphyseal dysplasia (SED) Spondyloepimetaphyseal dysplasia (SEMD)

Postgraduate Paediatric Orthopaedics, ed. Sattar Alshryda, Stan Jones and Paul A. Banaszkiewicz. Published by Cambridge University Press.
© Cambridge University Press 2014.

Radiographs

A skeletal survey will establish:

- The bones affected,
- The anatomic location (epiphysis, metaphysis or diaphysis).

Classification of bone dysplasia

Though Fairbank was the first to create a classification scheme, it is simpler to use Rubin's classification. Rubin grouped the dysplasias according to the anatomic distribution of the abnormalities (Table 13.2).

The dysplasias

There are a large number of skeletal dysplasias, many with a number of subtypes. Although these are relatively uncommon, it is important for the orthopaedic surgeon to have some knowledge of these conditions, as patients with them can present with many orthopaedic problems, from childhood and beyond. We have provided a summary of the salient features for some of the individual dysplasias that we consider most important for clinical practice and exams.

Achondroplasia

Achondroplasia is the most common form of short stature, with an incidence of between 1 per 10 000–100 000 live births.

Basic science

- Autosomal dominant inheritance with complete penetrance.
- 90% of cases are due to spontaneous mutations, which have been linked with paternal age greater than 36 years (suggesting that the mutation occurs on the paternal rather than the maternal chromosome).
- The risk of achondroplasia in offspring of two unaffected parents is 0.02%.
- The mutation is a glycine-arginine substitution in the gene encoding the fibroblast growth factor receptor-3 ($FGFR$-3) on chromosome 4p.

- $FGFR$-3 regulates linear growth by inhibiting physeal chondrocyte proliferation and differentiation, resulting in a failure of enchondral ossification.
- As the processes of intramembranous and periosteal ossification are unaffected, the clavicles and skull form normally, and while other long bones are shortened, they have a normal diameter.

Clinical features (Figure 13.1)

- Achondroplasia can be diagnosed using prenatal ultrasonography – short femora.
- The most noticeable clinical feature is disproportionate short stature with rhizomelia.
- The soft tissues of the limb, including the muscles, are relatively spared, giving the appearance that they are excessive for the length of the limbs. There is often also ligamentous laxity.
- The typical facies include frontal bossing, maxillary hypoplasia and a depression of the nasal bridge.
- There may be flexion contractures of the elbow, which can be the result of dislocation of the radial head.
- Relative shortening of the middle finger gives the appearance that all fingers are the same length ('starfish hand'). An abnormally increased separation of the middle and ring fingers gives the hand a 'trident' appearance.
- There is relative overgrowth of the fibula in relation to the tibia, believed to be the cause of tibia vara, genu varum and ankle varus.
- Foramen magnum hypoplasia can cause craniocervical stenosis, which may cause hypotonia, sleep apnoea or even sudden death.
- Thoracolumbar kyphosis is commonly seen in infants, but usually resolves with growth and maturity as muscle tone improves.
- While stenosis of the spinal canal occurs in all patients with achondroplasia (secondary to thickening of the pedicles, hypertrophy of the facets and enlarged

Table 13.2 Rubin classification of bone dysplasia

Location	Nature	Mechanism	Example
Epiphysis	Hypoplasia	Failure of articular cartilage	Spondyloepiphyseal dysplasia (SED)
		Failure of ossification centre	Multiple epiphyseal dysplasia (MED)
	Hyperplasia	Excess articular cartilage	Dysplasia epiphysealis hemimelica
Physis	Hypoplasia	Failure of proliferating cartilage	Achondroplasia
	Hyperplasia	Excess of hypertrophic cartilage	Enchondromatosis
Metaphysis	Hypoplasia	Failure to form primary spongiosa	Hypophosphatasia
		Failure to absorb primary spongiosa	Osteopetrosis
	Hyperplasia	Excessive spongiosa	Multiple exostoses
Diaphysis	Hypoplasia	Failure of periosteal bone formation	Osteogenesis imperfecta
	Hyperplasia	Excessive endosteal bone formation	Hyperphosphatasaemia

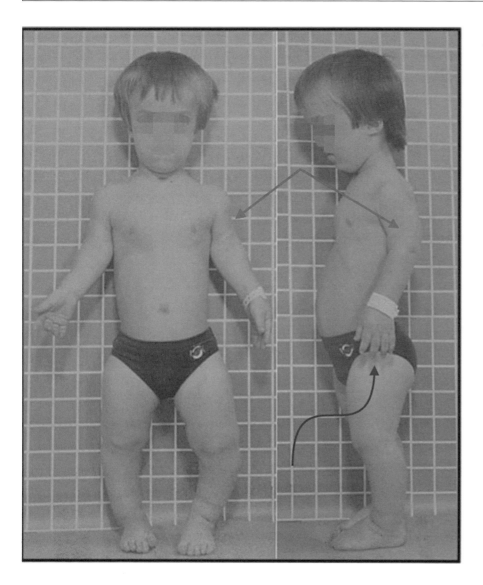

Figure 13.1 Child with classic features of achondroplasia: disproportionate short stature (limbs are short but trunk is of normal height); rhizomelic shortening (short proximal segments, straight arrows) and trident hand (curved arrow).

laminae), not all will develop symptoms due to this. Most of those who become symptomatic will do so by the third decade of life.

Radiographic features (Figure 13.2)

- The tubular bones (including those of the hand and feet) appear short, but with a relative increase in their density and diameter.
- The metaphyses are widened, with physes that are U- or V-shaped.
- The epiphyses are unaffected.
- Formed by intramembranous ossification, the pelvis appears broad and flat, with an inlet width that is greater than its depth ('champagne glass' pelvis).
- There is a relative overgrowth of the greater trochanters, causing the femoral neck appear to be in varus (but not true coxa vara).
- Premature fusion of the vertebral bodies with their arches results in increased narrowing of the spinal canal

from L1 to L5. Radiographically, this is manifest by short, broad pedicles with decreasing interpedicular distances (as opposed to the widening that is usually seen).

Management

- The role of limb lengthening in achondroplasia is controversial. Unlike the congenital deficiencies, lengthening is tolerated very well in achondroplasia because of the relative excess of soft tissues.
- A single lengthening can achieve a 35% increase in the original bone length (7–15 cm). This does not result in a height within the normal range. Even after multiple staged lengthening of both femora and tibiae, achondroplasia patients still had a more negative body image than normal control subjects, leading many to question the benefits of such complex reconstruction.
- The lower-limb angular deformities are rarely associated with degenerative changes in the knees, so surgery is

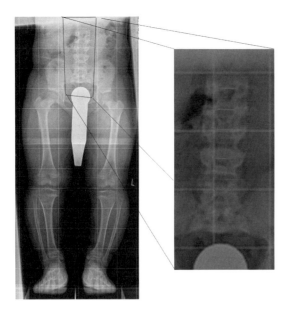
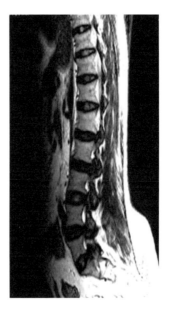

Figure 13.2 Left: Long leg alignment views of child with achondroplasia. Notice the varus knees and ankles with joint laxity. Centre: Spine radiograph shows decreasing interpedicular distance from top to bottom (normally should be increasing). Right: MRI of spine shows canal stenosis with very short pedicles.

recommended only for those with symptomatic or cosmetically unacceptable deformities.

- Spinal decompression may be required for those with symptomatic stenosis.
- Growth hormone has been shown to increase height in achondroplasia, but as it has a greater effect on the spine than the lower limbs, it accentuates the disproportionate stature.

Hypochondroplasia

- Hypochondroplasia is a rare form of short stature resembling achondroplasia, but it is generally less severe.
- It is 30 times less common than achondroplasia.
- Hypochondroplasia and achondroplasia are allelic disorders, as both are the result of defects at the same gene locus (the *FGFR-3* gene); the difference is the specific genetic mutation.
- It is inherited in an autosomal dominant fashion.
- Unlike achondroplasia, there is variability in the mutation that causes hypochondroplasia, and thus in the clinical expression (phenotype).

Pseudoachondroplasia

Unlike achondroplasia, pseudoachondroplasia (PSACH) affects the epiphyses and the metaphyses.

Those with the condition have short limbs, ligament laxity and often develop premature osteoarthritis. The prevalence is 4 per 1 million.

Basic sciences

- Although autosomal recessive forms are believed to exist, PSACH is usually transmitted as a dominant trait; both forms have mild and severe phenotypes.

- The defect affects the gene encoding cartilage oligomeric matrix protein (*COMP*), a large extracellular matrix protein expressed in cartilage, ligament and tendon.
- The mutation in the *COMP* gene results in intracellular retention of *COMP* within chondrocytes, which leads to:
  - Premature cell death, resulting in decreased physeal growth,
  - A deficiency of the extracellular COMP, which predisposes articular cartilage to degenerative changes.
- Similar mutations of the *COMP* gene are found in some forms of multiple epiphyseal dysplasia (MED).

Clinical features (Figure 13.3)

- The clinical features are not present at birth, and become apparent in the first 3 years of life with rhizomelic shortening.
- Unlike achondroplasia, the skull and faces are unaffected. This helps to differentiate the two conditions.
- Angular deformity of the lower limbs is a common feature, with both genu varum and valgum possible. There are often deformities in the distal femur, as well as in the proximal tibia.
- 'Windswept deformities' occur when genu valgum is present on one side and genu varum contralaterally (Figure 13.4).
- The ligamentous laxity associated with this condition can accentuate the deformities; this needs to be accounted for in considering corrective osteotomy.
- There is often incongruity between the femoral head, which is often flattened, and the acetabulum, which is often dysplastic.
- The epiphyseal deformities and joint incongruency often result in premature osteoarthritis.

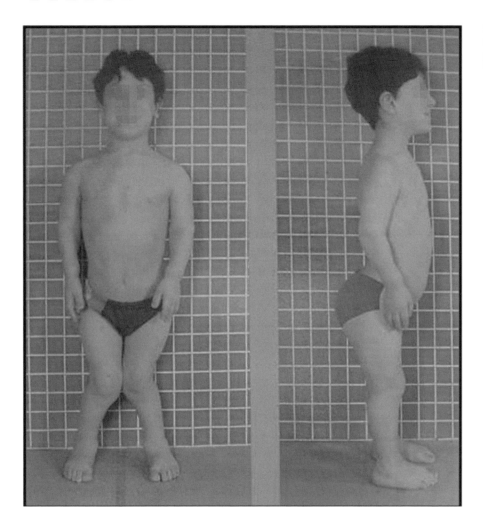

Figure 13.3 Child with pseudoachondroplasia, showing normal face and disproportionate short stature (limbs are short but trunk is of normal height).

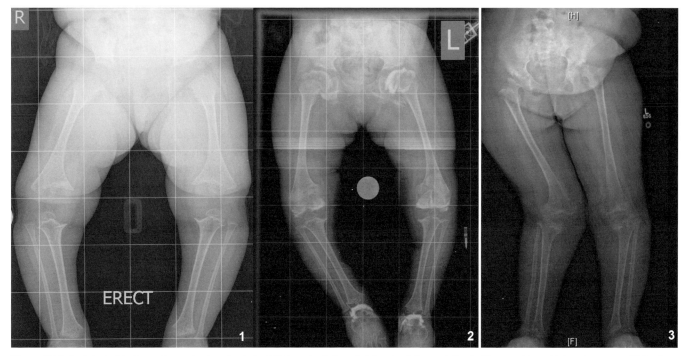

Figure 13.4 Radiological features of pseudoachondroplasia. 1, 2: Irregular flattened delayed epiphyses, delineated better with multiple arthrograms of joint. 3: Image of another child, showing a windswept deformity.

- Odontoid hypoplasia together with the ligamentous laxity can result in cervical atlantoaxial instability (AAI), which can cause symptoms ranging from increased fatigability to myelopathy.
- Radiographic investigations for C1–2 instability are therefore necessary in the pre-operative assessment of any child.

Radiographic findings (Figure 13.4)

Spine

- Platyspondyly, with anterior beaking and irregular endplates,
- Normal interpedicular distance,
- Odontoid hypoplasia,
- Atlantoaxial instability may be seen on flexion or extension views.

Extra-axial

- Delayed ossification of the epiphyses.
- Irregular and fragmented epiphyses, particularly affecting the hip or knee.
- Synchronous and symmetric involvement of the femoral epiphyses, without development of lucencies, differentiates this from Perthes disease.
- The femoral heads become flattened and enlarged, which may result in hip subluxation.
- Knees can demonstrate varus or valgus malalignment.

Management

- Atlantoaxial fusion for cervical instability when present.
- Corrective osteotomies are usually required for lower-limb malalignment.
- Valgus osteotomy of the proximal femur may improve both congruity of the joint, and abductor function.
- Salvage acetabular augmentation (e.g. shelf) may improve femoral head coverage.
- Arthroplasty is technically demanding due to the joint dysplasia and small bone sizes. Customized implants are usually required.

Spondyloepiphyseal dysplasia (SED)

This is a disproportionate short stature demonstrating progressive involvement of the spine and epiphyses of the long bones. The congenita (SEDC) type is present at birth, whereas the milder tarda (SEDT) type presents later in childhood.

Spondyloepiphyseal dysplasia congenita (SEDC)

Basic science

- Caused by a mutation in the *COL2A1* gene, which encodes the α1 chain of Type II procollagen.
- Inherited in an autosomal dominant fashion, but most cases are spontaneous mutations.

Clinical features

- Short trunk, rhizomelic and mesomelic dwarfism,
- Cervical spine instability (may cause myelopathy or respiratory problems),
- Wide-set eyes,
- Barrel chest,
- Hip flexion contractures with associated lumbar lordosis,
- Waddling gait secondary to coxa vara,
- Lower-limb malalignment, usually genu valgum,
- May have congenital talipes equinovarus (CTEV),
- The epiphyseal deformity predisposes to premature osteoarthritis,
- Non-skeletal associations include:
  - Cleft palate,
  - Myopia with retinal detachment,
  - Cataracts,
  - Deafness,
  - Herniae,
  - Nephrotic syndrome.

Radiographic findings (Figure 13.5)

- Delayed appearance of the epiphyses (femoral heads appear age 5 years),
- Flattened irregular epiphyses,
- Platyspondyly, possibly with a kyphoscoliosis,
- Odontoid hypoplasia,
- Atlantoaxial instability may be seen on flexion or extension views,
- Coxa vara, if severe, may result in femoral neck discontinuity.

Management

- Posterior cervical fusion for atlantoaxial instability.
- Scoliosis may require bracing, but the response is variable.
- Consider proximal femoral valgus osteotomy if:
  - Progressive varus deformity,
  - Neck-shaft angle less than 100°,
  - Hilgenreiner epiphyseal angle is greater than 60°,
  - Fairbank's triangle present,
  - Note that proximal femoral valgus osteotomy will increase the genu valgum deformity.
- Extension osteotomy of the proximal femur may be required for flexion deformities of the hips.
- Distal femoral varus osteotomies may be required for genu valgum.

It is unclear whether corrective osteotomies prevent the development of degenerative joint disease. In one study, almost all patients with SED reported activity-related pain, even though half had undergone previous orthopaedic surgical procedures.

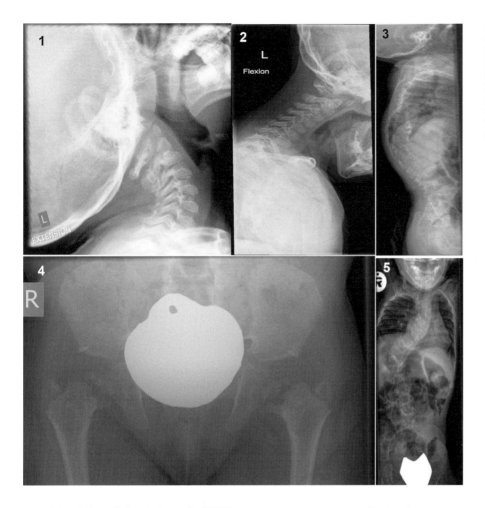

Figure 13.5 Radiological features of spondyloepiphyseal dysplasia. 1, 2: Odontoid hypoplasia and subtle anatomic axis instability. 4: Pelvis, showing delayed ossification and irregular epiphyses of the hips with overgrown trochanters. Fairbank's triangle is present (more evident on the right) as a triangular metaphyseal fragment being visible in the inferior part of femoral neck, the fragment is surrounded by an inverted Y pattern. 3, 5: Kyphoscoliosis with irregular vertebral epiphyses.

Spondyloepiphyseal dysplasia tarda (SEDT)

- This usually presents in later childhood or adolescence with mild short stature or hip pain.
- Inheritance is X-linked recessive (the *SEDL* gene) or autosomal recessive.
- The dysplasia of the femoral heads may be confused with Perthes disease. Symmetric, synchronous involvement of the hips, platyspondyly and abnormalities of the other epiphyses helps make the differentiation.
- Odontoid hypoplasia and consequent atlantoaxial instability may require posterior cervical fusion.
- Valgus proximal femoral osteotomy, with acetabular augmentation, aims to prevent premature arthritis, but the outcomes remain unknown.
- Hip arthroplasty with custom implants may be required, even in early adult life.

Multiple epiphyseal dysplasia (MED)

This was first described by Fairbank as dysplasia epiphysealis multiplex. It is characterized by a delay in the appearance of the epiphyses, which, once formed, are irregular.

Basic science

- Commonly, autosomal dominant inheritance (rarely, autosomal recessive).
- The predominant genetic mutation affects the *COMP* gene on chromosome 19 (similar to PSACH).
- The primary pathological abnormality in MED is irregular enchondral ossification of the epiphyses, with areas of degeneration. The articular cartilage becomes misshapen because of a lack of underlying osseous support.
- The femoral and humeral epiphyses are the most commonly affected, but the short tubular bones of the hands and feet may also be involved.

Clinical features

- Multiple epiphyseal dysplasia is not recognizable at birth, and is often not diagnosed until adolescence.
- Presenting features can include:
  - Delayed walking,
  - Pain,
  - Limp and waddling gait,
  - Joint stiffness or flexion contractures (especially hips, knees),
  - Short stature,

213

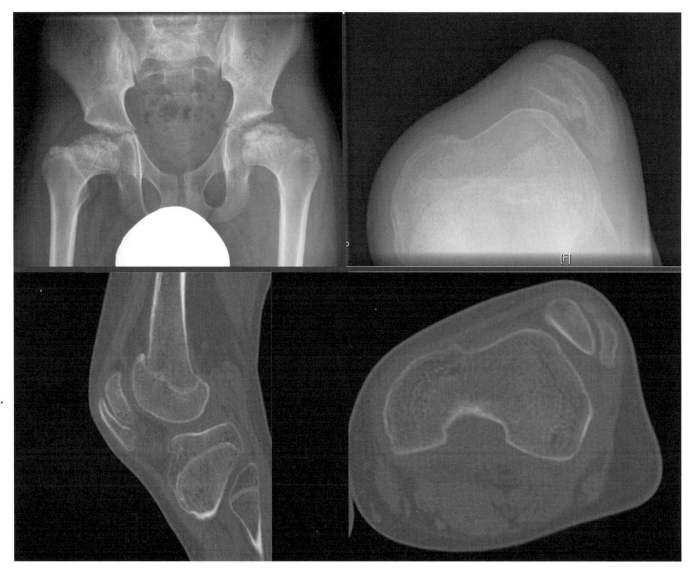

Figure 13.6 Multiple epiphyseal dysplasia. Top left: Radiograph of hips, showing metachronous appearance of epiphysis similar to Legg–Calvé–Perthes disease. Top right: Skyline view of knee, showing dislocated patella, and also the characteristic double-layered patella. Bottom: CT of patellae showing double-layered patella.

- Genu varum or valgum,
- Short stubby fingers and toes,
- Early osteoarthritis.

Radiographic findings (Figure 13.6)

- Delayed appearance of ossification centres, which, once apparent, are small and irregular.
- Reductions in epiphyseal and carpal height can help make the diagnosis.
- Changes are most commonly seen in the proximal femur, and need to be differentiated from bilateral Legg–Calvé–Perthes disease (LCPD). The following are suggestive of MED:

  - Symmetric, synchronous changes bilaterally,
  - Acetabular changes,
  - Absence of metaphyseal cysts (seen in LCPD),
  - Epiphyseal irregularities in the knees or shoulders.

- Avascular necrosis of the femoral epiphysis may be seen in LCPD and in MED. Neither MRI nor bone scan can differentiate between the two conditions.
- Angular deformities, such as coxa vara or genu varum or valgum, may be present.
- The 'double-layered' patella may be seen on a lateral radiograph of the knee, and is characteristic of MED.
- Short metacarpals and phalanges with irregular epiphyses.
- There may be mild vertebral endplate irregularities, but severe vertebral changes are not seen, differentiating MED from SED.

Management

- Physiotherapy, to maintain joint range of motion.
- Although the radiographic changes are similar to Perthes disease, there is no evidence to support containment orthoses or surgery in MED.

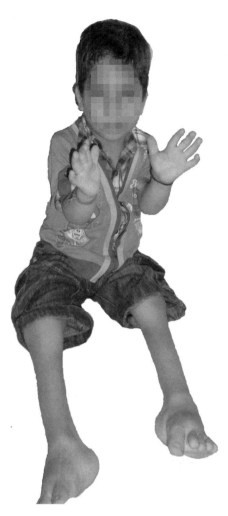

Figure 13.7 Diastrophic dysplasia, showing hitchhiker's thumb, though not classical. Note the club feet.

Clinical features (Figure 13.7)

- This condition is easily diagnosed at birth by:
  - 'Cauliflower ear',
  - 'Hitchhiker's thumb'.
- The newborn child is very short statured, with short limbs.
- A shortened triangular first metacarpal causes radial subluxation of the metacarpophalangeal joint of the thumb, causing it to lie almost perpendicular to the index finger ('hitchhiker's thumb').
- The CTEV deformities are marked and rigid.
- Most patients have stiff joints, often with flexion contractures of the hips, knees and elbows, but most patients are ambulatory.
- There is congenital dislocation of the hips in 25% of patients.
- Patellae and radial head dislocations are commonly seen.
- With increasing mobility, the child may develop a kyphoscoliosis, which is often rigid and progressive.

Radiographic features (Figure 13.8)

- Delayed appearance of the epiphyses, which, once formed, are flattened and irregular,
- Short broad long bones with flared metaphyses,
- Short triangular first metacarpals and metatarsals,
- A saucer-like indentation is often seen on the proximal femur,
- Coxa vara,
- Genu valgum.

Management

- The foot deformities are usually resistant to non-operative correction, and require open surgical release.
- The hip dislocations are teratologic; while open reduction can be performed, they may be best left alone.
- Flexion contractures of the knee and hip may require soft-tissue release, or even extension osteotomy.
- Severe and progressive spinal deformity may necessitate surgery during early childhood.

- Painful hinge abduction may require proximal femoral valgus osteotomy.
- Corrective osteotomies of the femur may be required to correct lower-limb malalignment.
- Osteoarthritis may require arthroplasty.

Diastrophic dysplasia

'Diastrophic' is derived from the Greek word for 'twisted'. This condition is associated with severe short stature, rigid congenital talipes equinovarus (CTEV), scoliosis and 'hitchhiker's thumb'.

Basic science

- Autosomal recessive inheritance.
- The mutation affects the diastrophic dysplasia sulfate transporter (*DTDST*) gene on chromosome 5.
- The impaired function of the sulfate transporter ultimately leads to:
  - Stunted enchondral growth,
  - Susceptibility of articular cartilage to early degenerative change.

Chondrodysplasia punctata

- Chondrodysplasia is a group of dysplasias characterized by multiple punctate calcifications within the unossified cartilage at the ends of the long bones, tarsal bones, pelvis and vertebrae (Figure 13.9).
- These calcifications disappear within the first year of life, making early diagnosis important.
- The most common form of this condition is Conradi–Hünermann syndrome, which is inherited as an X-linked dominant trait.
- There is a wide clinical spectrum; clinical features include:
  - Short stature, possibly with rhizomelic limb shortening,
  - Ichthyosiform erythroderma (dry, scaly skin),

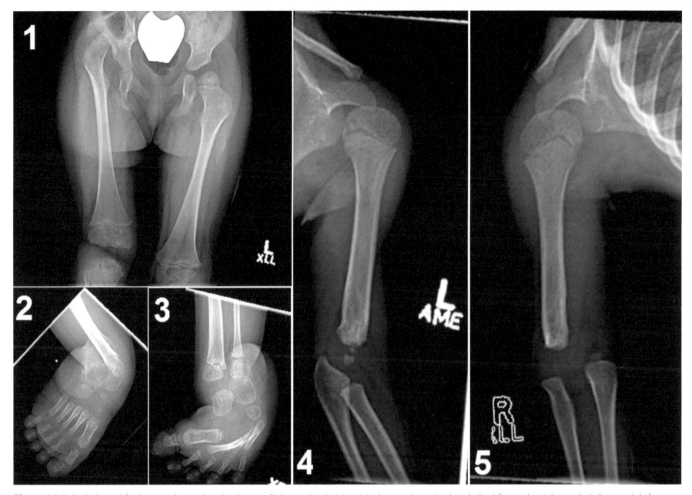

Figure 13.8 Radiological findings in diastrophic dysplasia. 1: Dislocated right hip with abnormal proximal and distal femoral epiphyses. 2, 3: Severe club foot deformities. 4, 5: Elbow contractures and radial head dislocation.

- Heart defects,
- Cataracts.

Metaphyseal chondrodysplasia

- In this group of bone dysplasias, failure of normal mineralization of the zone of provisional calcification leads to widened physes and enlarged, cupped metaphyses (similar to rickets).
- The physeal pathology interferes with normal longitudinal bone growth, causing short stature and angular deformities (particularly coxa vara and genu varum).
- The epiphyses are spared, so arthritis is not common.

There are several different types.

Jansen's type

- The rarest but most severe type; usually apparent at birth.
- It is due to a mutation of the parathyroid-hormone or parathyroid-hormone-related peptide receptor gene.

- It is associated with severe hypercalcaemia and hypophosphatasia despite normal parathyroid hormone (PTH) levels.

Schmid type

- The most common type of metaphyseal chondrodysplasia,
- Autosomal dominant inheritance,
- Genetic mutation on chromosome 6 affects type X collagen (*COL10A1*),
- Skeletal changes develop after weight-bearing at age 3–5 years.

Osteopetrosis

- Failure of osteoclasts to resorb enchondral bone, while new bone formation continues, results in osteosclerosis.
- The resulting immature bone has fewer collagen fibrils, making it brittle ('marble bone'), and therefore susceptible to fracture.

Clinically, this results in:

- Deformity (i.e. coxa vara),
- Bone pain,

- Osteomyelitis (commonly of the mandible),
- Pathologic fractures (slow to heal).

Radiographic features include (Figure 13.10):

- Increased radio-opacity of the bones,
- Loss of distinction between the cortex and medullary canal,
- 'Endobones', which are miniature radiodensities resembling tiny bones within the cortices of tubular bone; these are pathognomic for osteopetrosis,

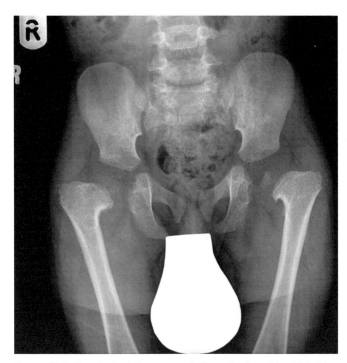

Figure 13.9 Chondrodysplasia punctata. Radiograph of an older child with Conradi–Hünermann syndrome shows speckled ossification features of right hip. This was associated with bilateral coxa vara.

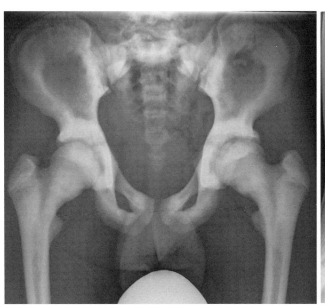

- 'Rugger-jersey' spine, with zones of osteosclerosis adjacent to the vertebral endplates, and a radiolucent space centrally.

There are two main types of this dysplasia.

Malignant osteopetrosis

- Autosomal recessive inheritance,
- Presents at birth or early infancy,
- Additional clinical features include:
  - Symptoms of pancytopaenia, caused by obliteration of the bone marrow space by the unresorbed bone,
  - Delayed dentition,
  - Blindness and deafness due to bony overgrowth of the cranial nerve foramina.

This type is rapidly progressive, and requires bone marrow transplant in early childhood. If successful, the 5-year disease-free survival rate is over 70%. The osteosclerosis resolves, and normal bone marrow function and bone modelling resume.

Benign osteopetrosis

- Autosomal dominant inheritance,
- About 40% of patients are asymptomatic and diagnosed incidentally,
- Two types:
  - Type I is not associated with increased fracture risk,
  - Type II is associated with mild anaemia and premature osteoarthritis.

A small proportion of patients have osteopetrosis related to renal tubular acidosis, in which there is carbonic anhydrase deficiency.

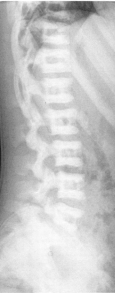

Figure 13.10 Osteopetrosis. There is increased radio-opacity of the bones, with loss of distinction between the cortex and medullary canal, a 'rugger-jersey' spine, with zones of osteosclerosis adjacent to the vertebral endplates, and a radiolucent space centrally. Spondylolytic spondylolisthesis, at L5, is seen as a feature in osteopetrosis.

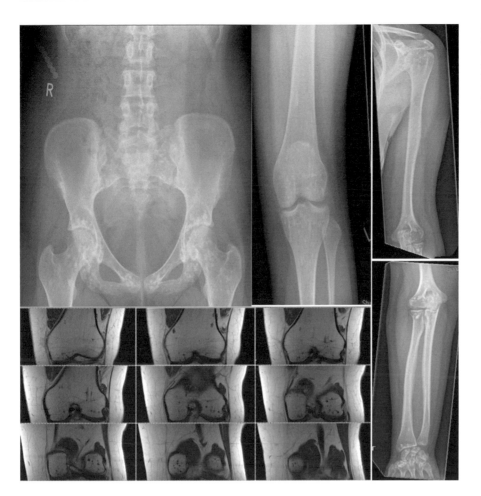

Figure 13.11 Osteopoikilosis. Plain X-radiographs and MRI show numerous white densities of similar size spread throughout all the bones. It must be differentiated from osteoblastic metastasis; it tends to present with larger and more irregular densities in less of a uniform pattern. Another differentiating factor is age, with osteoblastic metastasis mostly affecting older people, and osteopoikilosis being found in people of up to 20 years of age.

Osteopoikilosis

- An autosomal dominant condition, which is asymptomatic, and requires no treatment.
- Characterized by clusters of 2–10 mm oval radiodensities within cancellous bone (Figure 13.11).
- Approximately 10% of patients have associated yellow subcutaneous nodules (the skin and bone changes together are called dermatofibrosis lenticularis disseminata).
- Osteopoikilosis may be confused with bone metastases; bone scans cannot differentiate, as the lesions may show increased or no uptake.
- Over time, the bone lesions may increase in size or regress and disappear.
- Malignant change, though rare, has been described.

Melorheostosis

- This rare dysplasia is not thought to be a genetic disorder.
- It is characterized by a 'flowing' hyperostosis of the cortex, the radiographic appearance of which has been likened to a candle with dripping wax (Figure 13.12).

- It may affect one bone (monostotic), one limb or multiple sites (polyostotic).
- There are no reported cases of involvement of skull or facial bones.
- It is associated with osteopoikilosis, neurofibromatosis, tuberous sclerosis, scleroderma and rheumatoid arthritis.
- It usually presents in childhood or adolescence with bone pain and flexion tissue contractures.

Infantile cortical hyperostosis (Caffey disease)

- Caffey disease is a self-limiting condition mimicking infection.
- It usually presents before the age of 5 months:
  - Fever and irritability.
  - Localized deep soft-tissue mass, most often over the mandible, but also frequently over the ulna, tibia and clavicle.
  - Multifocal involvement is common.
  - Radiographs demonstrate periosteal new bone formation over the diaphysis of the affected bone (Figure 13.13).

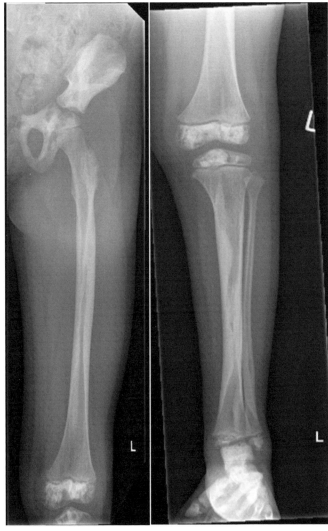

Figure 13.12 Melorheostosis. Notice thickening of bony cortex resembling 'dripping candle wax'. In this patient, only the left side was involved.

- The erythrocyte sedimentation rate (ESR) and level of alkaline phosphatase may be elevated.
- The condition may occur in the prenatal period, and if occurring before 35 weeks' gestation, can be fatal.
- Corticosteroids can be used in severe cases to treat the acute systemic symptoms, but do not affect the bony changes.
- Complete spontaneous recovery usually occurs within 6–9 months.

Cleidocranial dysostosis

- A dysplasia of the bones formed by intramembranous ossification (including clavicles, pelvis and cranium).
- The pattern of inheritance is autosomal dominant, but one-third of new cases are spontaneous mutations.

Clinical features

These are often present before the age of 2 years and include:

- Hypoplasia or absence of one or both clavicles (the lateral end is most commonly affected),
- There may be similar underdevelopment of the associated muscles (e.g. sternocleidomastoid and anterior deltoid),
- Abnormalities of the sternum, often with pectus excavatum,
- Hypoplastic scapula, which may demonstrate winging,
- Rarely, there may be upper-limb pain or numbness due to irritation of the brachial plexus,
- There are associations with syringomyelia and Wilms' tumour.

Radiographic features (Figure 13.14)

- Hypoplastic or absent clavicles,
- Multiple wormian bones in the skull,

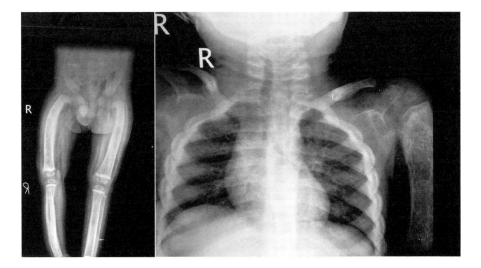

Figure 13.13 Infantile cortical hyperostosis. Radiographs show periosteal reactions and widening of bones seen in multiple segments. Other differential diagnoses need to be considered.

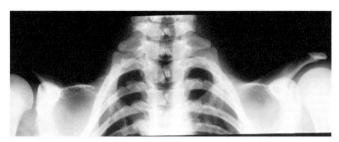

Figure 13.14 Cleidocranial dysostosis, showing an absent clavicle.

- Widened symphysis pubis and sacroiliac joints,
- Coxa vara,

- Scoliosis and spondylolysis,
- Hypoplastic/absent terminal phalanges,
- Increased length of the second metacarpals.

Orthopaedic management

- Proximal femoral valgus osteotomy,
- Excision of clavicular fragments to decompress the irritated brachial plexus,
- Scapulothoracic arthrodesis for painful scapular winging,
- Scoliosis treatment as per adolescent idiopathic scoliosis.

Chapter

14

Metabolic bone disease

Mubashshar Ahmad and Gavin De Kiewiet

Introduction

- The bone stores 98% of the body's calcium and 85% of its phosphorus, with only a small proportion present in the blood.
- The bony skeleton acts as a reservoir of stored calcium and can be drawn upon to maintain serum levels.
- Calcium haemostasis is closely linked to bone formation and resorption and is vital in its effects on the clotting cascade and in maintaining normal cell function, nerve conduction and muscle contraction.
- Calcium circulates in plasma in two main forms:
  - Free ionized calcium, which is physiologically active,
  - Inactive calcium, which is bound to albumin.

Disturbances in the metabolism of calcium (Ca) and phosphate (PO_4) can lead to metabolic bone disease (MBD) with inadequate mineralization of bone matrix. In children, the epiphyseal ends of the bones are the most active in osteogenesis, so the disease is more evident there.

The level of calcium in the serum is regulated by three hormones: vitamin D, parathyroid hormone (PTH) and calcitonin. The two main sources of vitamin D are:

1. Diet, which is a source of the inactive form of vitamin D2 (ergocalciferol) and D3 (cholecalciferol). The recommended dietary allowance of vitamin D for children is 400 IU.
2. The liver also produces 7-dihydrocholesterol (provitamin D), which is converted to vitamin D3 in the skin as a result of exposure to ultraviolet light. Melanin competes with 7-dihydrocholesterol, such that people who are heavily pigmented require a longer exposure to ultraviolet light to produce an equivalent quantity of vitamin D.

Inactive vitamin D undergoes hydroxylation in the liver (to form 25-hydroxycholecalciferol) and the kidney (to form 1,25-dihydroxycholecalciferol or 24,25-dihydroxycholecalciferol). 1,25-dihydroxycholecalciferol is also called calcitriol or the active form of vitamin D (Figure 14.1). Several medications, such as antiepileptics, can inhibit this process, leading to

vitamin D deficiency. Vitamin D acts on the intestine and bone and may have some action on the kidneys (Table 14.1).

Parathyroid hormone (PTH) is a polypeptide containing 84 amino acids and is secreted by the chief cells of the parathyroid gland. Its secretion is stimulated by low serum levels of Ca and PO_4 and inhibited by high serum levels of Ca, PO_4 and vitamin D. It acts on the intestine, bone and kidneys. Parathyroid hormone therapy is used to treat patients with severe osteoporosis (bone mineral density, T-score < -3) who cannot tolerate other treatment or patients with refractory osteoporosis; however, it is contraindicated in children with open physis, patients with metastatic bone diseases and patients at risk of developing osteosarcoma (Paget's disease and following bone irradiation).

Calcitonin is produced by the C cells of the thyroid gland. Although the exact physiological function of calcitonin is unknown, it has a powerful inhibitory effect on osteoclasts, causing flattening of their ruffled border and withdrawal of the osteoclasts from the bone surface. Salmon calcitonin is given intranasally as a treatment for osteoporosis. In addition to inhibiting bone resorption, there is a significant analgesic effect, especially in osteoporotic patients with vertebral fractures.

Although the regulation of osteoclasts has been the subject of extensive research, it is still not well understood. They are regulated by various molecular signals; the best studied one is probably the receptor activator for nuclear factor κB ligand (RANKL). This molecule is produced by osteoblasts and other cells (e.g. lymphocytes), and stimulates RANK (receptor activator of nuclear factor κB) on the osteoclasts' precursor cells, differentiating them into active osteoclasts. The RANK stimulation is the final common denominator of osteoclast activation. Numerous conditions, such as bone metastases, multiple myeloma, osteoporosis and hyperparathyroidism, result in osteoclast activation associated with increased expression and release of the RANKL from the surface of the osteoblasts. If the RANKL or RANK receptors are knocked out, then osteoclasts precursor cells cannot be activated and no bone resorption occurs.

Postgraduate Paediatric Orthopaedics, ed. Sattar Alshryda, Stan Jones and Paul A. Banaszkiewicz. Published by Cambridge University Press.
© Cambridge University Press 2014.

Table 14.1 Parathyroid hormone, vitamin D and calcitonin actions

Parameters		Parathyroid hormone	Vitamin D	Calcitonin
Origin		Chief cell, Parathyroid gland	Kidney	Parafollicular cells, Thyroid gland
Factors stimulating production		↓ Ca or PO$_4$	↑ Parathyroid hormone ↓ Ca or PO$_4$	↑ Ca
Factors inhibiting production		↑ Ca or vitamin D	↓ Parathyroid hormone ↑ Ca or PO$_4$	↓ Ca
Effects	Intestine	No direct effect, Indirectly through ↑ vitamin D	Strongly stimulate Ca and PO$_4$ absorption	?
	Kidney	Stimulate production of vitamin D, ↑ Ca absorption, ↓ PO$_4$ absorption	? ↑ Ca absorption, ↓ PO$_4$ absorption	?
	Bone	Osteoclastic bone resorption (which mobilizes Ca and PO$_4$ to the blood)	Dual actions: Direct: osteoclastic bone resorption Indirect: increase osteoid mineralization	Inhibit osteoclastic bone resorption
Net effects	Ca PO$_4$	↑ ↓	↑ ↑	↓ Transient

? Not fully understood.

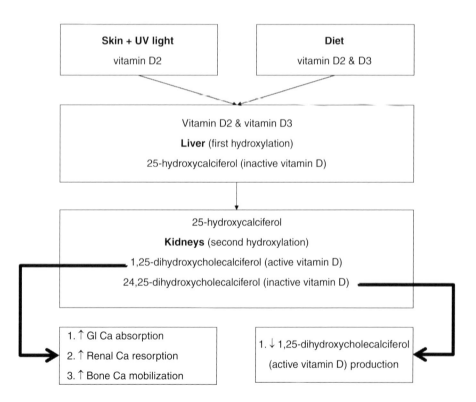

Figure 14.1 Vitamin D metabolism.

Rickets

Rickets is a defect in bone mineralization that occurs before the cessation of growth, whereas osteomalacia is a defect in bone mineralization after the cessation of growth (Figure 14.2). By contrast, osteoporosis (porous bone) is defined as a decrease in bone mass and density. The mineralization in osteoporosis can be normal.

The defect in bone mineralization can be caused by lack of calcium, phosphate or alkaline phosphatase.

Calcium deficiency

1. Nutritional rickets (prolonged breast feeding, vegetarian diets),
2. Gastrointestinal rickets (coeliac disease, Crohn's disease, ulcerative colitis),

3. Renal rickets:
    i. 1α-hydroxylase deficiency leads to a failure to convert 25-hydroxycholecalciferol to 1,25-dihydroxycholecalciferol. There is a high level of the former but a lower level of the

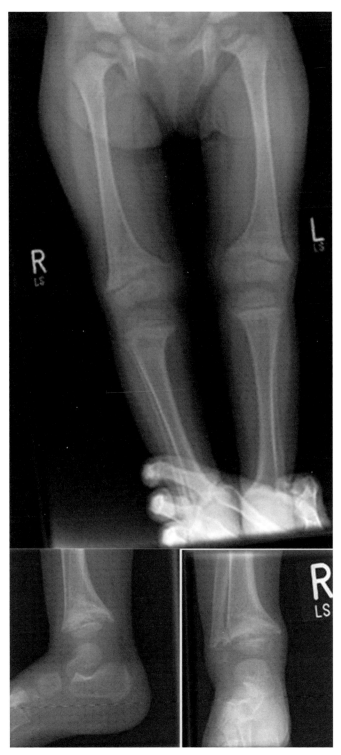

Figure 14.2 Radiograph of a child with rickets. The findings are very characteristic: the physes are widened, bulky and irregular (clearly visible in the ankle, distal and proximal femur). There is splaying ('cupping') of the bone at the junction of the metaphysis and physis. The widened growth plate is caused by lack of mineralization of the cartilage matrix; this weakens the growth plate.

latter. It can be treated with vitamin D supplement (dihydroxycholecalciferol).
    ii. Rickets of end-stage renal disease (renal osteodystrophy).
4. End-organ insensitivity to vitamin D (rare; there are very high levels of 1,25-dihydroxycholecalciferol; but the receptors are insensitive). Alopecia is a common feature.

Phosphate deficiency

X-linked hypophosphataemia

This is the most common form of inherited rickets, with a prevalence of 1 in 20 000 persons [1]. It is an X-linked dominant disorder. There is isolated renal phosphate wasting, leading to hypophosphataemia.

Renal tubular abnormalities

There is a failure of tubular reabsorption of phosphate, calcium, magnesium, bicarbonate, sodium, potassium, glucose, uric acid and small amino acids. The predominant cause of bone disease is hypophosphataemia from renal phosphate wasting, very similar to that seen in X-linked hypophosphatemic rickets. As a result, such patients are short and have a delayed bone age.

Alkaline phosphatase

Alkaline phosphatase deficiency is an autosomal recessive condition that causes hypophosphatasia and has a clinical overlap with rickets in children or osteomalacia in the adults. Additional clinical manifestations may include failure to thrive, increased intracranial pressure and craniosynostosis.

Renal osteodystrophy

This is common in children with renal failure secondary to diseases, such as chronic pyelonephritis or polycystic kidneys; especially those who develop it at a young age [2, 3].

Pathophysiology

Children with end-stage renal disease have:

- Impaired ability to excrete phosphorus; it precipitates with calcium, leading to hyperphosphataemia and a fall in serum calcium levels,
- Reduced production of 1,25-dihydroxyvitamin D (kidneys unable to hydroxylate 25-hydroxycholecalciferol),
- Low levels of vitamin D that lead to a decrease in calcium absorption from the small intestine,
- Hypocalcaemia increases the release of PTH (secondary hyperparathyroidism), leading to the demineralization of bone to increase the serum calcium level,
- Hyperphosphataemia can also directly lead to bone resorption,
- Parathyroid hormone also acts directly on stimulating osteoclasts, ultimately leading to osteitis fibrosa.

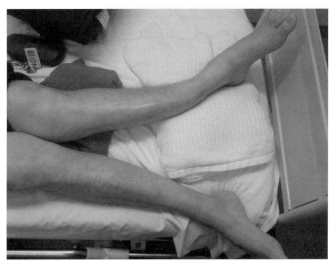

Figure 14.3 Lower-limb deformity in patient with renal osteodystrophy.

Presentation

- Renal disease precedes bone changes by several years. The presentation is similar to rickets or osteomalacia:
  - Failure to thrive,
  - Bone pain,
  - Listlessness, weakness, irritability, convulsions,
  - Delayed sitting, standing and walking.
- Short stature.
- Pathological fractures, SUFE.
- Lower-limb deformity. The poorly mineralized bone is soft and prone to bending with weight-bearing (genu valgum or varum and periarticular enlargement) (Figure 14.3).
- Trendelenburg gait secondary to muscle weakness or myopathy.

Biochemistry

- High serum levels of urea and creatinine,
- High serum levels of phosphate, alkaline phosphatase and parathyroid hormone,
- Low serum levels of calcium (may be corrected),
- Low vitamin D levels (rickets),
- Acidosis,
- Low urinary excretion rate of calcium and phosphate.

X-radiography

- The physes are widened and irregular.
- Physeal cartilage persists into the metaphysis, as a result of failure of calcification.
- Epiphysiolysis.
- Ground-glass appearance.
- Generalized osteopaenia, thinning of cortices, indistinct trabeculae.

- No physeal cupping, as seen in rickets.
- Salt-and-pepper appearance of the skull (coarse granular pattern).
- 'Rugger-jersey' spine (horizontal sclerotic bands adjacent to vertebral endplates giving a striped appearance). Note: this is also seen in osteopetrosis.
- Subperiosteal resorption (metacarpals, terminal aspect of distal phalanges and ulna, lateral end of clavicle and symphysis pubis).
- Soft-tissue calcification of periarticular tissues.
- Brown tumour (lytic defect within the pelvis and long bones containing multiple giant cells). Thinning of cortex, which may lead to pathological fractures.

Medical treatment

- Treatment of underlying renal disease.
- Replace vitamin D with 1,25-dihydroxyvitamin D.
- Administer sodium bicarbonate to reverse acidosis.
- Parathyroidectomy may be considered when medical treatment fails.

Orthopaedic treatment

- Multidisciplinary approach with renal specialist (electrolyte and fluid balance control in the perioperative period).
- Deformity correction to restore mechanical axis (only when renal disease under control):
  - Guided growth with hemiepiphysiodesis,
  - Multiple osteotomies (internal fixation or circular fixator correction).
- Treatment of SUFE; often bilateral, therefore prophylactic pinning of the contralateral hip should be considered (Figures 14.4 and 14.5).
- Physiolysis is seen in distal femur, proximal humerus, distal radius and ulna. Treatment is with cast immobilization of the physis.

Idiopathic juvenile osteoporosis
Background

Osteoporosis is defined as a bone density at least 2.5 standard deviations (SD) below peak bone mass (defined as the bone mass achieved by healthy adults aged 30 years). The T-score is defined as the number of SD above or below the mean for a healthy 30-year-old adult of the same sex and ethnicity as the patient, while the Z-score is defined as the number of standard deviations above or below the mean for the patient's age, sex and ethnicity. As children have not attained peak bone mass, the Z-score is more relevant to idiopathic juvenile osteoporosis and is now available for the lumbar spine, hip and total body. Idiopathic juvenile osteoporosis (IJO) is defined as a bone density Z-score below −2 SD, in combination with a fracture.

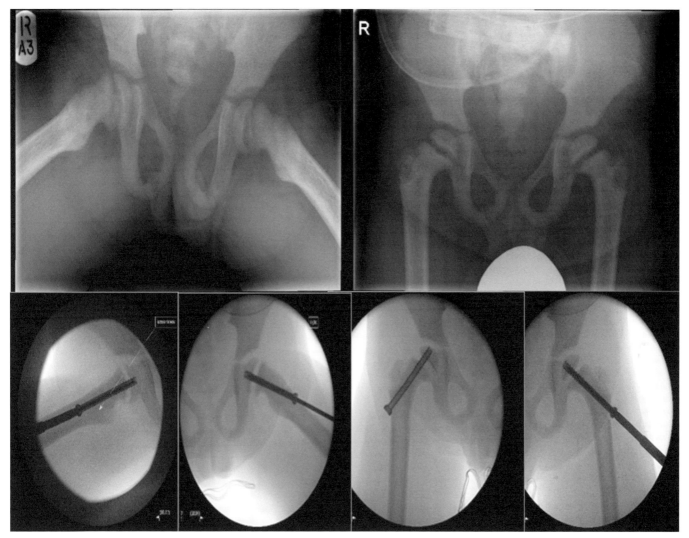

Figure 14.4 A patient with renal osteodystrophy developed bilateral SUFE and underwent pinning *in situ*. Notice the wide physes on both sides.

The average bone density is around $1500 \, \text{kg/m}^3$ ($1.5 \, \text{g/cm}^3$). Although density represents mass per unit volume (of bone tissue), it is currently measured in two dimensions (mass per unit area):

$$\text{average bone mineral density} = \frac{\text{bone mineral content (BMC)}}{\text{area in cm}^2}$$

Dual-energy X-ray absorptiometry (DEXA) is the most widely used test to measure bone density of selected bones (usually the spine, hip and wrist). The density of these bones is then compared with an average index based on age, sex and size (Figure 14.6).

Idiopathic juvenile osteoporosis (IJO) is rare in childhood. Although several conditions can cause osteoporosis in children (Table 14.2), the cause of IJO remains unknown and no genetic transmission has been implicated. There is usually a significant reduction in bone density secondary to an imbalance between bone formation and bone resorption. Bone is fully mineralized but its strength is less than normal for a child of similar age and sex.

Presentation

- M = F,
- Onset before puberty, average age = 7,
- Generalized back and leg pains,
- Limp,
- Increased fragility of bone with compression fractures (typically long bones and vertebrae),
- Formation of new but osteoporotic bone,
- Spontaneous recovery before skeletal recovery,
- Biochemical tests:
  - Serum calcium, phosphorus and vitamin D levels are normal.
  - Alkaline phosphatase and urinary hydroxyproline levels are also normal.

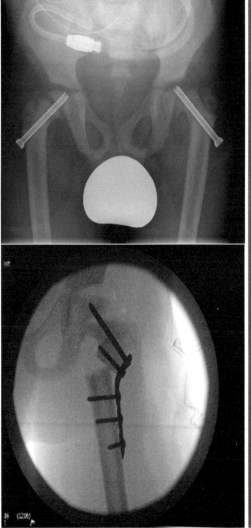

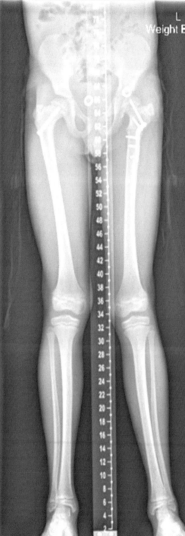

Figure 14.5 Renal osteodystrophy. The patient of Figure 14.3 developed a worsening slip and coxa vara in spite of adequate fixation (top left). This required revision fixation with a valgus osteotomy (bottom left). A few years later, the patient developed two problems: overgrowth on the right hip screw, risking slip progression, and left knee valgus.

X-radiography

- Diffuse generalized osteopaenia,
- Loss of trabecular pattern and thinning of the cortices,
- Spine: codfish appearance with anterior wedge fracture, leading to thoracolumbar kyphosis (Figure 14.7),
- Pathological fractures.

Diagnosis

- This is one of exclusion; all conditions listed in Table 14.2 should be excluded.
- The main differential is mild osteogenesis imperfecta. In osteogenesis imperfecta (OI):
  - Family history,
  - Blue sclera,
  - Dentinogenesis,
  - Ligamentous laxity,
- Easy bruising,
- Normal fracture callus in OI, whereas in osteoporosis the callus is osteopaenic,
- Bone biopsy:
  - OI: increased woven immature bone,
  - OP: increased osteoclastic resorption of bone.

Treatment
Medical

- Aimed at correcting any biochemical deficiencies,
- Antiresorptive agents (bisphosphonates).

Bisphosphonates have a similar structure to pyrophosphate, which has an affinity to attach to bone tissue. Bisphosphonate molecules preferentially bind to calcium. Bones have the largest store of calcium in the body. When osteoclasts ingest bisphosphonates, bound bone tissues die.

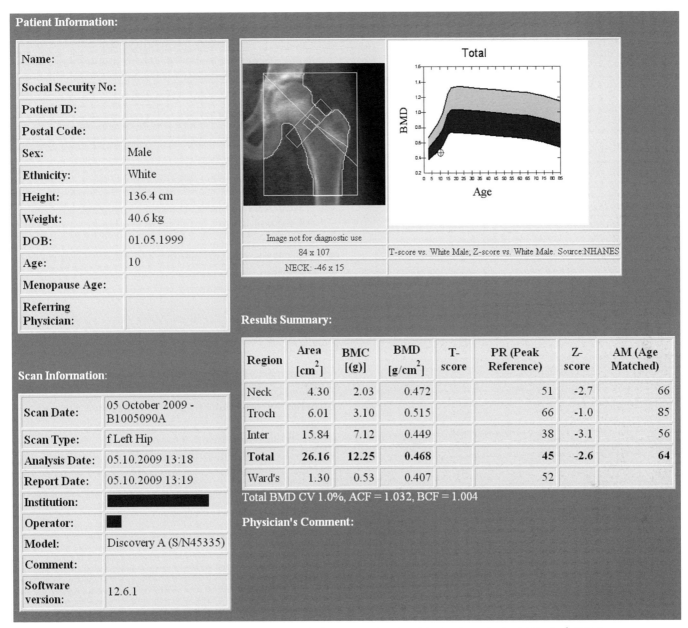

Patient Information:

Name:	
Social Security No:	
Patient ID:	
Postal Code:	
Sex:	Male
Ethnicity:	White
Height:	136.4 cm
Weight:	40.6 kg
DOB:	01.05.1999
Age:	10
Menopause Age:	
Referring Physician:	

Scan Information:

Scan Date:	05 October 2009 - B1005090A
Scan Type:	f Left Hip
Analysis Date:	05.10.2009 13:18
Report Date:	05.10.2009 13:19
Institution:	■■■■■■
Operator:	■
Model:	Discovery A (S/N45335)
Comment:	
Software version:	12.6.1

Image not for diagnostic use
84 x 107
NECK: -46 x 15

T-score vs. White Male; Z-score vs. White Male. Source:NHANES

Results Summary:

Region	Area [cm^2]	BMC [(g)]	BMD [g/cm^2]	T-score	PR (Peak Reference)	Z-score	AM (Age Matched)
Neck	4.30	2.03	0.472		51	-2.7	66
Troch	6.01	3.10	0.515		66	-1.0	85
Inter	15.84	7.12	0.449		38	-3.1	56
Total	**26.16**	**12.25**	**0.468**		**45**	**-2.6**	**64**
Ward's	1.30	0.53	0.407		52		

Total BMD CV 1.0%, ACF = 1.032, BCF = 1.004

Physician's Comment:

Figure 14.6 DEXA of the neck of femur in a child with IJO. Notice the low Z-score (−2.6) and the low bone density 0.468 g/cm^2. BMD, bone mineral density.

There are two classes of bisphosphonate:

1. Nitrogen-containing bisphosphonates (etidronate),
2. Non-nitrogen-containing bisphosphonates (pamidronate, risedronate, alendronate and zoledronate).

The two types of bisphosphonates work differently in killing osteoclast cells. The most common side effects of bisphosphonates are fever and myalgia. A rare but significant skeletal complication of bisphosphonate therapy is osteonecrosis of the jaw. This occurs more commonly in patients with metastatic bone disease who receive monthly treatment.

Others

Anabolic steroids (testosterone, oxandrolone) and growth hormone are under investigations. Parathyroid hormone is contraindicated in children because of the detection of osteogenic sarcoma in mice that were given very high test doses.

Surgical

- Stabilize any long bone fractures to prevent immobilization, as this leads to worsening of existing osteoporosis (Figure 14.8).
- Deformity correction.
- Brace spine for short period to relive back pain and prevent kyphosis.

Scurvy

- Nutritional deficiency of vitamin C (ascorbic acid),
- Rare but still occurs in such conditions as anorexia nervosa,
- Historically described in sailors.

Table 14.2 Some causes of childhood osteoporosis

Nutritional	Bone disorders
Malnutrition, Malabsorption, Scurvy	Osteogenesis imperfect, Turner's syndrome
Metabolic	**Endocrine**
Rickets of any cause, Liver disease, Chronic renal disease or dialysis, Homocystinuria	Hyperthyroidism, Hyperparathyroidism, Gonadal insufficiency, Anorexia nervosa, Cushing's disease
Malignant	**Iatrogenic**
Leukaemia, Lymphoma, Multiple myeloma	Steroid treatment, Heparin, Anticonvulsants
Miscellaneous	**Idiopathic**
Disuse, e.g. paralysis, Still's disease, Immobilization	Idiopathic juvenile osteoporosis

Pathology

- Vitamin C is necessary for hydroxylation of lysine to hydroxylysine and proline to hydroxyproline. Both of these amino acids are necessary for the cross-linkage of the triple helix of collagen.
- Collagen synthesis is impaired.
- Osteoblasts fail to produce new bone and osteoid tissue.
- Osteoclasts and chondroblasts function normally with normal mineralization.
- Osteoporosis occurs, especially in epiphyseal bone. Cortices and trabeculae become thin and fragile.
- Fractures are common. The provisional zone of calcification is weak, resulting in epiphyseal separation injuries.
- There is spontaneous bleeding secondary to abnormal collagen in blood vessels.
- Poor dental formation.

Presentation

- Loss of appetite, irritability, failure to thrive, anaemia.
- Spontaneous haemorrhages of gums, soft tissues, gut and skin, petechiae.
- Subperiosteal haemorrhage near large joints; this can present with pain, swelling and pseudoparalysis.
- Acute haemarthrosis.
- Poor wound healing.

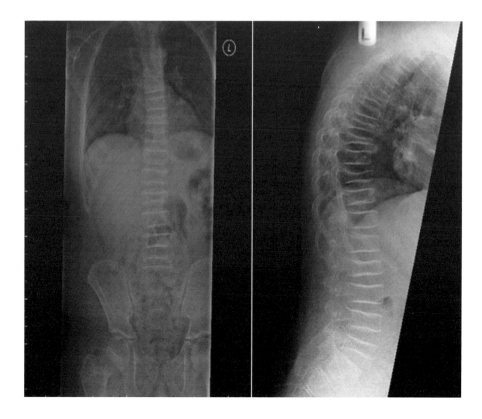

Figure 14.7 Idiopathic juvenile osteoporosis. There are multiple spontaneous vertebral fractures, giving the classical codfish appearance, with an anterior wedge fracture leading to thoracolumbar kyphosis.

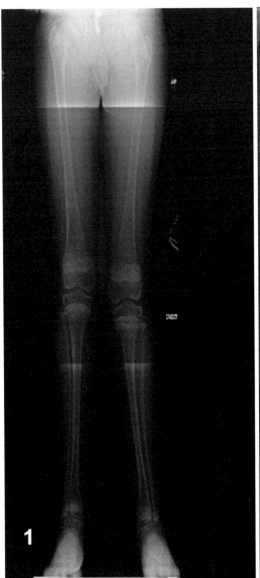
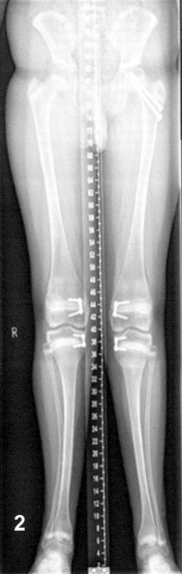

Figure 14.8 Idiopathic juvenile osteoporosis. The child of Figure 14.7 developed a left neck of femur fracture, which was fixed with cannulated screws. He also underwent guided growth using 8-plates over the medial distal femur and proximal tibia to correct a valgus deformity that he was developing.

Differential diagnosis

Osteomyelitis; however, in scurvy the level of C-reactive protein, erythrocyte sedimentation rate and white cell count are normal.

X-radiography

- Frankel's line: an opaque white line at the zone of provisional calcification.
- Wimberger's ring sign (ringing of the epiphysis): this represents increased sclerosis around the perimeter of secondary ossification centres as a result of continued mineral deposition despite compromised osteoid formation.

- Osteopaenia.
- Periosteal reaction secondary to subperiosteal haemorrhage.

Biochemistry

- Serum vitamin C levels are reduced.
- Absence of vitamin C in the buffy coat of centrifuged blood.

Treatment

- Vitamin C replacement.

References

1. Stans AA (2005) Osteomyelitis and septic arthritis. In *Lovell and Winter's Pediatric Orthopaedics*, 6th edition, volume 1, ed. Morrissy RT and Weinstein SL. Philadelphia: Lippincott Williams & Wilkins, pp. 440–80.

2. Herring JA (2008) *Tachdjian's Pediatric Orthopaedics*, 4th edition, volume 1. Philadelphia: Saunders Elsevier.

3. Dormans JP (2005) *Pediatric Orthopaedics. Core Knowledge in Orthopaedics*. Philadelphia: Elsevier Mosby.

Chapter

15

Physis and leg length discrepancy

Tim Nunn and Stan Jones

Physis and physeal injuries

Introduction

The paediatric skeleton is different from the adult's because the bones are more elastic and have growth plates (physes). In comparison with bone, the relative strength of the physis changes with age, becoming weaker as the child grows; hence, physeal injuries are more common in adolescence. The physis can be injured in many ways:

- Direct – fracture involving the physis,
- Fracture elsewhere in a limb segment (the result of ischaemia),
- Infection,
- Bone cyst,
- Tumour,
- Irradiation,
- Repetitive stress (sports injury).

An understanding of the anatomy and physiology of the physis is important to help one understand and thus manage these injuries properly.

The physis

Histology

Histologically, the physis consists of chondrocytes surrounded by an extracellular matrix (Figure 15.1). The chondrocytes are arranged in columns along the longitudinal axes of the respective bones, and directed toward the metaphysis where endochondral ossification takes place.

The physis is divided into four zones:

1. Reserve zone,
2. Proliferative zone,
3. Hypertrophic zone,
4. Zone of endochondral ossification (in the primary spongiosa of the metaphysis).

The reserve and proliferative zones have an abundance of extracellular matrix and thus resist shear forces easily. The hypertrophic zone has significantly less extracellular matrix than the reserve and proliferative zones and is therefore the weakest zone. It is believed that most physeal injuries occur in this zone, though any zone may be involved in high-energy injuries.

In the hypertrophic zone, chondrocytes increase in size, accumulate calcium in their mitochondria and degenerate.

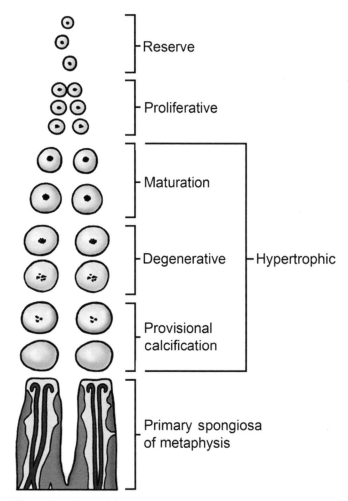

Figure 15.1 Zones of the physis.

Postgraduate Paediatric Orthopaedics, ed. Sattar Alshryda, Stan Jones and Paul A. Banaszkiewicz. Published by Cambridge University Press.
© Cambridge University Press 2014.

In addition, oxygen tension becomes progressively lower as cells pass through this zone. The zone is further subdivided into three zones:

1. Maturation,
2. Degeneration,
3. Provisional calcification.

The groove of Ranvier at the periphery of the physis contains an active group of chondrocytes and contributes to lateral growth (width) of the physis.

The physis is encircled by the perichondrial ring of LaCroix. This is a dense fibrous continuation of the periosteum and provides a strong mechanical support at the bone–physis interface.

The physes of long bones, such as that of the distal femur, have an undulating pattern with mamillary processes. These features provide greater shear strength.

Blood supply

The blood supply of the growth plate is provided by the:

1. Epiphyseal vessels,
2. Metaphyseal vessels,
3. Vessels from the perichondrial ring of LaCroix.

The epiphyseal vessels are the main source of blood. However, in the physes of the proximal femur and proximal humerus, where the epiphysis is fully covered by articular cartilage, the main source of vascularity is the metaphyseal vessels.

The blood supply to these physes can be significantly compromised in severe injuries that cause epiphyseal separation.

Physeal injuries

Eighteen per cent of all fractures in children are physeal. Boys are affected more than girls and the phalanges are most commonly involved. Over the years, various classification systems based on radiographs have been described: Salter–Harris [1], Ogden [2] and Peterson [3]. The Salter–Harris classification (Figure 15.2), which is based on five fracture patterns, is the one most widely used. This classification not only helps guide the choice of treatment but also predicts the prognosis.

Type I

This is characterized by the separation of the epiphysis from the metaphysis. These fractures are rare and are observed most frequently in infants, involving the proximal or distal humerus and the distal femoral physes. A slipped upper femoral epiphysis (SUFE) can be regarded as a Type I injury (Figure 3.1.3). Radiographs of undisplaced Type I fractures look normal except for soft-tissue swelling; hence, careful examination of the limb is required. Ultrasound, MRI or arthrography may be required to confirm the diagnosis. The aim of treatment is to maintain a satisfactory

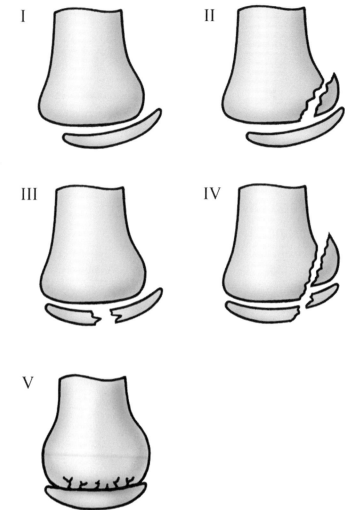

Figure 15.2 Salter–Harris classification.

alignment of the epiphysis and the metaphysis. The prognosis is generally excellent.

Type II

The fracture line extends across the physis and exits through the metaphysis (Thurston Holland fragment) at the opposite end of the fracture (Figure 4.16). This is the most common Salter–Harris fracture pattern. The treatment of choice for displaced fractures is careful gentle closed reduction and immobilization, though occasionally a flap of periosteum may be entrapped between the epiphysis and the metaphysis, blocking reduction. This requires careful surgical exploration to remove the entrapped periosteum. The prognosis is good.

Type III

The fracture line extends through the physis and epiphysis, creating an intra-articular injury, e.g. Tillaux fracture of the ankle (Figure 5.17). These fractures are usually the result of high-energy injuries and thus have a risk of growth disturbance and deformity due to physeal damage.

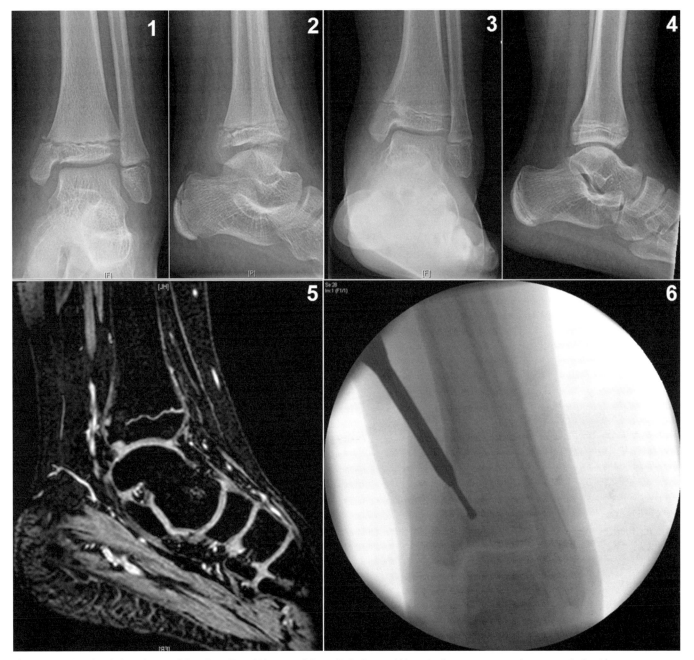

Figure 15.3 Peripheral physeal arrest. Salter–Harris Type IV fracture of the ankle in 8-year-old boy; the fracture was treated non-operatively with a cast. Subsequently, the boy developed a peripheral physeal arrest and distal tibial varus deformity. A bar resection was undertaken and the area packed with fat.

Anatomic open reduction and stabilization with screws is usually required to restore articular congruency. It is advisable to avoid penetration of the joint and the physis with the screws wherever possible.

Type IV

The fracture line extends from the metaphysis, crosses the physis and goes into the epiphysis (Figure 15.3).

This fracture pattern is frequently seen around the medial malleolus but may occur in other physes. Anatomic reduction and adequate stabilization with screws, etc., is required. If treated properly, the prognosis is good.

Type V

This is described as a compression injury to the physis. The initial radiographs are usually normal and these injuries are recognized in hindsight, when an angular deformity or a leg length discrepancy due to physeal fusion develops some time later. A classic example is a recurvatum deformity due to growth arrest affecting the proximal tibial physis.

Type VI (Rang modification)

This involves an injury to the perichondrial ring. Though the prognosis is good, there is a small risk of an angular deformity developing.

Complications

The complications associated with physeal fractures are no different from those of other fractures, except for the complication of physeal growth arrest, which may lead to angular deformity or limb length inequality.

The type and severity of deformity will depend upon:

1. The physis affected (from worst to best: distal femur, distal tibia, proximal tibia and distal radius),
2. The extent and type of physeal injury (from worst to best: Salter–Harris IV, III, I, II),
3. The cause of physeal injury (infection worse than trauma),
4. The size of the physeal bar (the larger, the worse: >50 of the surface area of the physis, 30–50%, <30%),
5. The site of the physeal bar (peripherally located bars are easier to excise than central or linear ones, see Figures 15.3 and 15.4, respectively),
6. The time lapse since injury,
7. The skeletal maturity of the patient.

Identification of the type of growth disturbance is important, as surgery may be required to correct or prevent deformity developing further. In addition to plain radiography, MRI and CT are usually required to define the size and position of a bony bar.

The treatment options are:

- Observation,
- Completion of a partial arrest by epiphysiodesis,
- Physeal bar resection,
- Correction of angular deformity or leg length inequality.

Observation

This is an acceptable option if the physeal bar involves the whole physis and the predicted limb length discrepancy or angular deformity at skeletal maturity is acceptable. This is usually the case in older children approaching maturity.

Completion of a partial arrest

This is done by drill epiphysiodesis and is usually undertaken for eccentric bars, to prevent the deformity worsening. Additional surgery may be required in these cases to correct deformities that are already present.

Resection

Resection of a physeal bar is usually undertaken if significant growth remains (>2 years) and the bar is less than 30% of the surface area of the physis. Following bar resection, it is advisable to fill the space created with autologous fat or polymethylmethacrylate, to prevent reformation of the bar (Figure 15.3).

Correction

Angular deformity can be corrected acutely using standard osteotomy techniques or distraction osteogenesis. The choice of technique depends on the surgeon's expertise, the patient's age and the severity of the deformity.

Leg length discrepancy
Introduction

Leg length inequality is a frequent cause of parental anxiety: 20% of asymptomatic adults have a leg length inequality averaging 5 mm. A variable amount of LLD has been implicated in the development of low back pain, sciatica, scoliosis, stress fractures and plantar fasciitis. The evidence, however, is not compelling.

The femoral head of the longer limb is relatively uncovered by the acetabulum (long leg dysplasia) and over the long term; osteoarthritis is more commonly seen on this side.

Limb length inequality may be due to hemihypertrophy (e.g. Beckwith–Wiedemann syndrome), causing a longer, larger limb, or hemiatrophy (e.g. Russell–Silver syndrome), causing a shorter, thinner limb (Table 15.1).

When managing children with LLD, one must be:

- Comfortable in assessing the patient clinically and radiologically,
- Familiar with the possible causes,
- Able to predict the discrepancy at skeletal maturity,
- Able to choose the most appropriate treatment options for each case.

Evaluation

- Evaluation commences with a history, in particular childhood illness: i.e. meningitis, injury or fracture and family history of skeletal dysplasia.
- Clinical examination should include a general assessment, looking for asymmetry, enlarged tongue and cutaneous manifestations, i.e. vascular anomalies. Be alert to such diagnoses as Proteus syndrome, Klippel–Trénaunay–Weber syndrome or Beckwith–Wiedemann syndrome. Examine for operative scars and café au lait spots.
- Gait may reveal compensatory mechanisms, including circumduction, persistent flexion of the knee of the longer limb, vaulting over the longer limb or toe walking on the shorter side. Characteristically, on the short side, the stance stride is shorter and there is reduced push-off. A shoulder dip is found if there is any vaulting.
- The degree of functional discrepancy is best assessed clinically by getting the patient to stand on graduated blocks under the shorter leg until the pelvis is level (Figure 2.4).
- With the patient supine, the pelvis is squared. Examination for flexion and adduction deformities in the hip and flexion of the knee and ankle can then be performed. The segment that is shorter is then ascertained (Galeazzi's test,

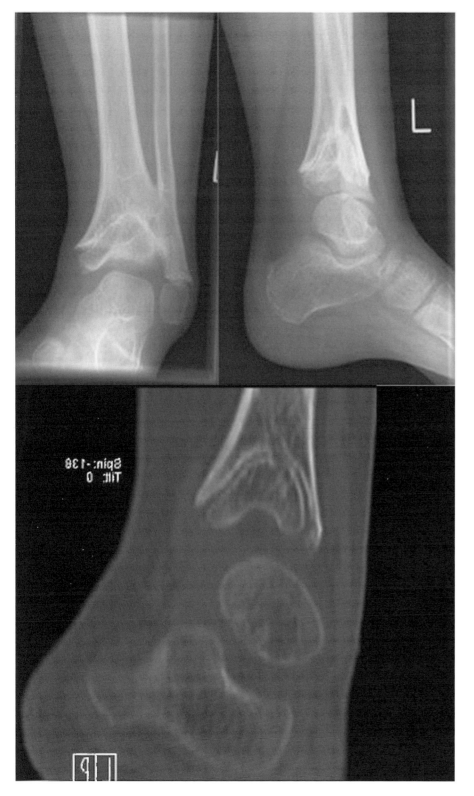

Figure 15.4 Central physeal arrest.

Figure 2.5). The size of the feet and any other abnormalities are noted.

- Neurological examination of the lower limbs and spinal examination completes the clinical assessment.

- Standing long leg radiographs of both lower limbs with an appropriate block under the short limb to level the pelvis are suggested. They are useful to quantify not only LLD but also any angular malformation.

- Computed tomography is also popular, with lower radiation exposure and great accuracy.
- Identifying the cause of LLD is important, as this will influence the prediction of LLD at maturity. Shapiro [4] analyzed LLD data in 803 patients and demonstrated that not all discrepancies increase at a constant rate over time. (Not all growth inhibition in growing children exhibits a linear pattern.)
- Shapiro described five basic patterns of leg length inequality (Table 15.2 and Figure 15.5).

Predicting leg length discrepancy

Being able to predict LLD at maturity is essential and helps one decide the best treatment option and when to intervene.

Table 15.1 Causes of leg length discrepancy (LLD)

Congenital	Dislocated hip (DDH), Longitudinal deficiency (congenital short femur, fibula or tibia hemimelia), Hemihypertrophy (Klippel–Trénaunay–Weber, Beckwith–Wiedemann or idiopathic), Hemiatrophy syndromes
Trauma	Diaphyseal fracture with either excessive shortening or overgrowth, epiphyseal injury with growth arrest
Infection	Septic arthritis, Meningococcal sepsis
Neuromuscular	Cerebral palsy, Spinal disorders
Neoplastic	Haemangiomas, Neurofibromatosis
Inflammatory	Juvenile idiopathic arthritis (leads to overgrowth)

Table 15.2 Shapiro's five basic patterns of LLD

Type	Description	Examples
I	Upward slope pattern There is a consistent rate of growth inhibition of the shorter leg.	Epiphyseal arrest, Ollier disease, proximal femoral focal deficiency.
II	Upward slope–deceleration pattern The rate of growth inhibition decreases over time.	Neuromuscular conditions.
III	Upward slope–plateau pattern After an initial constant growth inhibition, the legs grow at the same rate (plateau).	The overgrowth seen after femoral-shaft fractures.
IV	Upward slope–plateau–upward slope pattern A constant rate of growth inhibition is interrupted by a period of growth at the same rate.	Severe LCPD: there is an initial shortening due to collapse of the femoral head that leads to an LLD, which after some time increases again as a result of premature physeal arrest.
V	Upward slope–plateau–downward slope The slower-growing limb exhibits an initial growth deceleration, followed by symmetric growth and finally increased growth compared with the contralateral limb.	Juvenile idiopathic arthritis.

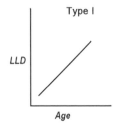

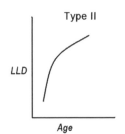

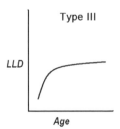

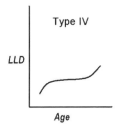

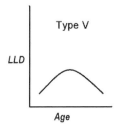

Figure 15.5 Shapiro's developmental patterns of LLD.

The methods available are:

1. Green–Anderson growth remaining chart [5],
2. Menelaus method,
3. The Moseley straight-line graph,
4. Paley's multiplier method.

All these methods assume that there is a constant (linear) rate of increase in LLD (Shapiro Type I) and that growth ends at 14 years in girls and 16 years in boys. In addition, knowledge of the percentage contribution of various physes to yearly increase in height is essential (Table 15.3).

Green–Anderson growth remaining chart

This predicts the growth remaining in the femur and the tibia (of each limb; the short and long) relative to the skeletal age of the patient (Figure 15.6). The skeletal age can be determined by taking wrist radiographs and comparing them with the Greulich and Pyle atlas.

Menelaus method

This method is also called the rule of thumb. During the last 2 years of growth, 9 mm of growth per year is from the femur and 6 mm of growth per year is from the tibia.

The Moseley straight-line graph

This method requires a special graph for each patient (Figure 15.7) and a number of radiological examinations (the lengths of the normal and shorter legs and the skeletal age) on at least three different occasions over a period of time.

Table 15.3 Contribution of various bones toward growth of entire limb

	Site	Contribution (%)
Lower limb	Proximal femur	15
	Distal femur	40
	Proximal tibia	30
	Distal tibia	15
Upper limb	Proximal humerus	40%
	Distal humerus	10%
	Proximal radius	10%
	Distal radius	40%

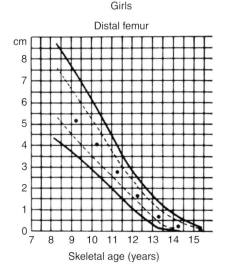

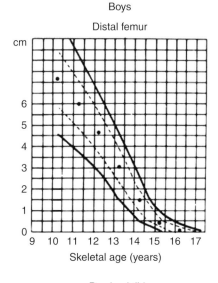

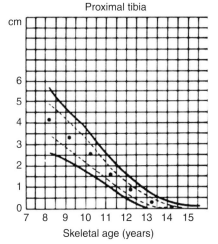

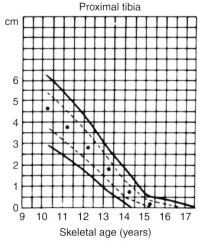

Figure 15.6 Green–Anderson graphs of remaining growth for girls and boys. Dashed line, 1 SD of the mean. Solid line 2 SD of the mean.

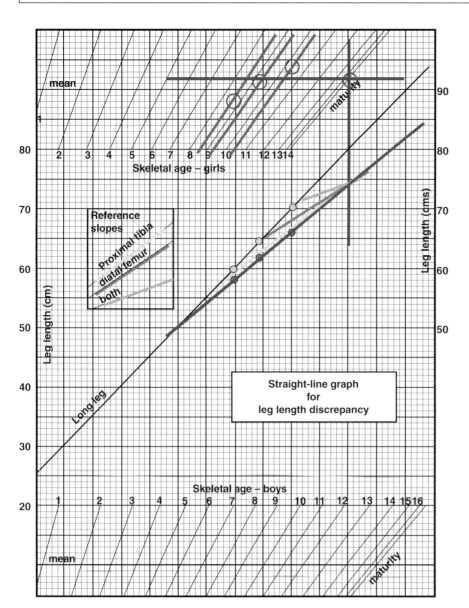

Figure 15.7 Moseley straight-line method for predicting LLD.

With this information, an estimate of the time of skeletal maturity can be made. The projected LLD can then be derived by drawing a straight line for each leg through the measured points. Using the reference slopes, one can then determine when epiphysiodesis could be done (see Chapter 19 for illustration).

Paley's multiplier method

Paley [6] introduced the multiplier method to estimate the LLD and patient's height at skeletal maturity. He identified an arithmetic factor (called it a multiplier) by dividing femoral and tibial lengths at skeletal maturity by the femoral and tibial lengths at different ages. The length of each leg at skeletal maturity can be calculated by multiplying the current length by the appropriate multiplier for the subject's age and sex:

mature (segment) length = present (segment) length × multiplier.

The segment could be tibia, femur, both or patient height. There is a multiplier for every patient age. This multiplier varies according to sex and the cause of the LLD (congenital or developmental). Online software and apps have been produced to help surgeons and parents to predict their children's height, LLD and foot size.

Treatment

The objective of treatment is to achieve near-equal leg lengths at skeletal maturity without excessive risk, morbidity or height reduction. The treatment algorithm generally used is depicted in Table 15.4 but the clinician must assess each case based on its own merits. In paralytic cases, such as cerebral palsy or myelomeningocele, it is advisable to undercorrect the LLD by

Table 15.4 Recommended treatment options according to LLD

Discrepancy	Treatment options
0–2 cm	No treatment if asymptomatic, shoe raise, epiphysiodesis
2–5 cm	Shoe raise, epiphysiodesis, limb lengthening, limb shortening
5–15 cm	Lengthening may be combined with epiphysiodesis or a shortening procedure
>15 cm	Lengthening and epiphysiodesis or shortening or ablative surgery and prosthetic use

leaving the weaker lower limb slightly shorter, thus facilitating clearance of the foot in the swing phase of gait.

Non-operative

Shoe raises are not easily accepted by all patients and tend to be used as a short-term measure, especially for the younger child. A raise of up to 1 cm can be fitted in the shoe, while a raise greater than 1 cm is best fitted to the sole of the shoe, to make it easier to walk.

Operative

Epiphysiodesis

Epiphysiodesis is the treatment of choice for smaller discrepancies (usually 2–5 cm) but may also be used in combination with other modalities for larger discrepancies.

The percutaneous drill technique (under X-ray guidance) is commonly used. This produces a permanent physeal growth arrest; it is important to time the surgery accurately using growth charts, as previously described.

Epiphysiodesis may be undertaken using 8-plates or staples. The effect is reversible and physeal growth resumes when the plates or staples are removed. This method is useful in situations when it is difficult to predict the timing of epiphysiodesis accurately, or in the younger child.

Acute bone shortening

This is usually undertaken in the skeletally mature patient for discrepancies of 2–5 cm.

There is a lower complication rate than lengthening procedures. Tibial shortening is undertaken less frequently than femoral shortening because it is technically more challenging and the complications, including vascular compromise and compartment syndrome, are more frequent and significant.

Femoral shortening may result in an extensor lag due to quadriceps muscle weakening and shortening should be limited to 10% or less of the original femoral length.

Lengthening

This is usually done gradually using external fixators, which may be circular or uniplanar.

In the skeletally mature patient, lengthening may be undertaken using a lengthening intramedullary rod.

Corticotomy for lengthening is done using a gigli saw or a drill and osteotomes.

Distraction is usually started 5–7 days after surgery. Lengthening is at the rate of 1 mm/day or slower, if the regenerate is poor.

In the presence of acetabular dysplasia, the hip joint may sublux during femoral lengthening and the dysplasia must be addressed surgically prior to lengthening.

In fibula hemimelia, it is important to span the knee joint with the fixator during femoral lengthening to prevent knee subluxation or dislocation.

Complications of limb lengthening include pin site infection, osteomyelitis, wire breakage, poor regenerate formation, premature regenerate consolidation, neurovascular injury, joint stiffness, joint subluxation or dislocation and regenerate fracture.

References

1. Salter R and Harris W (1963) Injuries involving the epiphyseal plate. *J Bone Joint Surg Am* **45A:** 587–622.

2. Ogden JA (1981) Injury to the growth mechanisms of the immature skeleton. *Skeletal Radiol* **6**(4):237–53.

3. Peterson CA and Peterson HA (1972) Analysis of the incidence of injuries to the epiphyseal growth plate. *J Trauma* **12**(4):275–81.

4. Shapiro F (1982) Developmental patterns in lower-extremity length discrepancies. *J Bone Joint Surg Am* **64**(5):639–51.

5. Anderson M, Green WT and Messner MB (1963) Growth and predictions of growth in the lower extremities. *J Bone Joint Surg Am* **45-A:**1–14.

6. Paley D, Bhave A, Herzenberg JE and Bowen JR (2000) Multiplier method for predicting limb length discrepancy. *J Bone Joint Surg Am* **82-A**(10): 1432–46.

Chapter

16

Deformity corrections

Farhan Ali and Alwyn Abraham

Introduction

A limb deformity can be defined as distortion from the normal form. Malalignment refers to loss of collinearity of the hip, knee and ankle. It is therefore possible to have a deformity without malalignment. Deformity and malalignment can lead to pain, abnormal gait, loss of function and cosmetic deformity. Accurate assessment of deformity, planning of correction and choice of the most appropriate management tool are the keys to success in managing these complex patients.

Our understanding of assessment and management of deformity has progressed significantly in the last century. In particular, the understanding of biomechanics of the musculoskeletal system aided by the development of sophisticated computerized gait analysis. The concept of distraction histogenesis was pioneered by Professor Gavriil Ilizarov. He used circular frames to treat non-unions by compression. He noted that bone had formed at a fracture site after distraction when one of his patients misunderstood the instructions and turned the nuts in the wrong direction, lengthening the fracture site rather than compressing it. He called this 'distraction histogenesis' and he subsequently used it for limb lengthening, for gradual correction of bony deformity and for bone transport to correct intercalary bone defects. Dror Paley deciphered the intuitive deformity assessment and planning performed by 'Ilizarov' surgeons, and developed an easy and systematic approach to understanding lower-limb deformity and planning treatment [1]. Dr Charles Taylor introduced the Taylor spatial frame, which is the external fixator most commonly used for deformity correction in the Western world.

Rationale for deformity correction
Cosmesis

A mild or gradually developing deformity may manifest initially with only a visible deformity. The cosmetic appearance in such cases may be alarming to parents and might be the initial reason for consultation. Even with startlingly obvious deformities, an infant often functions well and will easily adapt to physical activities. The absence of early joint degeneration precludes the presence of pain.

Loss of function

Gage lucidly describes the function of bones as levers. With joints functioning as pivots and muscles generating force, the femur and tibia provide mechanical advantage for the generation of torque (principle of moments) and to facilitate an energy efficient gait cycle. With a deformed and therefore less efficient lever, the amount of torque generated is suboptimal and muscle fatigue occurs during gait. The objective of deformity correction is to restore the anatomical alignment of the femur and tibia, such that a child's efficient gait and exercise tolerance is restored.

Joint pain and progressive osteoarthritis

In spite of severe longstanding deformities, it is rare to encounter radiological osteoarthritis, even in adolescents. Joint pain, if reported, is likely to be due to synovitis, abnormal joint shear stresses or joint instability secondary to deformity. There is evidence to associate a distal femoral valgus deformity with lateral compartment osteoarthritis of the knee. Likewise, distal femoral varus and proximal tibial varus are associated with medial compartment osteoarthritis of the knee. Related data implicate the effects of distal tibial varus and valgus with subsequent ankle and subtalar osteoarthritis.

Assessing limb deformity
History

A comprehensive history will determine symptoms and functional loss. It is important to understand the patient's expectations for surgery. Obtain a detailed history of previous treatments, including non-operative and operative interventions. Where appropriate, obtain a specific history, dependent on the underlying diagnosis; for example, a patient with achondroplasia may have sleep apnoea, while congenital pseudarthrosis of tibia is most probably a feature of Type I

Postgraduate Paediatric Orthopaedics, ed. Sattar Alshryda, Stan Jones and Paul A. Banaszkiewicz. Published by Cambridge University Press. © Cambridge University Press 2014.

Table 16.1 Causes of limb deformity

Congenital	Acquired
Proximal femoral focal deficiency, Postero medial tibial bowing, Fibular hemimelia, Tibial pseudarthrosis, Blount's disease, Skeletal dysplasias, e.g. multiple hereditary exostosis	Malunion, Infection, Metabolic bone disease, Physeal arrest, Neurological condition (cerebral palsy and polio), Joints diseases and contractures (DDH, LCPD)

neurofibromatosis. Hypophosphataemic rickets runs in the family, as it has an X-linked inheritance. Some diagnoses are listed in Table 16.1.

Clinical assessment

This should include the following:

1. Segment and site of deformity; this is generally obvious from the history and clinical examination findings.
2. Congenital vs acquired causes (Table 16.1): congenital causes are occasionally not detected at birth.

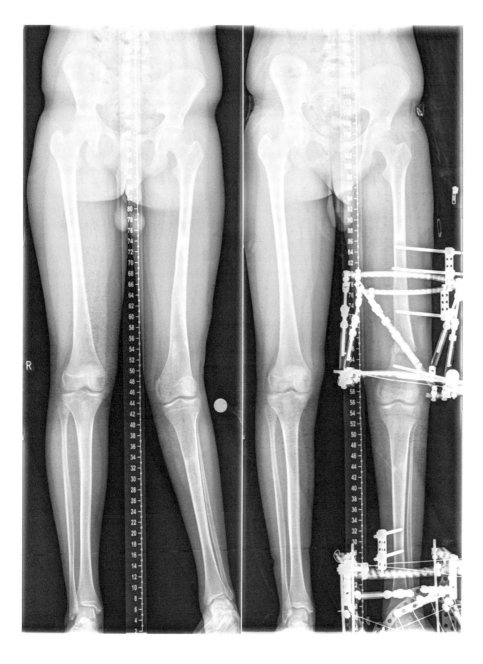

Figure 16.1 Distal femoral deformity with distal subtalar fixed deformity. A 14-year-old who had previous foot surgery presented with genu valgum. He was noticed to have plantigrade feet but with fixed supination. Isolated correction of the knee deformity would uncouple the foot deformity, so both were addressed together.

3. Leg length discrepancy: lower-limb deformity is often associated with LLD (axial deformity) and, in some cases, LLD may be the presenting symptom.

Gait

Clinical assessment begins with examination of gait. For genu varum deformities, it is important to look for a lateral thrust at the knee, to give an idea of instability or laxity.

Examine the deformity, paying attention to rotational or torsional abnormalities. Also, assess the limb for any compensatory deformities, e.g. varus deformity at the ankle is compensated by eversion at the subtalar joint and supination at the forefoot. If any of these deformities is fixed, this would need to be addressed at the time of treatment (Figure 16.1).

Joints

Examine joints both above and below the deformity for range of motion, to rule out fixed contractures. It is important to assess for any joint laxity or instability. Uncorrected fixed joint contracture, either below or above the deformity, will lead to secondary difficulties after surgery. Joint contractures and laxity can be part of the deformity. If unrecognized, they may lead to under- or overcorrection. For example, a patient with a recurvatum bony deformity of the ankle may also have a planter flexion deformity of the ankle, and if this is not addressed at the time of surgery, it will lead to an equinus contracture of the foot. A lax lateral collateral ligament in a child with achondroplasia may give rise to a genu varum deformity. Any joint instability will put the joint at risk of subluxation or dislocation following deformity correction and lengthening.

Leg length discrepancy

Both apparent and true LLD should be assessed clinically and radiologically. Estimates of height and limb length discrepancy at maturity should be made (see Chapter 15).

Neurovascular status

Carry out a careful examination of neurovascular status. In children with hereditary multiple exostosis and achondroplasia, it is important to rule out spinal stenosis, to prevent neurological injury following treatment of deformities.

Radiological assessment

The effect of body weight on lower-limb alignment is seen on standing radiographs. The patellae should be 'neutral' (facing forward) and blocks should be used to square the pelvis, as this will remove possible compensatory errors from hip or knee flexion. The superimposition of a metric ruler allows calibration to measure the LLD.

There are three methods in common use to obtain long leg alignment views [2]:

Teleoroentgenography:	A long film and a ruler are placed under the patient, and a single exposure is made, centred over the limbs.
Orthoroentgenography:	A long film and a ruler are placed under the patient. Several exposures are made at the hip, knee and ankle levels, without moving the patient or the film. These exposures are stitched together.
Scanography:	The film is advanced under the joint to be radiographed and exposed sequentially.

The state of the physes should be noted. Occasionally, it will be important to obtain special X-rays to estimate bone age. The most commonly used method is that described by Greulich and Pyle, where radiographs of the left hand are used to estimate the bone age. This is particularly important if planning to address the deformity correction using hemiepiphysiodesis.

Steps for radiological assessment of deformity

1. Ensure good quality X-rays.
2. Mechanical axis deviation test: A line is drawn from the centre of the femoral head to the centre of the ankle joint in the coronal plane. This should pass within 8 mm of the centre of the knee joint.
3. Joint orientation angles: The mechanical axis line connects the centre of a proximal joint to the centre of the distal joint. The anatomic axis line is the mid-diaphyseal line. The mechanical axis is a feature of the coronal plane only, while the anatomic axis line is used in both coronal and sagittal planes. The orientation of each joint can be measured using angles (named joint orientation angles) created by these lines and the joint surface lines (JOLs). Table 16.2 lists, and Figure 16.2 shows, these angles. Their nomenclature is standardized: axis (m, mechanical; a, anatomical), side (M, medial; L, lateral), site (P, proximal; D, distal), bone (F, femur; T, tibia).

Table 16.2 Joint orientation angles (°)

Mechanical		Anatomical	
mLPFA	90 (85–95)	MPFA	84 (80–89)
mLDFA	87 (85–90)	NSA	124–136
JLCA	0–2	aLDFA	81 (79–83)
MPTA	87 (85–90)	JLCA	0–2
mLDTA	89 (86–92)	MPTA	87 (85–90)
		LDTA	89 (86–92)

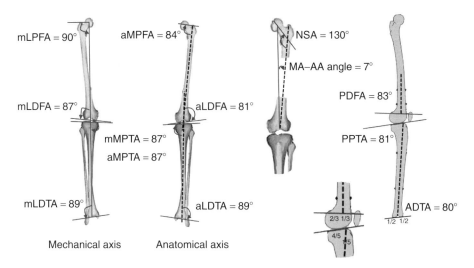

mLPFA = 90°   aMPFA = 84°   NSA = 130°

MA–AA angle = 7°

mLDFA = 87°   aLDFA = 81°   PDFA = 83°

mMPTA = 87°   PPTA = 81°
aMPTA = 87°

mLDTA = 89°   aLDTA = 89°   ADTA = 80°

2/3 1/3   1/2 1/2
4/5
4/5

Mechanical axis   Anatomical axis

Figure 16.2 Lower-limb alignment in the frontal and sagittal planes. Mechanical lateral proximal femoral angle (mLPFA), 90°; mechanical lateral distal femoral angle (mLDFA), 87°; mechanical lateral distal tibial angle (mLDTA), 89°; anatomical medial proximal femoral angle (aMPFA), 84°; anatomical lateral distal femoral angle (aLDFA), 81°. Note the difference of 7° between the anatomical and mechanical femoral angles, reflecting the angle between the femoral mechanical axis (MA) and the anatomic axis (AA). The tibial mechanical and anatomical angles are the same, because the axes are the same. In the sagittal plane, only the anatomical axis is used; this represents the mid-diaphyseal lines of the bones; these intersect the joint edge lines at the junction between the anterior third and the posterior two-thirds at the femur, the junction between the anterior fifth and posterior four-fifths at the proximal tibia, and the junction halfway along the distal tibia.

The mechanical lateral distal femoral angle (mLDFA) and medial proximal tibial angle (MPTA) should each be around 87°. The mechanical lateral proximal femoral angle (mLPFA) and mechanical lateral distal tibial angle (mLDTA) should be around 90°. A joint line convergence angle (JLCA) greater than 2° would be considered abnormal laxity of the joint, which would contribute to mechanical axis deviation.

4. Rule out knee subluxation in the coronal plane: The midpoints of the femoral and tibial joint lines at the knee should be within 3 mm of each other.

5. Rule out a condylar deficiency at the knee: Any deficiency of either the femoral condyles or tibial hemiplateau should be noted, as this may be the source of mechanical axis deviation.

Pitfalls

- It is possible to have a normal mechanical axis with deformities in the hip or close to the ankle joint.
- It is possible to have a normal mechanical axis with malorientation of the joint lines around the knee.

Radiological planning for the management of the deformity

Femoral deformities can have either mechanical axis or anatomic axis planning, depending on the mode of correction. Generally, it is safer to use mechanical axis planning and this is most commonly used when gradual correction is performed using external fixators. Anatomic axis planning is used for diaphyseal deformities that are being corrected with an intramedullary nail.

Pitfall

Rotational deformity cannot be assessed on an X-radiograph. Clinical assessment should be supplemented with CT examination.

Concept of CORA

Mechanical and anatomic axes are straight lines; however, when there is a deformity, these lines are no longer straight

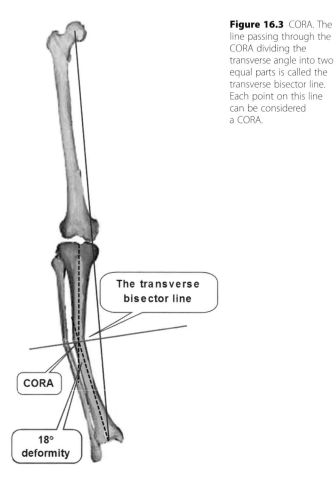

The transverse bisector line

CORA

18° deformity

Figure 16.3 CORA. The line passing through the CORA dividing the transverse angle into two equal parts is called the transverse bisector line. Each point on this line can be considered a CORA.

and create an angle. The CORA (centre of rotation of angulation) is the intersection points of the anatomical or mechanical axes when there is a deformity (Figure 16.3). A simple malunited fracture usually has one CORA but a bone with congenital bowing may have several CORAs. If the CORA does not coincide with an obvious deformity, there may be a hidden deformity.

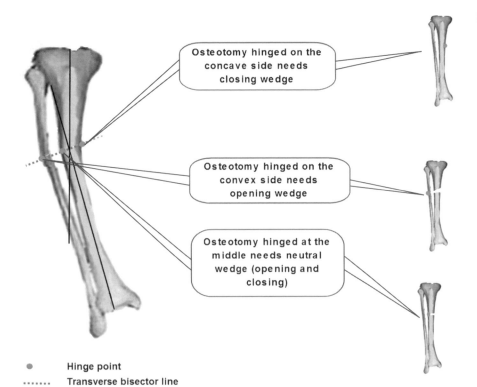

Figure 16.4 Osteotomy rule 1.

Osteotomy hinged on the concave side needs closing wedge

Osteotomy hinged on the convex side needs opening wedge

Osteotomy hinged at the middle needs neutral wedge (opening and closing)

●   Hinge point

······   Transverse bisector line

Osteotomy rules

To correct a deformity, the bone is divided (osteotomy). Careful planning of the osteotomy and the hinge around which the bone will be rotated is vital for good correction. The following rules are useful:

Rule 1

The osteotomy should pass through the transverse bisector line. If the hinge is placed on the convex side, an opening wedge is needed; if on the concave side, a closing wedge; and if at the centre, a half-closing and half-opening (neutral) wedge (Figure 16.4).

Rule 2

If the osteotomy is performed at a different level from the CORA, then translation occurs.

Rule 3

If the osteotomy is performed at a different level from the CORA but a hinge is placed at the osteotomy site, the mechanical axis becomes parallel but anatomical axis becomes zigzagged (Figure 16.5).

Rule 4

The point where the mechanical axes of the proximal and distal segments meet is termed the resolved CORA. If an

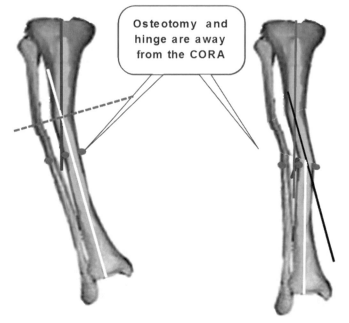

Osteotomy and hinge are away from the CORA

Figure 16.5 Osteotomy rule 3.

osteotomy is performed at the resolved CORA, the limb is functionally normal; this avoids multiple osteotomies.

Rule 5

If the osteotomy is performed through the resolution CORA, rather than the true multiple apices, the mechanical axis and joint orientation will be corrected with a residual alteration in the anatomic axis of the bone. This may be a cosmetic problem but it does not affect joint orientation or mechanical axis alignment.

Techniques to correct deformity

Acute correction

Mild to moderate deformities can be corrected acutely and then stabilized, either internally or using external fixators (Figure 16.6). Generally, deformities greater than 30° carry a risk of neurovascular injury and compartment syndrome and acute correction should be avoided. Acute correction can be stabilized using either plates and screws or intramedullary nails.

Plates and screws

Advantage: Ideally suited for peri-articular deformities, where external fixation carries a risk of spreading infection into the joint and is also likely to cause stiffness.

Disadvantage: Generally more invasive.

Intramedullary nail

Advantages: Minimally invasive techniques, percutaneous osteotomy. Ideally suited for diaphyseal and rotational deformities.

Disadvantages: Osteotomy rule 1 is applicable, as there is very limited scope for correction with translation.

Gradual correction

Hemiepiphysiodesis

This is a technique to inhibit growth on one side of the physis to correct the deformity. Inhibition of growth can be temporary or permanent. Older techniques using a Phemister bone block and drill epiphysiodesis can only be used toward the end of growth. Temporary epiphysiodesis can be done using staples and 8-plates and is particularly useful in younger patients.

Temporary: 8-plates, staples, etc.

Permanent: Drill hemiepiphysiodesis, Phemister bone block technique.

Distraction osteogenesis

This utilizes Ilizarov's principles to correct deformities using external fixators. These can be summarized as:

- Stable construct,
- Low-energy osteotomy (preservation of blood supply),
- Latency period of 5 to 7 days,

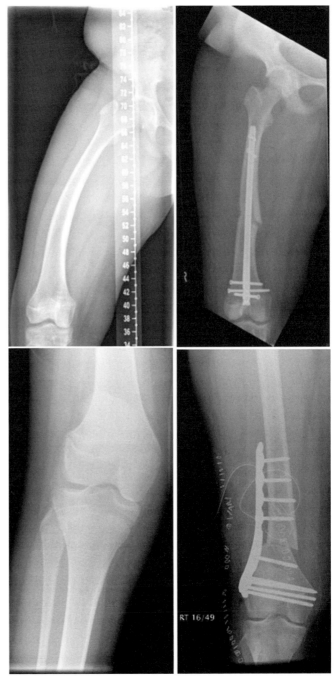

Figure 16.6 Acute deformity corrections.

- Rate and rhythm of 1 mm distraction per day in four divided stages.

External fixators used for distraction osteogenesis can be monolateral or circular.

Monolateral fixator

Advantages: Patient comfort; causes minimal interference with joint range of motion.

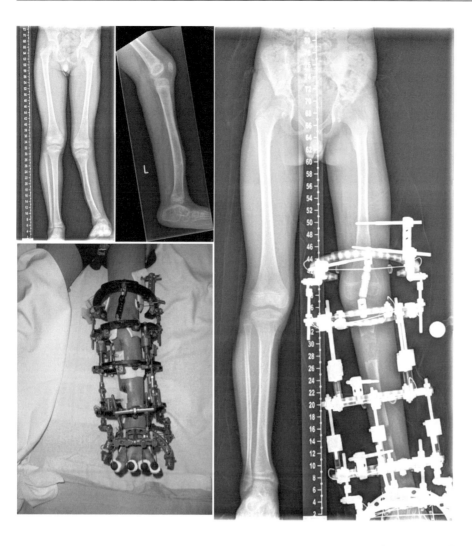

Figure 16.7 Fibular hemimelia deformity correction.

Disadvantages: Often rotational deformities are corrected acutely at the time of surgery. Generally less margin of error and less manoeuvrability than circular fixator.

Circular fixators

These are versatile deformity correction tools; all aspects of deformity can be corrected gradually with this fixator. They are broadly of two types – the traditional Ilizarov type fixators and hexapod fixators. Of the hexapod fixators, the Taylor spatial frame is most popularly used in the UK and North America (Figure 16.7).

Advantages: All aspects of the deformity can be corrected gradually. It is mechanically more stable.

Disadvantages: Fine wire fixation around the joints can cause patient discomfort, joint stiffness and are prone to infection. Techniques using half pins can give these fixators the advantage of monolateral fixators with the versatility of circular fixators.

Taylor spatial frame

To correct a deformity using a Taylor spatial frame (Figure 16.8), the following are required:
1. The type and magnitude of the deformity,
2. The shape of the frame and its mounting parameters to the bone,
3. Structures at risk (such as common peroneal nerve when correcting valgus leg),
4. The safe duration of deformity correction.

The type and magnitude of the deformity

Whether dealing with a fracture or deformity, there are two bony fragments, traditionally called proximal and distal. In the language of the Taylor spatial frame, these become the 'reference' and 'moving' fragments. Either can be the proximal or the distal fragment. There are six deformity measurements of the moving fragment in relationship to the reference fragment to be identified (Figure 16.9):
1. AP view angulation,
2. AP view translation,

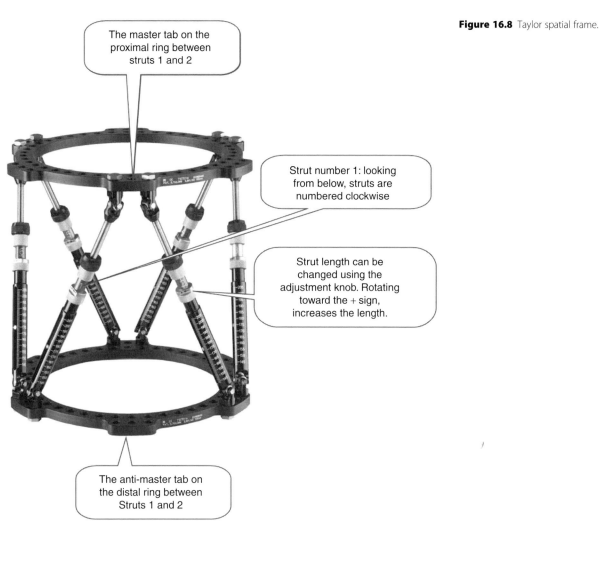

The master tab on the proximal ring between struts 1 and 2

Strut number 1: looking from below, struts are numbered clockwise

Strut length can be changed using the adjustment knob. Rotating toward the + sign, increases the length.

The anti-master tab on the distal ring between Struts 1 and 2

Figure 16.8 Taylor spatial frame.

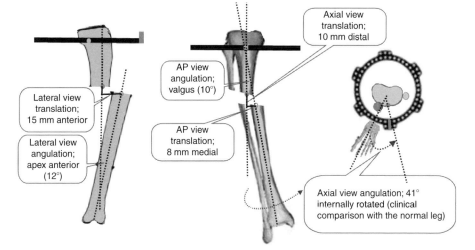

Axial view translation; 10 mm distal

AP view angulation; valgus (10°)

AP view translation; 8 mm medial

Lateral view translation; 15 mm anterior

Lateral view angulation; apex anterior (12°)

Axial view angulation; 41° internally rotated (clinical comparison with the normal leg)

Figure 16.9 Deformity description in the Taylor spatial frame. There are six deformity measurements; angulation and translation for each view (AP, lateral and axial).

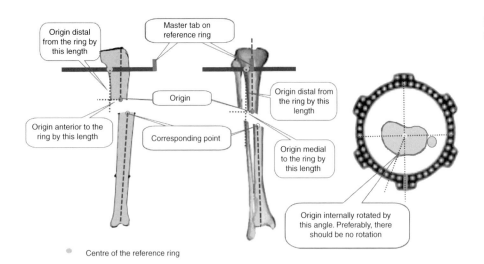

Figure 16.10 Mounting parameters for Taylor spatial frame.

Centre of the reference ring

3. Lateral view angulation,
4. Lateral view translation,
5. Axial view angulation,
6. Axial view translation.

The shape of the frame and its mounting parameters to the bone

To identify any object in space, three points are needed. In the context of the Taylor spatial frame, each fragment is identified by a ring (two points) and another point in that particular fragment. This third point is called the 'origin' on the reference fragment and the 'corresponding point' on the moving fragment. The best choices for origin and corresponding points are points that are coincident in the anatomic (reduced) state. In fractures, these are the broken ends of the bone. In congenital deformity correction, the choice may be slightly more complicated and is beyond the scope of this chapter. To identify a fragment to the software, the position of the origin to the centre of the reference ring must be known. This is usually measured on radiographs in three dimensions (Figure 16.10).

Theoretically, rings can be mounted anywhere; provided we know the exact mounting parameters, we should be able to correct the deformity. However, in practice, we tend to mount the ring in a way to minimize mounting parameters, measurements and errors. Rings should be mounted parallel to a nearby joint line and as close as possible to the origin. Although, only the mounting parameters of the reference ring are important, it is still good practice to mount both rings as if they were reference rings (to allow flexibility to use either as a reference ring if it is needed).

The reference ring carries what is called 'the master tab', which is the tab between Strut 1 and Strut 2 that denotes the ring (and the frame) rotation. Ideally, the ring should be mounted so that the reference ring rotation is 0° (not always practical).

The size and type of the proximal and distal rings, the size of the struts and their lengths should be identified for the software in order to produce the 'prescription' for deformity correction.

Structures at risk and the rate of safe distraction

The structure at risk, if there is any, can be identified by providing its distance from the origin on the AP, lateral and axial views. Finally, the maximum safe distraction rate must be entered. One mm per day is generally accepted.

References

1. Paley D and Herzenberg JE (2003) *Principle of Deformity Correction*, volume 2. Berlin: Springer.

2. Herring JA (2008) *Tachdjian's Pediatric Orthopaedics*, 4th edition, volume 1. Philadelphia: Saunders Elsevier.

Miscellaneous paediatric conditions

Kathryn Price and Akinwanda Adedapo

Non-accidental injury
Background

Ambrose Tardieu first reported non-accidental injury (NAI) in 1860, noting the correlation between cutaneous lesions, fractures, subdural haematomas and death [1]. Caffey again highlighted the association between long bone fractures and subdural haematomas in 1946 [2]. However, it was Henry Kempe who raised the profile of NAI in 1962 when he coined the term 'battered-child syndrome' [3]. He described the association between multiple fractures, subdural haematomas, failure to thrive, soft-tissue swelling or bruising and sudden unexplained death. He also highlighted the importance of situations in which the type or degree of injury did not correlate with the history. The US Child Abuse Prevention and Treatment Act (CAPTA) defines child abuse and neglect as:

> Any act or failure to act resulting in imminent risk of death, serious physical or emotional harm, sexual abuse or exploitation of a child by a parent or caretaker who is responsible for a child's welfare.

Child abuse is more common than most would expect; it is estimated that 7% of children suffer serious physical abuse. Studies suggest that 25% of fatally abused children had been seen recently by a healthcare provider [4].

Predisposing factors

It has been postulated that three common factors exist where child abuse has taken place. These include [5, 6]:

- A child with provocative qualities.
- Abuse is more common in the first-born child, unplanned pregnancies, premature delivery, stepfamilies, multiple births and children with special needs.
- A carer with a psychological predisposition.
- Young, poor, single, violent or unemployed carers as well as those having a personal history of abuse.
- A stressful event that triggers a violent reaction.

There is a clear connection between drug or alcohol abuse and child abuse.

Injury patterns

The following patterns should raise a suspicion of child abuse:

- Injuries that are multiple, frequent, or of different ages.
- Injury that is not consistent with the stated history or the developmental age of child.
- Delayed presentation, reluctance to seek help or fear of medical examination.
- Attendance at different surgeries or departments (to avoid detection of repeated injuries).
- Unexplained denial or aggression.
- No explanation for the injuries, a story that changes on repetition or child's story that differs from the carer's.
- Bruising in the shape of a hand, ligature, stick, tooth mark, grip, fingertips or implement. Bruises at sites where accidental bruising is unusual: face, eyes, ears (bruising around the pinna may be subtle), neck and top of shoulder, anterior chest, abdomen.
- Petechiae (tiny red or purple spots) not caused by a medical condition – these may be due to shaking or suffocation.
- The following fractures should raise suspicions:

1. Metaphyseal fractures (Figure 17.1),
2. Rib fractures (Figure 17.2),
3. Complex or wide (diastatic) skull fractures,
4. Digital fractures,
5. Any scapular fracture,
6. Fractures of different ages (Figure 17.3),
7. Bilateral or multiple diaphyseal fractures.

Clinical assessment

Careful detailed documentation is absolutely essential in suspected cases of NAI. It can be extremely difficult to distinguish deliberate from accidental injury and often it is only

Postgraduate Paediatric Orthopaedics, ed. Sattar Alshryda, Stan Jones and Paul A. Banaszkiewicz. Published by Cambridge University Press.
© Cambridge University Press 2014.

inconsistencies in the history that reveal the underlying problem. A careful history must be taken, detailing the events leading to injury. Very close attention must be paid to the timing of events. Delayed presentation is very common in NAI. It is also important to get a clear story relating to the mechanism of injury, so that this can be compared with injury patterns. In NAI there is commonly a discrepancy between the type or degree of injury sustained and the suggested mechanism. It is also vital to record any unusual behaviour on the part of the child or carer and ideally, in older patients, to obtain a history directly from the child.

A careful past medical and developmental history needs to be obtained and documented. It can be very important to note previous injuries, as well as any family history of multiple fractures that suggests an underlying condition, such as osteogenesis imperfecta. The achievement of developmental milestones is important, particularly ambulatory status.

For children who are ambulatory, the likelihood of fractures being due to NAI is markedly reduced.

It is important to examine presenting injury carefully, with meticulous documentation of findings. In suspected cases of NAI, it is vital to examine the whole child thoroughly, looking for other injuries. Multiple injuries at various stages of healing are strongly associated with NAI. All injuries must be catalogued, including the site, size and colour of any skin lesions for comparison at a later date. Ideally, clinical photographs should be taken from two different views for adequate documentation. Similarly, any fractures must be clearly documented, including fracture site, presumed mechanism of injury, level of displacement and stage of healing [5].

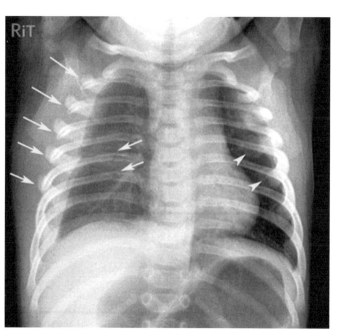

Figure 17.1 Metaphyseal fracture of distal femur. Metaphyseal corner fractures are considered pathognomic for non-accidental injury, and are commonly called classical metaphyseal lesions (CML). They are caused by indirect gripping and twisting forces on the limb.

Figure 17.2 Multiple rib fractures. Rib fractures have a very high specificity for non-accidental injury in the absence of a history of major trauma, such as a road traffic accident. In a child with proven NAI, there were multiple rib fractures of different healing stages (note the callus formation on the left side and its absence on the right).

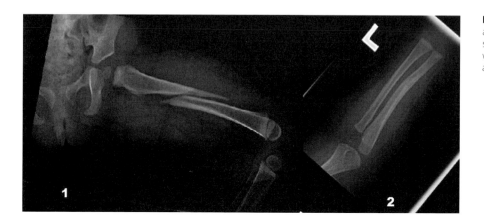

Figure 17.3 Multiple bone fractures of different ages in a 9-month-old child with Down's syndrome. He was brought in by his grandparents with a left femoral fracture. Skeletal survey showed a healed forearm fracture without medical input.

Table 17.1 Average times for radiological signs of healing

Sign	Average time to appearance
Resolution of soft tissues	4–10 days
Subperiosteal new bone formation	10–14 days
Loss of fracture line delineation	14–21 days
Soft callus formation	14–21 days
Hard callus formation	21–42 days
Remodelling	1 year

Radiological assessment

Radiological assessment is necessary for all identified injuries. Fracture type and stage of healing can be very helpful in corroborating a history or refuting it. Radiological dating of injuries is not an exact science but is very helpful in allowing one to date injuries roughly; see Table 17.1. Interval radiographs are required to ensure that no undisplaced fractures are missed and to date events more accurately [7].

Standards for radiological investigations of suspected NAI were published by the Royal College of Radiologists and the Royal College of Paediatrics and Child Health in March 2008.

In children under 2 years with suspected NAI, a full skeletal survey is indicated (ideally after discussion among senior members of the child medical protection team). This involves the following series of images:

1. AP skull,
2. Lateral skull,
3. AP chest,
4. Oblique left ribs,
5. Oblique right ribs,
6. AP abdomen and pelvis,
7. Lateral spine,
8. PA both hands,
9. PA both feet,
10. AP left humerus,
11. AP right humerus,
12. AP left forearm,
13. AP right forearm,
14. AP left femur,
15. AP right femur,
16. AP left tibia and fibula,
17. AP right tibia and fibula.

In children older than 2 years, this should be guided by the history and physical examination. A skeletal survey for NAI is different from a skeletal survey performed for other conditions, such as dysplasia or neoplasia.

Although bone scanning has been used as an alternative to skeletal survey for injuries, it may miss metaphyseal lesions due to increased uptake in that region. Moreover, spinal fractures and old or new injuries may not show up on the bone scan. For these reasons, it is not commonly employed. CT of the head is very commonly required, to allow identification of subtle skull fractures and to screen for subdural haematomas.

Differential diagnosis [5, 7, 8]

Osteogenesis imperfecta (OI):	Mild forms of OI may present with multiple fractures occurring at low levels of trauma; many children will have white sclera and show no other signs. Family history and skin testing can be helpful in making this diagnosis.
Accidental trauma:	The majority of injuries that occur as a result of abuse are the same as those that occur accidentally. The history and ambulatory status are extremely important in differentiating the two.
Normal variants:	Nutrient vessels, metaphyseal beaking and physiological subperiosteal new bone formation (SPNBF) can all be confused with fractures. Physiological SPNBF is seen in 30–50% of children between 1 and 6 months of age, usually involves the tibia and femur, never extends to the metaphysis and very rarely exceeds 2 mm; it is indistinguishable from fracture healing on X-ray.
Obstetric trauma:	These fractures will usually have SPNBF by 11 days after birth and are associated with difficult births and large babies.
Skin disorders:	Impetigo and blue spots can be confused with skin lesions.
Haematological conditions:	Myelodysplasia, leukaemia and other bleeding disorders may present with easy bruising and fractures.
Infection:	Osteomyelitis may present with SPNBF, confused with healing fractures.
Other rare diagnoses:	Rickets, scurvy, vitamin A intoxication leading to raised intracranial pressure, Caffey disease (also called infantile cortical hyperostosis; a rare, benign, proliferating bone disease affecting infants), copper deficiency, skeletal dysplasias.

Management

Reporting suspected NAI is a legal and ethical requirement [9]. The consequences of failing to identify and report abuse are high. The re-injury rate of battered children is between 30% and 50% and the risk of death between 5% and 10% [6].

Most hospitals have developed a multidisciplinary team to deal with suspected child abuse which usually includes paediatricians, social workers, chaplains, and, when indicated, specialists, such as orthopaedic surgeons or radiologists.

Marfan syndrome

Background

Marfan syndrome is caused by a mutation in the *FBN1* gene, on the long arm of chromosome 15, which codes for the connective tissue protein fibrillin. Its incidence is 1 in 10 000 live births and it is autosomal dominant, although 15–30% of cases are a result of sporadic mutations. Variable penetrance and a spectrum of phenotypic severity can make diagnosis difficult. Fibrillin is a large glycoprotein closely associated with elastin and commonly found in the aortic media, the suspensory ligament of the lens of the eye and the skin, tendons, cartilage and periosteum. It can cause extracellular growth factors to become more readily available to cell receptors, contributing to tall stature and arachnodactyly [5, 6, 10].

At present, there is no generic treatment for Marfan syndrome; appropriate management of conditions as they arise is required. Cardiovascular issues are the leading cause of premature death in this group, with 81% demonstrating cardiovascular abnormalities.

Diagnosis

Patients with Marfan syndrome encompass a diverse group, and have skeletal, cardiac and ocular manifestations. This is one of very few syndromes associated with tall stature. Skeletal findings include tall stature with dolichostenomelia (long, narrow limbs), and arachnodactyly, scoliosis, protrusio acetabula, ligamentous laxity, patellofemoral joint instability and planovalgus feet. They classically have a high, arched palate with a long, narrow face (Figure 17.4). Pectus deformities may be present, owing to overgrowth of the ribs, and striae are usually seen in the skin.

Although the defective gene has been identified, the diagnosis remains a clinical one, and is based on the fulfilment of diagnostic criteria, such as the Berlin or Ghent criteria [11]. These criteria have been widely debated and there is no consensus on the minimum absolute criteria for diagnosis. Table 17.2 summarizes the Ghent criteria. A diagnosis of Marfan syndrome requires major criteria in two systems and involvement in a third. If a mutation known to cause Marfan syndrome is present, diagnosis requires one major criterion in one organ system and involvement in a second.

Differential diagnosis

A few conditions present with a similar phenotypical appearance to Marfan syndrome:

Homocysteinuria:	This has a very similar appearance to Marfan syndrome but demonstrates mental retardation and high levels of homocysteine in the urine.
Congenital contractural arachnodactyly:	Children have marked arachnodactyly from birth but present with contractures as opposed to laxity. This is always a sporadic mutation.
Stickler syndrome (hereditary progressive arthro-ophthalmopathy):	Children have distinctive facial abnormalities, ocular problems, hearing loss and joint problems. It is also autosomal dominant, so a family history is often found. However, Stickler syndrome has features of a skeletal dysplasia radiographically.

Management

Patients with Marfan syndrome are commonly seen by orthopaedic surgeons, as approximately 76% having musculoskeletal issues.

Cardiovascular abnormalities, such as dilation of the ascending aorta, aneurysm and subsequent dissection, are the leading cause of death in this group. Mitral and aortic valve incompetence are also common, resulting in a cardiac murmur on examination. Cardiac screening has been the biggest single factor in reducing mortality, raising average life expectancy from 45 to 72 years. It is particularly important to be aware of Marfan syndrome as a potential diagnosis; early referral to a cardiologist can be instrumental in preventing sudden cardiac death.

Scoliosis is commonly the first presentation; this has been reported in 30–100% of children with Marfan syndrome. Patients may also develop spondylolisthesis or dural ectasia. Those presenting with scoliosis often have short curves with associated anomalies of the vertebrae. There is often a kyphoscoliosis, particularly when it affects the lumbar region of the spine. Scoliosis in Marfan syndrome should be treated in a similar fashion to adolescent idiopathic scoliosis (see Chapter 6). Bracing is not well tolerated and does not commonly halt progression. Surgery should be considered for those with curves over 50° or those with rapidly progressive curves.

There is a higher rate of complications (10–20%) following surgery, including a higher rate of pseudarthrosis, instrumentation failure and postoperative curve decompensation in comparison with idiopathic scoliosis. Segmental posterior fixation is usually adequate [5, 6].

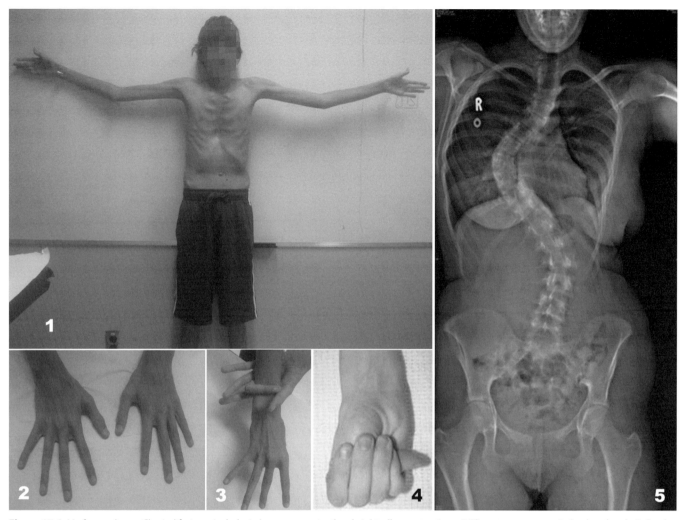

Figure 17.4 Marfan syndrome. Classical features include: 1. Arm span greater than height, elbow extension <170°, pectus excavatum. 2: Arachnodactyly. 3: Overlap of little finger and thumb when clasping. 4: Steinberg sign: the thumb extends beyond the ulnar border of the palm when held in a fist. 5: Scoliosis and hip protrusio.

Patellofemoral joint instability occurs frequently and can be extremely difficult to manage. Non-operative treatment is preferred, as recurrence of instability following attempted surgical correction is common due to the underlying soft-tissue disorder.

Protrusio acetabuli has been demonstrated in approximately one-third of patients with Marfan syndrome and is commonly an incidental finding on X-ray. No correlation has been found between bone mineral density and protrusio acetabuli in these patients, and also no clear correlation between radiographic parameters and symptoms. It has therefore been recommended that prophylactic surgery is unnecessary as the development of arthritis is not universal. Treatment should be based on symptoms, as with any other group of patients.

Bladder exstrophy

Background

Bladder exstrophy is a congenital condition affecting approximately 1 in 10 000–50 000 live births. It is part of a wider spectrum of anomalies affecting the closure of the anterior abdominal structures, ranging from epispadias at one end to cloacal exstrophy at the other (Table 17.3).

Classical bladder exstrophy is characterized by a failure of closure of the anterior abdominal wall, resulting in pelvic diastasis and an open bladder. It is believed that bladder exstrophy is caused by failure of the cloacal membrane to be reinforced by ingrowth of mesoderm. It is more commonly seen in boys than girls, with a ratio of 2.5:1, and carries a 1 in 100 risk of occurrence in subsequent pregnancies.

Studies of the pelvis by CT and MRI and dissection of anatomic specimens showed that in classic exstrophy the pubic bones are foreshortened by about one-third, the iliac wings are normal in size but externally rotated by approximately 13° and the acetabulae are retroverted but femoral version is normal. The sacroiliac joints are also externally rotated and the pelvis is angled caudally. The bladder itself is small and fibrotic and the external genitalia are hypoplastic. In cloacal exstrophy, there may be absence, hypoplasia or asymmetry of the sacroiliac joint, as well as a dislocation of the hips [5].

Table 17.2 Ghent criteria

Systems	Major criteria	Minor criteria	Notes
Cardiovascular	1. Dilation of ascending aorta and sinuses of Valsalva, 2. Aortic dissection	1. Mitral valve prolapse, 2. Annulus mitralis calcification in patients <40 years, 3. Pulmonary artery dilation, 4. Descending or abdominal aorta dilation or dissection in patients <50 years	One major or one minor criterion to confirm cardiovascular system (CVS) involvement
Dura	Lumbosacral dural ectasia (detected by MRI or CT)	N/A	One major criterion
Family and genetic history	1. First-degree relative with Marfan syndrome, 2. Presence of the *FBN1* mutation known to cause Marfan syndrome	N/A	One major criterion
Musculoskeletal	1. Pectus carinatum, 2. Pectus excavatum requiring surgery, 3. Arm span:height ratio >1.05 or upper segment: lower segment ratio <0.86, 4. Wrist and thumb signs, 5. Scoliosis >20° or spondylolisthesis, 6. Elbow extension <170°, 7. Pes planus, 8. Protrusio acetabuli	1. Typical facies (dolichocephaly, malar hypoplasia, enophthalmos, retrognathia, down-slanting palpebral fissures, 2. Joint hypermobility, 3. Pectus excavatum not requiring surgery, 4. High-arched palate with crowded teeth	Two of the eight major criteria or one of these plus two minor criteria
Eye	Lens dislocation	1. Myopia, 2. Flat cornea, 3. Iris or ciliary muscle hypoplasia	Two minor criteria
Pulmonary	N/A	1. Pneumothorax, 2. Apical blebs (seen on chest X-ray)	One minor criterion
Skin	N/A	1. Atrophic striae not secondary to pregnancy or weight change, 2. Recurrent or incisional hernia	One minor criterion

Table 17.3 Spectrum of bladder exstrophy

Condition	Genitalia	Bladder	Hindgut	Pubic symphysis	Others
Epispadias	Open	Intact	Intact	Diastasis common	Rare
Classic bladder exstrophy	Open	Open	Intact	Wide diastasis common	Rare
Cloacal exstrophy	Open	Open	Open	Wide diastasis common	Renal, McKusick–Kaufman syndrome and neural anomalies in 50%

Clinical features

Classic findings on examination are a midline defect in the anterior abdominal wall at the level of the pubic symphysis, exposing an open bladder and urethra (Figure 17.5). This defect is approximately 3–4 cm. The legs are externally rotated but the hips are usually stable. For those with cloacal exstrophy, the defect will be much larger. There may be anomalies of the bladder and bowel and also of the spinal column (Figure 17.5). Neurological defects are much more common, with associated hip dislocation and foot deformities.

Radiographic features

The pubic bones are foreshortened by about one-third and separated by about 4–5 cm at birth (normal being 1 cm) and

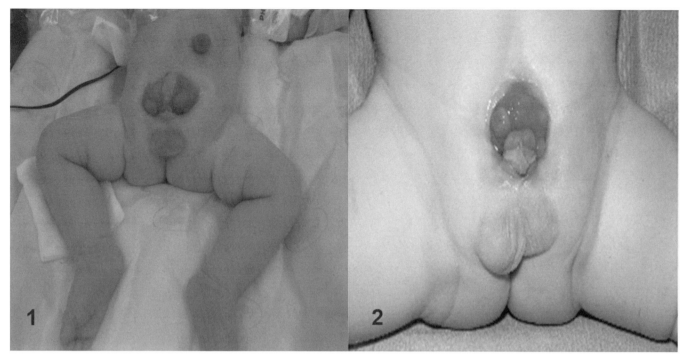

Figure 17.5 Bladder exstrophy. 1: Patient with cloacal exstrophy, who had had ileostomy shortly after birth and came for definitive surgical correction. 2: Patient with classic bladder exstrophy.

increases with age (differential diagnosis is cleidocranial dysplasia). The iliac bones are of normal size but externally rotated. The acetabuli are retroverted but rarely dysplastic (Figure 17.6).

Natural history

Patients with bladder exstrophy do not commonly develop orthopaedic issues requiring surgery. They have normal athletic capabilities and are not increasingly affected by hip osteoarthritis, despite the acetabular retroversion. Pelvic osteotomy is usually only indicated if needed as part of a urological reconstruction procedure.

Children can have marked external rotation affecting their gait, but this typically resolves over time without surgical intervention. Patients may present with patellofemoral instability due to their abnormal rotational profile but this rarely requires surgery. The only other common orthopaedic manifestation is sacroiliac joint pain [12, 13].

Treatment

The treatment objective in bladder exstrophy is urological reconstruction, commonly obtained in staged procedures. The prioritics are to close the bladder, gain continence, reconstruct the genitalia and achieve an acceptable appearance. Pelvic osteotomy may be required to assist with the urological reconstruction. Various surgical techniques have been recommended, each with pros and cons. The osteotomized pelvis may be immobilized using cast, traction, external fixation or internal fixation (Figure 17.7).

If a pelvic osteotomy is performed, complications occur in approximately 4% of cases. These include all of the routine complications, but specifically nerve palsies are common, owing to traction during the surgery.

Neurofibromatosis
Background

Neurofibromatosis (NF) is the most common hereditary hamartomatous condition affecting the peripheral and central nervous systems. This condition comprises neurofibromatosis Type 1 (NF-1) and neurofibromatosis Type 2 (NF-2).

Neurofibromatosis Type 1 is the more common peripheral form; it is often called Von Recklinghausen disease. It affects 1 in 2500–4000 live births and follows an autosomal dominant pattern of inheritance. It is a single gene disorder relating to a mutation on chromosome 17. This affects neurofibromin-1, a tumour-suppressor gene with an important role in the regulation of cell growth and differentiation. There is nearly complete penetrance for transmission; however, the clinical severity is extremely variable, even within families, making it impossible to predict the outcome of future pregnancies. It is important to note that approximately 50% of cases represent sporadic mutations, meaning that a family history is not necessary for diagnosis.

Diagnosis

The diagnostic criteria for NF-1, as agreed by the Consensus Development Conference on neurofibromatosis at the National Institute for Health (NIH) in 1987, are shown in

255

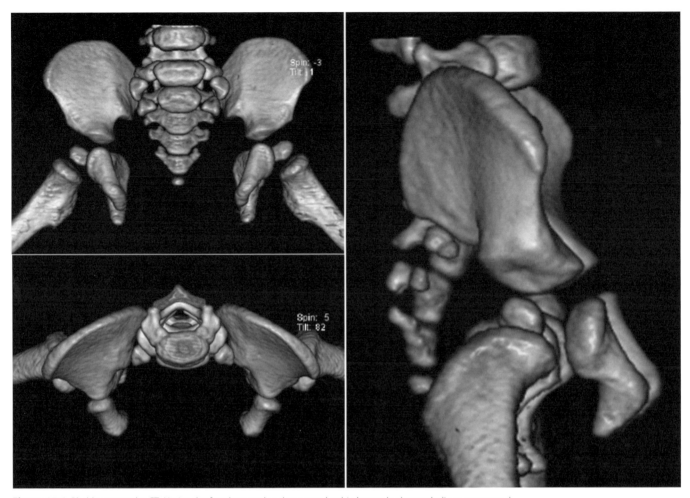

Figure 17.6 Bladder exstrophy CT. Notice the foreshortened and separated pubic bones; both acetabuli are retroverted.

Table 17.4. If two or more of these signs are present, a diagnosis can confidently be made.

Clinical features

Neurofibromatosis Type 1 affects multiple systems, including the nervous system, skeleton, skin, deeper connective tissues and endocrine system. However, it is estimated that 50% of cases will have significant musculoskeletal manifestations of disease, with 10–70% requiring surgical treatment. Patients are commonly of short stature with a disproportionately large head and experience precocious puberty as a result of hypothalamic dysfunction. Hypertension may be caused by renal artery stenosis or pheochromocytoma and is a risk factor for early mortality.

Café au lait spots are the most common clinical finding in neurofibromatosis, affecting >90% of cases. They are areas of hyperpigmentation of the skin with a smooth border, in contrast to those seen in fibrous dysplasia (Figure 12.5). They are usually present by 2 years of age and increase in size and number with age. Axillary and inguinal freckling affects >80% of cases by the age of 6 years. This is very specific to NF-1 and is rarely seen in other conditions (Figure 17.8).

Cutaneous neurofibromas typically do not occur until pre-adolescence. They are composed of Schwann cells and fibrous tissue and increase in size and number with age. Cutaneous neurofibromas do not undergo malignant transformation but may be excised if they become particularly symptomatic, although this is rare. Surgical excision is often complicated by bleeding.

Plexiform neurofibromas are very sensitive subcutaneous neurofibromas that are painful to palpation and are present from birth. They are large infiltrative masses that usually arise from major nerve trunks and follow the course of peripheral nerves. They are described as feeling like a 'bag of worms' and may be associated with overlying skin pigmentation. Plexiform neurofibromas extend much deeper than their cutaneous counterparts and may cause overgrowth or deformity, potentially leading to functional impairment and serious morbidity. They carry a 1–4% risk of malignant transformation to neurofibrosarcoma. If excision is required, the surgery can be extremely challenging. The goal of resection is to partially restore normal function and appearance, reduce pain and prevent malignant transformation. These structures can be highly infiltrative, leading to excessive bleeding and frequent neurological deficit when they are excised, particularly when a tourniquet cannot be used, owing to position.

Lisch nodules are domed elevations of the iris, which are considered to be pathognomic of NF-1.

Table 17.4 Diagnostic criteria for NF-1

Sign	Requirement
Café au lait spots	6 or more, >5 mm in children, >15 mm in adults
Cutaneous neurofibromas	2 or more
Plexiform neurofibroma	1 or more
Axillary or inguinal freckling	Any
Optic glioma	1 or more
Lisch nodules	2 or more
Distinctive bone lesions	Sphenoid dysplasia; cortical thinning of long bone with or without pseudarthrosis
First-degree relative	Must have documented NF-1 as per these criteria

There is a disproportionate overgrowth of the soft tissues in comparison with the bone in NF-1. Hemihypertrophy can occur in NF-1 and may be associated with haemangiomas, lymphangiomas, elephantiasis or numerous beaded plexiform neurofibromas. The hemihypertrophy typically follows a nerve root distribution, suggesting a neural origin as opposed to a

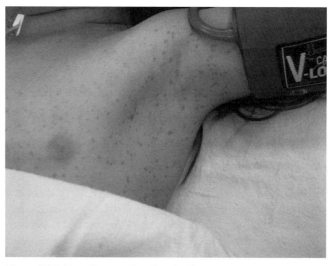

Figure 17.8 Neurofibromatosis: axillary freckles.

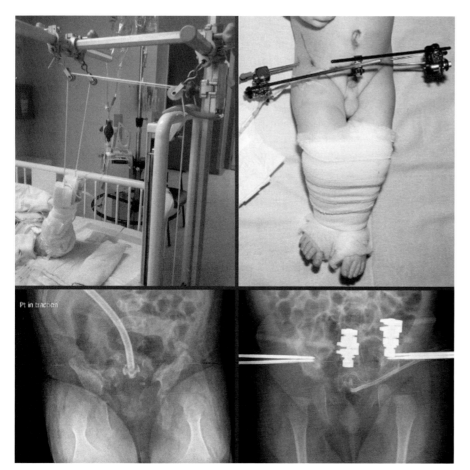

Figure 17.7 Bladder exstrophy postoperative stabilization. Patients of Figure 17.5. Left: Bilateral pelvic osteotomy was required to allow urological repair. Although no stabilization was required, traction for 3 weeks is often necessary. Right: Pelvic osteotomy was immobilized using external fixators and mermaid bandage.

primary bone dysplasia. The bone is elongated with a thickened cortex and there may be macrodactyly with disproportionately elongated digits.

Pseudarthrosis of the tibia and scoliosis are discussed in more detail later. Other orthopaedic manifestations include patella hypoplasia, coxa vara, coxa valga and protrusio acetabuli in 20% of cases.

Scoliosis is seen in 10–60% of patients with NF-1; this is covered in Chapter 6. Pseudarthrosis of any long bone can occur in NF-1, however the most common site is the tibia; this is discussed in Chapter 4.

There is an increased risk of malignancy associated with neurofibromatosis; this has been quoted as being between 1% and 20% greater than normal [6]. Tumours are commonly of neural crest origin and occur at an early age. Multiple primary tumours have been described. The most common malignancy is transformation of a neurofibroma to a neurofibrosarcoma. This is most frequently seen in severe cases with increasing age. Any lesion that is rapidly increasing in size or suddenly changes should be investigated for malignant transformation.

Plexiform neurofibromas are present in 25% of cases and carry a 1–4% risk of malignant transformation. The lifetime risk of developing peripheral malignant nerve sheath tumours (PMNSTs) is 8–13%; however, neurofibromatosis accounts for up to 70% of all PMNSTs. When these malignancies do occur in patients with neurofibromatosis, they are more likely to be advanced and the prognosis is poor [14, 15].

Other malignancies are also more common in patients with NF-1. They frequently develop central nervous system tumours, such as optic glioma, acoustic neuroma, astrocytoma or spinal cord tumours. They are also prone to developing leukaemia, Wilms' tumour and rhabdomyosarcoma of the urogenital tract. Therefore, these patients and their management teams need to be aware of the increased risk of developing any malignancy, not just those affecting the peripheral nerves.

Neurofibromatosis Type 2

Neurofibromatosis Type 2 is a central form of the disease, affecting 1 in 40 000 live births. It is an autosomal dominant condition, with almost complete penetrance caused by a mutation on the long arm of chromosome 22. Nearly all individuals develop vestibular schwannomas, with progressive hearing loss and ambulation difficulties. Spinal cord tumours occur in more than 80% of individuals but are rarely symptomatic. Some 50% of patients will have meningiomas, and may develop diminished vision and chronic pain. It is unusual for these patients to present to the orthopaedics department as there is no peripheral involvement.

Osteogenesis imperfecta
Background

Osteogenesis imperfecta (OI) is a genetic disorder of connective tissue, resulting in defective Type 1 collagen metabolism. Type 1 collagen is the most common protein in bone and is the major structural component of bone, tendons and ligaments.

Defects may be quantitative or qualitative. Quantitative defects result in lower levels of structurally normal collagen, while qualitative defects occur when glycine residues are substituted for other amino acids, leading to an abnormality in the folding of the triple helix. The severity of the phenotype is dependent on the location of the defect in the collagen molecule, with more severe phenotypes being associated with abnormalities near the N-terminal of the molecule [6, 16].

Osteogenesis imperfecta affects 1 in 15 000–20 000 live births. More than 90% of cases are caused by mutations in the COL1A1 and COL1A2 genes. The COL1A1 gene is located on chromosome 7q, while COL1A2 is found on chromosome 17q. The diagnosis can be made in most cases by culturing skin fibroblasts to analyze the Type 1 collagen, or by isolating DNA from white cells to identify the COL1A1 and COL1A2 gene.

Approximately 10–15% of cases do not have the classic mutations in collagen and will not be identified by these tests. This means that a positive test for OI confirms the diagnosis, but a negative test does not exclude it. Bone markers are normal, with the exception of alkaline phosphatase level, which is elevated as a result of increased bone turnover.

Presentation

Osteogenesis imperfecta is characterized by generalized osteopaenia of bone, leading to fragility fractures, multiple spinal wedge fractures resulting in scoliosis and long bone deformity. It is particularly associated with fractures in preschool age children; these fractures may be multiple and recurrent. This makes it an extremely important diagnosis to consider when investigating suspected cases of non-accidental injury. Fractures will typically heal but are very prone to refracture. Bones are narrow, with thin cortices contributing to their fragility. Skeletal deformity results from microfractures of the bone and asymmetrical growth from the physis.

Children may present to the orthopaedics department with bone pain, muscle weakness or ligamentous hyperlaxity. Patients have thin, translucent skin with easy bruising and subcutaneous haemorrhages. They may have blue sclerae and dentinogenesis imperfecta (fragile opalescent teeth). There is an increased tendency to develop hernias, and any surgical scars are likely to be wide. It is common to present with presenile hearing loss starting in the patient's twenties, and there is frequently a history of excessive sweating, owing to the hypermetabolic state.

Radiological features vary considerably with the level of disease. Bone deformity from microfractures and plastic deformation are seen in the more severe types. Patients undergoing pamidronate therapy will have the classic transverse sclerotic lines associated with each dose. Coxa vara and protrusio acetabuli are sometimes seen on hip radiographs. Patella, hip and radial neck dislocations are occasionally present. In the spine there may be scoliosis, kyphosis, spondylolisthesis, platyspondyly and biconcave vertebrae. Hyperplastic callus formation can be an alarming finding after fracture or surgery, and is discussed later (Figure 17.9).

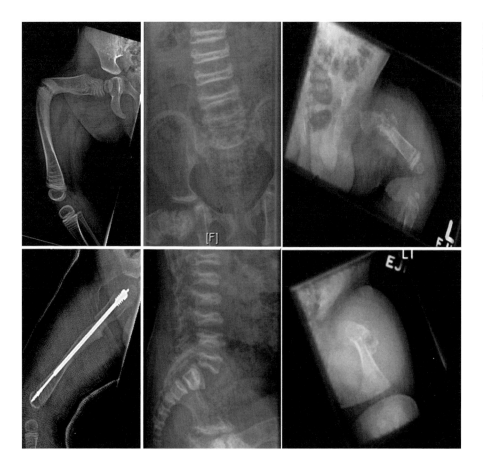

Figure 17.9 Osteogenesis imperfecta radiographs. Left: Femoral deformity and fracture treated with growing rod (Fassier–Duval rod). Notice the transverse sclerotic lines associated with pamidronate treatment. Middle: Platyspondyly and biconcave vertebrae. Right: Hyperplastic callus formation.

Classification

The best-known classification of OI is the Sillence classification, which divides patients into four groups based on clinical features. An additional three groups of patients have subsequently been identified (Types V–VII), which do not fit within this traditional model. There is no defect in Type 1 collagen in this condition (see Table 17.5).

Spinal involvement

Scoliosis occurs in 40–100% of cases of OI as a result of ligamentous laxity and multiple spinal wedge fractures. The severity of the scoliosis is related to the severity of the bone fragility, with six or more biconcave vertebrae indicating the potential for development of severe kyphosis. Curves less than 50° should be observed for progression. Bracing has been attempted in some cases but can lead to severe rib fractures and does not commonly prevent progression. Patients with curves greater than 50° usually require surgical fixation, with posterior segmental fixation usually being sufficient. During any surgical procedure there is a high risk from anaesthesia and also from excessive bleeding.

Spondylolisthesis and basilar impression may also be seen. In basilar impression, the relatively soft bone of the foramen magnum migrates into the posterior cranial fossa. The upper cervical spine compresses the spinal cord leading to headaches, facial spasm, numbness, bulbar palsy and long tract signs.

Medical management

There is no specific therapy for the underlying cause of OI, but various therapies have been tried to treat the consequences. Growth hormone has been used with little success in the past, and there is some evidence that mesenchymal stromal cell transplant may partially correct the OI phenotype. This is an area of research for the future, but is not widely used therapeutically at this time.

Bisphosphonates are the mainstay of medical therapy. These drugs inhibit osteoclastic resorption of bone, thus inhibiting bone resorption and increasing bone mass. They reduce bone turnover rates and increase the bone mineral density. In some cases, this has been shown to reduce the occurrence of fractures but this has not been the case in other series. Bisphosphonates have also been shown to improve muscle strength, mobility and give a sense of well-being. They are particularly effective when used in children under the age of 3 years. For those with the more severe types of OI, early administration of bisphosphonates can help to reduce the occurrence of the severe phenotypes.

The most common regime reported is three-monthly cycles of intravenous pamidronate. For each cycle of bisphosphonate therapy, a classic transverse line of sclerosis is seen on X-ray, allowing monitoring of growth between cycles (Figure 17.9).

The side effects of bisphosphonates include an influenza-like reaction after the first pamidronate infusion with

Table 17.5 Sillence classification for osteogenesis imperfecta

Type	Subtypes	Teeth	Sclerae	Clinical features	Prognosis
I	IA	Normal	Blue	Autosomal dominant, mildest form with less severe fragility fractures, short stature	Normal life expectancy
	IB	Dentinogenesis imperfecta	Blue	Less severe, fragility fractures, short stature	Normal life expectancy
II	II	Normal	Blue	Autosomal recessive and autosomal dominant, the worst type, associated with perinatal death	Perinatal or early infant death
III	III	Dentinogenesis imperfecta	Bluish at birth, white by puberty	Autosomal recessive and autosomal dominant, the worst survivable type. Progressive deformity, multiple fractures, scoliosis, severe limitation of function	Will usually require wheelchair, premature death
IV	IVA	Normal	White	Autosomal dominant, fragility fractures, short stature, moderate deformity of long bones, kyphoscoliosis	Fair
	IVB	Dentinogenesis imperfecta	White	Fragility fractures, short stature, moderate deformity of long bones, kyphoscoliosis	Fair
Beyond Sillence classification					
V				Autosomal dominant, moderate to severe bone fragility, accounting for 4–5% of cases. Patients develop calcification of the interosseous membrane of the forearm with severe restriction of hand movement and dislocation of the radial head. They may develop hyperplastic callus formation after minor trauma, fractures or surgery (Figure 17.9). Difficult to differentiate from osteosarcoma.	
VI				Radiologically mimic rickets with Looser's zones commonly seen; however, the growth plate is not involved in OI and biochemistry is normal.	
VII				Autosomal recessive, affecting specific communities, such as those of Native American, Northern Quebec or Irish descent. There is a mutation affecting chromosome 3, leading to bone fragility and rhizomelic limb shortening. There is no discernible defect in Type 1 collagen.	

vomiting, fever and a rash. This can be associated with a transient decrease in serum calcium levels, and a transient increase. There is delayed healing after osteotomies but not fractures.

Surgery

This focuses on treating fractures, correcting long bone deformity and scoliosis. The majority of fractures can be managed without surgery; however, in some cases, this is not practical. Olecranon fractures are very common in OI and are treated well with tension band wiring. Intramedullary fixation using telescopic rods (Fassier–Duval or Sheffield rod) is generally recommended where appropriate to prevent issues with recurrent fractures, progressive deformity or the rods becoming short with growth.

Ideally, long bone deformity should be prevented, or corrected where deformity has already occurred for a number of reasons. Restoring the mechanical axis prevents progressive deformity through continued microfractures, allows bracing and increases ambulatory capacity.

References

1. Tardieu, A (1860) Etude médico-légale sur les sévices et mauvais traitements exercés sur des enfants. *Annales d'hygiène publique et de médecine légale* **13**:361–98.

2. Caffey J (1946) Multiple fractures in the long bones of infants suffering from chronic subdural hematoma. *Am J Roentgenol Radium Ther* **56**(2):163–73.

3. Kempe CH, Silverman FN, Steele BF, Droegemueller W and Silver HK (1962) The battered-child syndrome. *JAMA* **181**:17–24.

4. Lucas, DR, Wezner KC, Milner JS *et al.* (2002) Victim, perpetrator, family, and incident characteristics of infant and child homicide in the United States Air Force. *Child Abuse Negl* **26**(2):167–86.

5. Morrissy RT and Weinstein SL (2005) *Lovell and Winter's Pediatric Orthopaedics*, 6th edition, volume 1. Philadelphia: Lippincott Williams & Wilkins.

6. Herring JA (2008) *Tachdjian's Pediatric Orthopaedics*, 4th edition, volume 1. Philadelphia: Saunders Elsevier.

7. Jayakumar P, Barry, M and Ramachandran M (2010) Orthopaedic aspects of paediatric non-accidental injury. *J Bone Joint Surg Br* **92**(2):189–95.

8. Wheeler DM and Hobbs CJ (1988) Mistakes in diagnosing non-accidental injury: 10 years' experience. *Br Med J (Clin Res Ed)* **296**(6631): 1233–6.

9. General Medical Council (2012) *Protecting Children and Young People: The Responsibilities of All Doctors.* Manchester: GMC.

10. Judge DP and Dietz HC (2005) Marfan's syndrome. *Lancet* **366**(9501):1965–76.

11. De Paepe A, Devereux RB, Dietz HC, Hennekam RC and Pyeritz RE (1996) Revised diagnostic criteria for the Marfan syndrome. *Am J Med Genet* **62**(4):417–26.

12. Kantor R, Salai M and Ganel A (1997) Orthopaedic long term aspects of bladder exstrophy. *Clin Orthop Relat Res* **335**:240–5.

13. Yazici M, Kandemir U, Atilla B and Eryilmaz M (1999) Rotational profile of lower extremities in bladder exstrophy patients with unapproximated pelvis: a clinical and radiologic study in children older than 7 years. *J Pediatr Orthop* **19**(4):531–5.

14. Canavese F, Krajbich JI (2011) Resection of plexiform neurofibromas in children with neurofibromatosis Type 1. *J Pediatr Orthop* **31**(3):303–11.

15. Ferrari A, Bisogno G, Macaluso A *et al.* (2007) Soft-tissue sarcomas in children and adolescents with neurofibromatosis type 1. *Cancer* **109**(7):1406–12.

16. Stans AA (2005) Osteomyelitis and septic arthritis. In *Lovell and Winter's Pediatric Orthopaedics*, 6th edition, volume 1, ed. Morrissy RT and Weinstein SL. Philadelphia: Lippincott Williams & Wilkins, pp. 440–80.

MCQs and EMQs

18

Paul A. Banaszkiewicz and Manish Changulani

Children's Orthopaedics multiple-choice questions

Part 1 of the FRCS (Tr & Orth) is the written part of the exam and consists of two papers. The first paper is sat in the morning while the second paper takes place in the afternoon. The Joint Committee on Intercollegiate Examinations endeavours to provide a minimum of 30 minutes between each paper.

It is considered the easiest part of the exam to pass, the clinicals and vivas being the difficult hurdles. This can lead to a false sense of security and some candidates may not apply themselves in their reading preparation as much as needed. The other issue is that candidates are not expected to fail this section, and this may increase expectations and pressures on candidates. The UK In-Training exam acts as a dress rehearsal and should be completed yearly by orthopaedic trainees. Your score should improve yearly and ideally peak the year before you sit the real exam. From 2013, the pass mark for the Part 1 exam has been increased by the Examination Board. This was unpredicted and means that candidates have to 'up' their exam preparation to avoid falling at this hurdle.

Paper 1: Single best answer MCQs (2 hours 15 minutes – including 15 minutes reading time for published paper)

The first paper is multiple-choice and it is one-best choice from five. There are 110 questions, the first 12 relate to a published paper. There are unconfirmed reports that the published paper section will be scrapped some time in 2014. Please check the official JCIE site for confirmation.

The examination committee meet every 3 months to choose new questions for inclusion in the exam. The content of both examination papers is mapped to the curriculum. Writing these MCQs is a long and arduous process. There should be no ambiguity in the question; it should act as a good differentiator of candidates and test relevant useful clinical knowledge required for a practising orthopaedic surgeon. A large number of questions get rejected as they do not meet all these criteria. If the question gets past the committee stage and finds its way into the exam, it's still not home. If the question is flagged up by candidates as poor or misleading, it may get eliminated from the paper and, therefore the candidates' scores. This occurs on average with about two to four questions per exam.

Paper 2: Extended matching item format (2 hours 30 minutes)

The second paper has 135 multiple-choice questions in an extended matching item format.

These questions are favoured by some candidates as being more straightforward. There can be issues with time, as it may take a candidate longer to read the introduction to the questions.

We believe may be there too much reliance now placed on MCQ books. Some FRCS (Tr & Orth) books are poor quality and way off the exam standard. To base your revision on these books is to invite trouble. The *Orthobullets* and *Hyperweb* sites are an excellent source of practice MCQs. The MCQs should be used as a guide to those areas of orthopaedics in which you are weak and need to read up on in the relevant book. Yes, standard textbooks should still be used as reading material for the exam. We do not think covering the 2000 or so MCQ questions on these websites and reading the provided answer gives you enough information to tackle Part 1.

There are exam tactics to refine with MCQ and EMQ papers. Be careful with time, do not leave too many questions initially unanswered, finish the paper, do not leave any questions unanswered.

We recommend you visit www.postgraduateorthopaedics.com and then go to the material on *Postgraduate Orthopaedics*, 2nd edition, Chapter 2, for a more detailed discussion of the Part 1 paper.

Postgraduate Paediatric Orthopaedics, ed. Sattar Alshryda, Stan Jones and Paul A. Banaszkiewicz. Published by Cambridge University Press. © Cambridge University Press 2014.

Children's Orthopaedics MCQs

1. Which of the following statements is true for adolescent idiopathic scoliosis?
   1. Right thoracic curves are rare and the spinal cord should be evaluated by MRI.
   2. A curve magnitude of $>20°$ is a risk factor for progression.
   3. The spinous processes swing round toward the convexity of the curve.
   4. Curves are commonly associated with an increased thoracic kyphosis.
   5. It is more common in boys.

2. A patient presenting with slipped upper femoral epiphysis:
   1. Is unlikely to be going through the pubertal growth spurt.
   2. Is less likely to develop avascular necrosis of the femoral head if closed anatomical reduction is achieved at operation.
   3. Gives a history of trauma in less than half of cases.
   4. Will develop avascular necrosis of the femoral head if bearing weight at presentation.
   5. Under the age of 10 may have an underlying endocrine abnormality.

3. You are seeing a 5-year-old girl with in-toeing due to excessive femoral anteversion. She is otherwise normal and healthy, and her mobility is unimpaired. Her parents are greatly concerned by the cosmetic appearance and possible future disability, and request that she be treated. You recommend which one of the following?
   1. Observation,
   2. Medial shoe wedges,
   3. Torque heels,
   4. Sleeping in a Denis Browne splint for 6 months,
   5. Derotational osteotomy of the femur.

4. In Legg–Calvé–Perthes disease, group B patients (according to the Herring lateral pillar classification) have a prognosis best described by which of the following statements?
   1. Uniformly good outcome in all age groups.
   2. Uniformly poor outcome in all age groups.
   3. Better than group A but worse than group C.
   4. Worse outcome in patients with bone age more than 6 years at presentation.
   5. Worse outcome in patients with bone age more than 4 years at presentation.

5. Which one of the following statements is FALSE about trigger thumbs in childhood?
   1. Under 9 months of age, 30% resolve spontaneously.
   2. Over the age of 1 year, less than 10% resolve spontaneously.
   3. 30% are bilateral.
   4. Surgical release of the A1 pulley is the treatment of choice in children over the age of 1 year.
   5. There is a strong familial inheritance pattern.

6. A 15 year old presents with back pain. Plain radiographs show vertebra plana at L1. Which is the most likely diagnosis?
   1. Discitis,
   2. Eosinophilic granuloma,
   3. Osteoblastoma,
   4. Scheuermann's,
   5. Rickets.

7. Which of the following is NOT a common cause for spasmodic torticollis?
   1. Sternocleidomastoid trauma during delivery,
   2. Peritonsillar abscess,
   3. Retropharyngeal abscess,
   4. Spinal haematoma,
   5. Cervical trauma.

8. A patient, who underwent *in-situ* pinning for SUFE and was asymptomatic following surgery, develops pain, stiffness and flexion deformity. The most likely diagnosis is:
   1. AVN,
   2. Chondrolysis,
   3. Further slip,
   4. Normal,
   5. Pin penetration.

9. In developmental dysplasia of the hip (DDH), which of the following statements is true regarding the Ortolani test?
   1. It is a provocative test for DDH that attempts to subluxate the femoral head.
   2. It is often positive in the walking child.
   3. It consists of pushing down the greater trochanter while simultaneously adducting the hip.
   4. It consists of lifting up the greater trochanter while simultaneously abducting the hip.
   5. It is always positive in the infant with DDH.

10. A 12-year-old boy walks into the accident and emergency department with a month-long history of right knee pain. Radiographs show a slipped capital femoral epiphysis (Southwick angle 20°). Which of the following is true?
    1. There is at least a 50% chance that this child will develop a slip on the contralateral side.
    2. Safe surgical dislocation and subcapital realignment osteotomy is a reasonable treatment option.
    3. When pinning *in situ*, screw entry should be proximal to the lesser trochanter.

4. Ultrasound of the hip should be considered.
5. This child has a high risk of developing avascular necrosis.

11. With regards to the anterior approach (Smith-Petersen) to the hip, which of the following statements is true?
    1. The superficial dissection is between the gracilis and the sartorius.
    2. The internervous plane is between the obturator nerve and the femoral nerve.
    3. The medial femoral circumflex artery is a structure commonly at risk.
    4. The internervous plane is between the femoral nerve and the superior gluteal nerve.
    5. The superficial dissection is between the rectus femoris and the sartorius.

12. Which of the following is INCORRECT regarding valgus proximal femoral osteotomy?
    1. The limb is inevitably lengthened.
    2. At least 15° of pre-operative abduction is necessary.
    3. It is indicated for post-Perthes-disease deformity.
    4. It involves a medially based closing wedge.
    5. The abductor lever arm is lengthened.

13. Which of the following statements is true about adductor tenotomy in a child with cerebral palsy?
    1. Usually involves division of adductor longus.
    2. Usually involves division of adductor magnus.
    3. Usually involves division of adductor brevis.
    4. Should include a neurectomy of the anterior branch of the obturator nerve.
    5. Is a common cause of hip subluxation.

14. At what age does the proximal femoral epiphysis usually ossify?
    1. *In utero*,
    2. 1–3 months,
    3. 4–6 months,
    4. 6–12 months,
    5. After 12 months.

15. Which of the following statements is true of Syme's amputation?
    1. It allows for easy application of a prosthesis.
    2. It can be performed in the absence of a viable heel pad.
    3. It can only be performed in the presence of a patent posterior tibial artery.
    4. It is preferred more in girls than boys.
    5. It is not a good operation for children with congenital foot deformities.

16. The most common cause of in-toeing in the preschool age group is:
    1. Internal tibial torsion,
    2. Metatarsus adductus,
    3. Developmental dysplasia of the hip,
    4. Excessive femoral anteversion,
    5. Club foot.

Children's Orthopaedics EMQs

1. **Physeal pathology:**
   A. Maturation zone,
   B. Zone of provisional calcification,
   C. Primary spongiosa,
   D. Secondary bony epiphysis,
   E. Degenerative zone,
   F. Zona reticularis,
   G. Reserve zone,
   H. Secondary spongiosa,
   I. Proliferative zone.

   1. Achondroplasia affects which zone of the growth plate?
   2. Rickets affects which zone of the growth plate?
   3. Acute haematogenous osteomyelitis affects which zone of the growth plate?

2. **Basic science:**
   A. Hyperparathyroidism,
   B. Renal osteodystrophy,
   C. Rickets,
   D. Postmenopausal osteoporosis,
   E. Scurvy,
   F. Paget's disease,
   G. Osteopetrosis,
   H. Pseudohypoparathyroidism,
   I. Hypoparathyroidism.

   1. Vitamin C deficiency, leading to defective collagen synthesis.
   2. Decreased oestrogen levels, leading to reduced bone mass.
   3. Genetic disorder, caused by a lack of effect of parathyroid hormone at the target cells.

3. **Lower-limb anatomy:**
   A. The medial femoral circumflex artery,
   B. The inferior gluteal nerve,
   C. The femoral nerve,
   D. The superior gluteal nerve,
   E. The sciatic nerve,
   F. The obturator artery,
   G. The lateral femoral circumflex artery,
   H. The inferior gluteal artery,
   I. The superior gluteal artery,
   J. The femoral artery.

   1. During a direct lateral (Hardinge) approach to the hip, which neurovascular structure may be injured by excessive retraction of the gluteus medius muscle?
   2. The artery of the ligamentum teres (foveal artery) is a branch of which vessel?

   3. The anterior (Smith-Petersen) approach to the hip utilizes the internervous plane between muscles supplied by the superior gluteal nerve and which other nerve?

4. **Radiological features:**
   A. Developmental dysplasia of the hip,
   B. Congenital coxa vara,
   C. Slipped upper femoral epiphysis,
   D. Osteomyelitis of the hip,
   E. Transient synovitis,
   F. Legg–Calvé–Perthes disease.

   1. Southwick angle greater than 15°.
   2. Triangular ossification defect in inferomedial femoral neck.
   3. Acetabular index less than 25°.

5. **Diagnosis:**
   A. Developmental dysplasia of the hip,
   B. Slipped capital femoral epiphysis,
   C. Achondroplasia,
   D. Down's syndrome,
   E. Turner's syndrome,
   F. Coxa plana,
   G. Coxa vara,
   H. Tibial torsion,
   I. Femoral anteversion.

   1. A child with trident hand and inability to approximate extended middle and ring fingers.
   2. A 6-year-old boy with hip pain and decreased abduction and internal rotation; crescent sign on radiograph.
   3. A 2-year-old child with in-toeing gait and internal rotation of feet, with patella facing forward.

6. **Radiographic angles:**
   A. Slipped upper femoral epiphysis,
   B. Perthes disease,
   C. Developmental dysplasia of the hip,
   D. Adolescent idiopathic scoliosis,
   E. Supracondylar fracture of the humerus,
   F. Lateral mass fracture of the distal humerus,
   G. Club foot,
   H. Tibia vara,
   I. Coxa vara.

   1. The radiographic measurement of the Baumann angle is useful for which condition?
   2. The radiographic measurement of the Southwick angle is useful for which condition?

3. The radiographic measurement of the centre edge angle of Wiberg is useful for which condition?

7. **Management of DDH:**
   A. Pavlik harness,
   B. MRI arthrogram,
   C. X-ray imaging,
   D. Ultrasound imaging,
   E. Conservative management,
   F. Closed reduction and casting,
   G. Open reduction and casting,
   H. Repeat clinical examination,
   I. Open reduction and acetabular osteotomy.

   1. A 5-week-old baby with a positive Ortolani test is best assessed with which imaging?
   2. Primary treatment of dislocations presenting at the age of 18 months should be:
   3. A 14-year-old child presenting with painless bilateral dislocations should have treatment with:

8. **Regarding the Ponseti method of correction of congenital talipes equinovarus deformity:**
   A. Depression of the first ray,
   B. Correction of equinus,
   C. Correction of varus,
   D. Correction of valgus,
   E. Lengthening of the Achilles tendon,
   F. Elevation of the first ray,
   G. Tibialis posterior tendon transfer,
   H. Tibialis anterior tendon transfer,
   I. Achilles tenotomy,
   J. Plantar fascia release.

   1. The first step in deformity correction with this technique.
   2. The surgical procedure required in approximately 90% of cases.
   3. Surgical procedure required in up to 20% of cases for correction of residual deformity.

9. **Which component of the physis is affected in each of the following conditions?**
   A. Perichondrial ring of LaCroix,
   B. Hypertrophic layer,
   C. Reserve zone,
   D. Zone of provisional calcification,
   E. Proliferative layer,
   F. Groove of Ranvier.

   1. Rickets,
   2. Gaucher's disease,
   3. Achondroplasia.

10. **Treatment of DDH:**
    A. Pavlik harness,
    B. Double nappies,
    C. Medial open reduction and hip spica,
    D. Salter's innominate osteotomy,
    E. Dega osteotomy,
    F. Chiari osteotomy,
    G. Ganz osteotomy,
    H. Total hip replacement,
    I. Broomstick plaster.

    1. A 6-week-old girl with a reducible hip dislocation.
    2. A 5-year-old with a concentric hip and an acetabular index of 35°.
    3. A 14-year-old girl with a lateralized, spherical but non-concentric hip.

11. **Approximate age at which each of the following ossification centres appears:**
    A. 2 months,
    B. Birth,
    C. 10 years,
    D. 6 months,
    E. 3 years,
    F. 1 year,
    G. Fifth week of gestation,
    H. 16 years.

    1. Olecranon,
    2. Clavicle,
    3. Greater tuberosity of the humerus.

12. **The following pathologies are associated with which of these clinical conditions?**
    A. Cerebral palsy,
    B. Rett syndrome,
    C. Poliomyelitis,
    D. Guillain–Barré syndrome,
    E. Charcot–Marie–Tooth disease,
    F. Friedreich's ataxia,
    G. Spinal muscular atrophy,
    H. Duchenne muscular dystrophy,
    I. Becker dystrophy,
    J. Werdnig–Hoffmann disease.

    1. Genetically determined demyelination or axonal degeneration in peripheral nerves,
    2. Periventricular leucomalacia,
    3. Autoimmune mediated demyelination or axonal destruction in peripheral nerves.

13. **A 10-year-old boy presents with symptomatic rigid pes planus requiring excision of a tarsal coalition.**
    A. Sural nerve,
    B. Extensor digitorum longus,
    C. Superficial peroneal nerve,
    D. Talus and calcaneum,
    E. Extensor digitorum brevis,
    F. Sustentaculum tali,
    G. Calcaneum and cuboid,

H. Calcaneum and navicular,
I. Medial malleolus and talus,
J. Deep peroneal nerve.

1. Through Ollier's approach, which structure(s) is/are most at risk?
2. An osseous bar between which structures is most likely?
3. Interposition of which structure(s) completes the procedure?

14. **With congenital constriction ring syndrome in the hand:**
    A. Simple constriction rings,
    B. Rings and distal deformity,

C. Rings and distal fusion,
D. Amputations,
E. Urgent surgical treatment,
F. Delayed surgical treatment,
G. Staged surgical treatment,
H. Z-plasty.

1. Acrosyndactyly implies:
2. Tight constrictions on the digits or extremities with vascular compromise:
3. When two rings are adjacent the preferred option is:

Children's Orthopaedics MCQs – answers

1. **Which of the following statements is true for adolescent idiopathic scoliosis?**
   1. Right thoracic curves are rare and the spinal cord should be evaluated by MRI.
   2. A curve magnitude of >20° is a risk factor for progression.
   3. The spinous processes swing round toward the convexity of the curve.
   4. Curves are commonly associated with an increased thoracic kyphosis.
   5. It is more common in boys.

   1. False,
   2. True,
   3. False,
   4. False,
   5. False.

Adolescent idiopathic scoliosis is present in 2–4% of children between 10 and 16 years of age. It is defined as a lateral curvature of the spine greater than 10°, accompanied by vertebral rotation. It is thought to be a multigene dominant condition with variable phenotypic expression. Scoliosis can be identified by the Adam's forward bend test during physical examination. Severe pain, a left thoracic curve or an abnormal neurologic examination are red flags that point to a secondary cause for the spinal deformity.

Specialty consultation and magnetic resonance imaging are needed if red flags are present. Of adolescents diagnosed with scoliosis, only 10% have curves that progress and require medical intervention. The main risk factors for curve progression are a large curve magnitude, skeletal immaturity and female sex. The likelihood of curve progression can be estimated by measuring the curve magnitude using the Cobb method on radiographs and by assessing skeletal growth potential using Tanner staging and Risser grading.

References

Reamy BV and Slakey JB (2001) Idiopathic scoliosis is lordoscoliotic, resulting in a hypokyphosis. *Am Fam Physician* **64**:111–16.

Solomon L, Warwick DJ and Nayagam S (2001) *Apley's System of Orthopaedics*, 8th edition. London: Arnold, pp. 374–82.

2. **A patient presenting with slipped upper femoral epiphysis:**
   1. Is unlikely to be going through the pubertal growth spurt.
   2. Is less likely to develop avascular necrosis of the femoral head if closed anatomical reduction is achieved at operation.
   3. Gives a history of trauma in less than half of cases.
   4. Will develop avascular necrosis of the femoral head if bearing weight at presentation.
   5. Under the age of 10 may have an underlying endocrine abnormality.

   1. False,
   2. False,
   3. False,
   4. False,
   5. True.

In SUFE, the age at presentation is 12–14 years for boys and 10–13 years for girls. Most patients have a relatively uniform skeletal age, i.e. younger children are advanced and older children are borderline immature. The slip appears to occur in a narrow skeletal age range. In girls, SUFE almost exclusively occurs before the menarche. Predisposing factors are obesity, rapid growth, endocrinopathies such as hypothyroidism, renal rickets, pituitary deficiency, growth hormone deficiency when treated with growth hormones. Classification on presentation: acute (3 weeks), chronic (>3 weeks), acute-on-chronic. Loder classification: stable and unstable, based on weight-bearing status; severity, based on Southwick angle (head–shaft angle in lateral view); 1, 30°; 2, 30–60°; 3, >60°.

Reference

Solomon L, Warwick DJ and Nayagam S (2001) *Apley's System of Orthopaedics*, 8th edition. London: Arnold, pp. 374–82.

3. **You are seeing a 5-year-old girl with in-toeing due to excessive femoral anteversion. She is otherwise normal and healthy, and her mobility is unimpaired. Her parents are greatly concerned by the cosmetic appearance and possible future disability, and request that she be treated. You recommend which one of the following?**
   1. Observation,
   2. Medial shoe wedges,
   3. Torque heels,
   4. Sleeping in a Denis Browne splint for 6 months,
   5. Derotational osteotomy of the femur.

   1. True,
   2. False,
   3. False,
   4. False,
   5. False.

In-toeing is often evident in 3–6 year olds and is due to excessive internal rotation of the femur. Clinically, there is increased internal rotation and decreased external rotation. The patella is internally rotated. Children sit in the 'W' position. Long-term patellofemoral joint problems can occur but most cases resolve by the age of 10. If less than 10°

external rotation is present, a femoral derotational osteotomy is often utilized (best when performed in intertrochanteric region to allow adequate correction). Medial shoe wedges would worsen internal rotation; torque heels would not help. Denis Browne boots are for CTEV and a derotational osteotomy is best performed at a later date.

4. **In Legg–Calvé–Perthes disease, group B patients (according to the Herring lateral pillar classification) have a prognosis best described by which of the following statements?**
   1. Uniformly good outcome in all age groups.
   2. Uniformly poor outcome in all age groups.
   3. Better than group A but worse than group C.
   4. Worse outcome in patients with bone age more than 6 years at presentation.
   5. Worse outcome in patients with bone age more than 4 years at presentation.

1. False,
2. False,
3. False,
4. True,
5. False.

The outcome of Herring group B hips can vary with age. Overall, children with a bone age over 6 years at presentation do worse.

Group B hips do better than group C but worse than group A because the extent of epiphyseal involvement is less than group C but more than group A.

5. **Which one of the following statements is FALSE about trigger thumbs in childhood?**
   1. Under 9 months of age, 30% resolve spontaneously.
   2. Over the age of 1 year, less than 10% resolve spontaneously.
   3. 30% are bilateral.
   4. Surgical release of the A1 pulley is the treatment of choice in children over the age of 1 year.
   5. There is a strong familial inheritance pattern.

1. False,
2. False,
3. False,
4. False,
5. True.

There is no familial inheritance pattern; the other statements are correct. Trigger digits, however, are seen with neurologic syndromes (trisomy 18) and mucopolysaccharidoses.

Transverse incision in the digital crease is to be preferred for a better scar.

Reference

Waters PM (2005) The upper limb. In *Lovell and Winter's Pediatric Orthopaedics*, 6th edition, volume 2, ed. Morrissy RT and

Weinstein SL. Philadelphia: Lippincott Williams & Wilkins, pp. 921–86.

6. **A 15 year old presents with back pain. Plain radiographs show vertebra plana at L1. Which is the most likely diagnosis?**
   1. Discitis,
   2. Eosinophilic granuloma,
   3. Osteoblastoma,
   4. Scheuermann's,
   5. Rickets.

1. False,
2. True,
3. False,
4. False,
5. False.

Reference

Floman Y, Bar-On E, Moshieff R *et al.* (1997) Eosinophilic granuloma of the spine. *J Pediatr Orthop B* **6**(4): 260–5.

7. **Which of the following is NOT a common cause for spasmodic torticollis?**
   1. Sternocleidomastoid trauma during delivery,
   2. Peritonsillar abscess,
   3. Retropharyngeal abscess,
   4. Spinal haematoma,
   5. Cervical trauma.

1. True,
2. False,
3. False,
4. False,
5. False.

Sternocleidomastoid trauma at birth is thought to be the mechanism for congenital muscular torticollis.

Reference

Tao K, McStay CM, Bowman JG *et al.* (2013) *Acute Torticollis.* New York: Medscape, http://emedicine.medscape.com/article/794191.

8. **A patient, who underwent *in-situ* pinning for SUFE and was asymptomatic following surgery, develops pain, stiffness and flexion deformity. The most likely diagnosis is:**
   1. AVN,
   2. Chondrolysis,
   3. Further slip,
   4. Normal,
   5. Pin penetration.

1. False,
2. True,
3. False,
4. False,
5. False.

Although rare, chondrolysis is one of the recognized complications of SUFE. It usually presents as pain and significant restriction of the joint movement.

Reference

Tachdjian MO (1990) *Pediatric Orthopaedics*, 2nd edition, volume 2. Philadelphia: Saunders Elsevier, p. 1066.

9. **In developmental dysplasia of the hip (DDH), which of the following statements is true regarding the Ortolani test?**
   1. It is a provocative test for DDH that attempts to subluxate the femoral head.
   2. It is often positive in the walking child.
   3. It consists of pushing down the greater trochanter while simultaneously adducting the hip.
   4. It consists of lifting up the greater trochanter while simultaneously abducting the hip.
   5. It is always positive in the infant with DDH.

1. False,
2. False,
3. False,
4. True,
5. False.

The Barlow and Ortolani tests are used to diagnose DDH in neonates and infants. The Barlow test is the provocative test for the dislocatable hip, while the Ortolani test is the relocating test for the already 'out' hip. (Remember: Ortolani for Out!)

The 'clunk' of Ortolani is a sensation of relocation of the head that is seen or felt but not heard. Nevertheless, the 'clicky' baby hip always needs further investigation via ultrasonography.

Reference

Herring JA and Sucato DJ (2008) Developmental dysplasia of the hip. In *Tachdjian's Pediatric Orthopaedics*, 4th edition, volume 1, ed. Herring JA. Philadelphia: Saunders Elsevier, pp. 637–770.

10. **A 12-year-old boy walks into the accident and emergency department with a month-long history of right knee pain. Radiographs show a slipped capital femoral epiphysis (Southwick angle 20°). Which of the following is true?**
    1. There is at least a 50% chance that this child will develop a slip on the contralateral side.
    2. Safe surgical dislocation and subcapital realignment osteotomy is a reasonable treatment option.
    3. When pinning *in situ*, screw entry should be proximal to the lesser trochanter.
    4. Ultrasound of the hip should be considered.
    5. This child has a high risk of developing avascular necrosis.

1. False,
2. False,
3. True,
4. False,
5. False.

The chances of a slip on the contralateral side are between 20% and 30%. Surgical dislocation and realignment osteotomy is increasing in popularity for severe slips, but would not be appropriate for a mild slip. It is best to avoid the lateral cortex with screw placement through the anterior cortex to avoid the risk of fracture. Ultrasound would not contribute to management in this case. This is a stable slip, so there is a low risk of AVN.

References

Uglow MG and Clarke NMP (2004) The management of slipped capital femoral epiphysis. *J Bone Joint Surg Br* **86-B**:631–5.

Loder RT, Richards BS, Shapiro PS, Reznick LR and Aronson DD (1993) Acute slipped capital femoral epiphysis: the importance of physeal stability. *J Bone Joint Surg Am* **75**(8):1134–40.

Southwick WO (1967) Osteotomy through the lesser trochanter for slipped capital femoral epiphysis. *J Bone Joint Surg Am* **49-A**:807–35.

11. **With regards to the anterior approach (Smith-Petersen) to the hip, which of the following statements is true?**
    1. The superficial dissection is between the gracilis and the sartorius.
    2. The internervous plane is between the obturator nerve and the femoral nerve.
    3. The medial femoral circumflex artery is a structure commonly at risk.
    4. The internervous plane is between the femoral nerve and the superior gluteal nerve.
    5. The superficial dissection is between the rectus femoris and the sartorius.

1. False,
2. False,
3. False,
4. True,
5. False.

This approach takes advantage of the interneural plane between the sartorius (femoral nerve) and tensor fasciae latae (superior gluteal nerve). It is useful for such operative procedures as open reduction of the congenitally dislocated hip. The lateral femoral cutaneous nerve is retracted anteriorly, and the ascending branch of the lateral femoral circumflex artery (which lies superficial to the rectus) is ligated. For deeper dissection, approach the interval between the gluteus medius and rectus femoris. Detach the origin of both heads of the rectus femoris. Reflection of the conjoined rectus tendon too distally can risk injury to the descending branch of the lateral femoral circumflex artery. Retract the rectus medially and the gluteus medius laterally. Dissect any attachments of the iliopsoas to the inferior capsule and perform a capsulotomy. There is a risk to the lateral femoral cutaneous nerve, which is located anterior or medial to the sartorius about 6–8 cm below the anterior superior iliac spine. The superficial circumflex artery penetrates the tensor fasciae latae just anterior to the lateral femoral cutaneous nerve. The femoral nerve and vessels can sometimes be injured by aggressive medial retraction of the sartorius.

12. **Which of the following is INCORRECT regarding valgus proximal femoral osteotomy?**
    1. The limb is inevitably lengthened.
    2. At least 15° of pre-operative abduction is necessary.
    3. It is indicated for post-Perthes-disease deformity.
    4. It involves a medially based closing wedge.
    5. The abductor lever arm is lengthened.

1. False,
2. False,
3. False,
4. True,
5. False.

This is a common operation for post-Perthes deformity. One residual of Legg–Calvé–Perthes disease is a malformed femoral head with resulting hinged abduction. Hinged abduction of the hip is an abnormal movement that occurs when the deformed femoral head fails to slide within the acetabulum. A trench is formed laterally, adjacent to a large uncovered portion of the deformed head anterolaterally.

Raney *et al.* described a lateral closing wedge valgus subtrochanteric osteotomy for malformed femoral heads with hinge abduction. All were Catterall Types III and IV with previous failed treatment. At 5-year follow-up, 62% had satisfactory results.

References

Bulstrode C, Wilson-MacDonald J, Eastwood DM *et al.* (2011) *Oxford Textbook of Trauma and Orthopaedics*, 2nd edition, volume 1. Oxford: Oxford University Press, pp. 991–4.

Canale ST and Beatty JH (2008) *Campbell's Operative Orthopaedics*, 11th edition, volume 2. Philadelphia: Elsevier Mosby, Part IX.

Raney EM, Grogan DP, Hurley ME and Ogden MJ (2002) The role of proximal femoral valgus osteotomy in Legg–Calvé–Perthes disease. *Orthopedics* **25**(5):513–17.

13. **Which of the following statements is true about adductor tenotomy in a child with cerebral palsy?**
    1. Usually involves division of adductor longus.
    2. Usually involves division of adductor magnus.
    3. Usually involves division of adductor brevis.
    4. Should include a neurectomy of the anterior branch of the obturator nerve.
    5. Is a common cause of hip subluxation.

1. True,
2. False,
3. False,
4. False,
5. False.

Adductor myotomy is one of the oldest and most commonly performed operations in children with cerebral palsy. It usually involves the gracilis and adductor longus. In severe deformities, the surgeon may choose to divide the brevis and rarely, if ever, the adductor magnus. Anterior branch obturator neurectomy is usually avoided.

Reference

Morrissy RT and Weinstein SL (2005) *Atlas of Paediatric Orthopaedic Surgery*. Philadelphia: Lippincott Williams & Wilkins, p. 379.

14. **At what age does the proximal femoral epiphysis usually ossify?**
    1. *In utero*,
    2. 1–3 months,
    3. 4–6 months,
    4. 6–12 months,
    5. After 12 months.

1. False,
2. False,
3. True,
4. False,
5. False.

The femoral epiphysis usually ossifies between 4 and 6 months of age; this can be delayed in cases of DDH, either as a result of the condition or as a consequence of the treatment; in the latter case this most probably represents AVN.

15. **Which of the following statements is true of Syme's amputation?**
    1. It allows for easy application of a prosthesis.
    2. It can be performed in the absence of a viable heel pad.
    3. It can only be performed in the presence of a patent posterior tibial artery.
    4. It is preferred more in girls than boys.
    5. It is not a good operation for children with congenital foot deformities.

1. False,
2. False,
3. True,
4. False,
5. False.

Syme's amputation is indicated for congenital foot deformities, fibular hemimelia and severe injury to the foot, as long as the heel pad remains viable.

The posterior tibial artery must be preserved since it provides a blood supply to the heel flap. The tough durable skin of the heel flap provides normal weight-bearing skin. The two most common causes of an unsatisfactory Syme's stump are posterior migration of the heel pad and skin sloughing.

The prosthesis used for a classic Syme's stump consists of a moulded plastic socket and a solid ankle, cushioned heel foot (SACH). The prosthesis used must accommodate the flair of the distal tibial metaphysis and is thus large and bulky. Therefore, this amputation is not recommended for women.

References

Canale ST and Beatty JH (2008) *Campbell's Operative Orthopaedics*, 11th edition. Philadelphia: Elsevier Mosby, p. 590.

Gaine WJ and McCreath SW (1996) Syme's amputation revisited a review of 46 cases. *Bone Joint Surg Br* **78-B**:461–7.

16. **The most common cause of in-toeing in the preschool age group is:**
    1. Internal tibial torsion,
    2. Metatarsus adductus,
    3. Developmental dysplasia of the hip,
    4. Excessive femoral anteversion,
    5. Club foot.

1. True,
2. False,
3. False,
4. False,
5. False.

Children's orthopaedics EMQs – answers

1. **Physeal pathology:**
   A. Maturation zone,
   B. Zone of provisional calcification,
   C. Primary spongiosa,
   D. Secondary bony epiphysis,
   E. Degenerative zone,
   F. Zona reticularis,
   G. Reserve zone,
   H. Secondary spongiosa,
   I. Proliferative zone.

   1. Achondroplasia affects which zone of the growth plate?
   Correct answer: I – proliferative zone. It leads to a deficiency of cell proliferation.
   2. Rickets affects which zone of the growth plate?
   Correct answer: B – zone of provisional calcification. There is a deficiency of calcium or PTH, leading to abnormal calcification of the matrix.
   3. Acute haematogenous osteomyelitis affects which zone of the growth plate?
   Correct answer: C – primary spongiosa. Bacteria settle in the slow moving, poorly oxygenated blood in the terminal branches of the metaphyseal arteries.

2. **Basic science:**
   A. Hyperparathyroidism,
   B. Renal osteodystrophy,
   C. Rickets,
   D. Postmenopausal osteoporosis,
   E. Scurvy,
   F. Paget's disease,
   G. Osteopetrosis,
   H. Pseudohypoparathyroidism,
   I. Hypoparathyroidism.

   1. Vitamin C deficiency, leading to defective collagen synthesis.
   Correct answer: E.
   2. Decreased oestrogen levels, leading to reduced bone mass.
   Correct answer: D.
   3. Genetic disorder, caused by a lack of effect of parathyroid hormone at the target cells.
   Correct answer: H.

3. **Lower-limb anatomy:**
   A. The medial femoral circumflex artery,
   B. The inferior gluteal nerve,
   C. The femoral nerve,
   D. The superior gluteal nerve,
   E. The sciatic nerve,
   F. The obturator artery,
   G. The lateral femoral circumflex artery,
   H. The inferior gluteal artery,
   I. The superior gluteal artery,
   J. The femoral artery.

   1. During a direct lateral (Hardinge) approach to the hip, which neurovascular structure may be injured by excessive retraction of the gluteus medius muscle?
   Correct answer: D.
   2. The artery of the ligamentum teres (foveal artery) is a branch of which vessel?
   Correct answer: F.
   3. The anterior (Smith-Petersen) approach to the hip utilizes the internervous plane between muscles supplied by the superior gluteal nerve and which other nerve?
   Correct answer: C.

4. **Radiological features:**
   A. Developmental dysplasia of the hip,
   B. Congenital coxa vara,
   C. Slipped upper femoral epiphysis,
   D. Osteomyelitis of the hip,
   E. Transient synovitis,
   F. Legg–Calvé–Perthes disease.

   1. Southwick angle greater than 15°.
   Correct answer: C.
   2. Triangular ossification defect in inferomedial femoral neck.
   Correct answer: F.
   3. Acetabular index less than 25°.
   Correct answer: A.

5. **Diagnosis:**
   A. Developmental dysplasia of the hip,
   B. Slipped capital femoral epiphysis,
   C. Achondroplasia,
   D. Down's syndrome,
   E. Turner's syndrome,
   F. Coxa plana,
   G. Coxa vara,
   H. Tibial torsion,
   I. Femoral anteversion.

   1. A child with trident hand and inability to approximate extended middle and ring fingers.
   Correct answer: C.
   2. A 6-year-old boy with hip pain and decreased abduction and internal rotation; crescent sign on radiograph.
   Correct answer: F.
   3. A 2 year-old child with in-toeing gait and internal rotation of feet, with patella facing forward.
   Correct answer: H.

6. **Radiographic angles:**
   A. Slipped upper femoral epiphysis,
   B. Perthes disease,
   C. Developmental dysplasia of the hip,
   D. Adolescent idiopathic scoliosis,
   E. Supracondylar fracture of the humerus,
   F. Lateral mass fracture of the distal humerus,
   G. Club foot,
   H. Tibia vara,
   I. Coxa vara.

   1. The radiographic measurement of the Baumann angle is useful for which condition?

Correct answer: E.

   2. The radiographic measurement of the Southwick angle is useful for which condition?

Correct answer: A.

   3. The radiographic measurement of the centre edge angle of Wiberg is useful for which condition?

Correct answer: C.

7. **Management of DDH:**
   A. Pavlik harness,
   B. MRI arthrogram,
   C. X-ray imaging,
   D. Ultrasound imaging,
   E. Conservative management,
   F. Closed reduction and casting,
   G. Open reduction and casting,
   H. Repeat clinical examination,
   I. Open reduction and acetabular osteotomy.

   1. A 5-week-old baby with a positive Ortolani test is best assessed with which imaging?

Correct answer: D.

   2. Primary treatment of dislocations presenting at the age of 18 months should be:

Correct answer: F.

   3. A 14-year-old child presenting with painless bilateral dislocations should have treatment with:

Correct answer: E.

8. **Regarding the Ponseti method of correction of congenital talipes equinovarus deformity:**
   A. Depression of the first ray,
   B. Correction of equinus,
   C. Correction of varus,
   D. Correction of valgus,
   E. Lengthening of the Achilles tendon,
   F. Elevation of the first ray,
   G. Tibialis posterior tendon transfer,
   H. Tibialis anterior tendon transfer,
   I. Achilles tenotomy,
   J. Plantar fascia release.

   1. The first step in deformity correction with this technique.

Correct answer: F.

   2. The surgical procedure required in approximately 90% of cases.

Correct answer: I.

   3. Surgical procedure required in up to 20% of cases for correction of residual deformity.

Correct answer: H.

Reference

Changulani M, Garg NK, Rajagopal TS *et al.* (2006) Treatment of idiopathic club foot using the Ponseti method: initial experience. *J Bone Joint Surg Br* **88**(10):1385–7.

9. **Which component of the physis is affected in each of the following conditions?**
   A. Perichondrial ring of LaCroix,
   B. Hypertrophic layer,
   C. Reserve zone,
   D. Zone of provisional calcification,
   E. Proliferative layer,
   F. Groove of Ranvier.

   1. Rickets,

Correct answer: D.

   2. Gaucher's disease,

Correct answer: C.

   3. Achondroplasia.

Correct answer: E.

Osteomalacia results from inadequate mineralization of bone matrix (osteoid). In rickets there is inadequate mineralization of cartilage matrix (chondroid) and this affects the provisional zone of calcification in the physis. Rickets is caused by a lack of serum calcium and phosphate, insufficient to allow mineralization of the newly formed chondroid matrix. This may be seen on plain radiographs as a widened, thickened physis with metaphyseal flaring due to the persistence of metaphyseal cartilage.

10. **Treatment of DDH:**
    A. Pavlik harness,
    B. Double nappies,
    C. Medial open reduction and hip spica,
    D. Salter's innominate osteotomy,
    E. Dega osteotomy,
    F. Chiari osteotomy,
    G. Ganz osteotomy,
    H. Total hip replacement,
    I. Broomstick plaster.

    1. A 6-week-old girl with a reducible hip dislocation.

Corrcct answer: A.

    2. A 5-year-old with a concentric hip and an acetabular index of 35°.

Correct answer: D.

    3. A 14-year-old girl with a lateralized, spherical but non-concentric hip.

Correct answer: F.

The Pavlik harness is the treatment of choice for a child 1–6 months of age with DDH. The harness must hold the hip in more than 90° of flexion, with the proximal femoral metaphysis pointed toward the triradiate cartilage. If reduction is not obtained or maintained (clinically and ultrasonographically) within 3–4 weeks, the harness is discontinued. If reduction is confirmed, the harness is continued for 6 weeks after stability has been established.

Salter's or Pemberton osteotomy is recommended for patients younger than 8 years with concentric but dysplastic hips. After 2 years of age, an acetabular index over 30° is definitely abnormal. There is good evidence that acetabular dysplasia persisting beyond 5 years of age does not adequately correct and requires a pelvic osteotomy.

A Chiari osteotomy or a shelf procedure (e.g. Staheli) is warranted in non-concentric hips. These are salvage procedures, since the femoral head is eventually covered by fibrocartilage and not repositioned acetabular cartilage.

Reference

Herring JA and Sucato DJ (2008) Developmental dysplasia of the hip. In *Tachdjian's Pediatric Orthopaedics*, 4th edition, volume 1, ed. Herring JA. Philadelphia: Saunders Elsevier, pp. 637–770.

11. **Approximate age at which each of the following ossification centres appears:**
    A. 2 months,
    B. Birth,
    C. 10 years,
    D. 6 months,
    E. 3 years,
    F. 1 year,
    G. Fifth week of gestation,
    H. 16 years.

    1. Olecranon,
Correct answer: C.
    2. Clavicle,
Correct answer: G.
    3. Greater tuberosity of the humerus.
Correct answer: E.

12. **The following pathologies are associated with which of these clinical conditions?**
    A. Cerebral palsy,
    B. Rett syndrome,
    C. Poliomyelitis,
    D. Guillain–Barré syndrome,
    E. Charcot–Marie–Tooth disease,
    F. Friedreich's ataxia,
    G. Spinal muscular atrophy,
    H. Duchenne muscular dystrophy,
    I. Becker dystrophy,
    J. Werdnig–Hoffmann disease.

    1. Genetically determined demyelination or axonal degeneration in peripheral nerves,
Correct answer: E.
    2. Periventricular leucomalacia,
Correct answer: A.
    3. Autoimmune mediated demyelination or axonal destruction in peripheral nerves.
Correct answer: D.

CMT has been classically divided into demyelinating and axonal forms. However, research indicates that demyelination renders the axon susceptible to degeneration; hence, the two pictures can coexist.

Periventricular leucomalacia and intra- and periventricular haemorrhages are frequent MRI findings in cerebral palsy. The former results from an ischaemic insult to the arterial watershed area close to the ventricular walls.

Guillain-Barré syndrome is now the commonest cause of acute flaccid paralysis in children in the West. It is characterized by symmetric motor and sensory paresis of the limbs and, at times, the trunk. The disease is autoimmune and directed against peripheral nervous system myelin, axon or both. It is triggered by a preceding bacterial or viral infection.

Reference

Herring JA (2008) *Tachdjian's Pediatric Orthopaedics*, 4th edition, volume 2. Philadelphia: Saunders Elsevier, Section VI.

13. **A 10-year-old boy presents with symptomatic rigid pes planus requiring excision of a tarsal coalition.**
    A. Sural nerve,
    B. Extensor digitorum longus,
    C. Superficial peroneal nerve,
    D. Talus and calcaneum,
    E. Extensor digitorum brevis,
    F. Sustentaculum tali,
    G. Calcaneum and cuboid,
    H. Calcaneum and navicular,
    I. Medial malleolus and talus,
    J. Deep peroneal nerve.

    1. Through Ollier's approach, which structure(s) is/are most at risk?
Correct answer: C.
    2. An osseous bar between which structures is most likely?
Correct answer: H.
    3. Interposition of which structure(s) completes the procedure?
Correct answer: E.

References

Canale ST and Beatty JH (2008) *Campbell's Operative Orthopaedics*, 11th edition, volume 2. Philadelphia: Elsevier Mosby.

Jahss MH *Disorders of the Foot and Ankle: Medical and Surgical Management*, volume 1. Philadelphia: WB Saunders, Chapter 38.

14. **With congenital constriction ring syndrome in the hand:**
    A. Simple constriction rings,
    B. Rings and distal deformity,
    C. Rings and distal fusion,
    D. Amputations,
    E. Urgent surgical treatment,
    F. Delayed surgical treatment,
    G. Staged surgical treatment,
    H. Z-plasty.

    1. Acrosyndactyly implies:
Correct answer: C.
    2. Tight constrictions on the digits or extremities with vascular compromise:

Correct answer: E.
    3. When two rings are adjacent the preferred option is:
Correct answer: G.

This is a rare condition. Constriction ring syndrome is classified into four types: simple constriction rings; rings with distal deformity; rings with distal tethering and amputations. Acrosyndactyly refers to rings with distal tethering. Early release of the tethering prevents development of deformity but formal correction is delayed until the child is older.

Reference

Wolfe SW, Hotchkiss RN, Pederson WC and Kozin SH (2011) *Green's Operative Hand Surgery*, Philadelphia: Elsevier, Chapter 40.

Chapter

19

Viva and clinical practice

Mohamed O. Kenawey and Paul A. Banaszkiewicz

Topic 1: Club foot

Viva practice 1

Congenital talipes equinovarus (CTEV), or club foot, is a fairly common topic for the viva. There is more than enough material to cover in a 5-minute slot with room to spare. The treatment method has significantly changed in the last 10 years with the introduction of the Ponseti technique. This is something that you must be familiar with and in an ideal world have seen performed. That way you should be able to confidently describe the technique to the examiners, leaving them with the impression that you have actually seen the procedure being done.

In the clinical examination you might be shown a case of old club foot with residue deformities in a young adult. This can be challenging, as you will have to piece together what surgery has been performed previously and what further surgical options are available.

Examiner: You have been called to the paediatric ward because the doctors are unhappy with the appearance of this baby's right foot. What do you see? What is the diagnosis?
Candidate: These are clinical photographs of a newborn child, showing a deformed right foot: the heel is turned in (varus), the forefoot is deviated toward the midline (adductus), and

there are posterior and medial creases. Although it is not very clear from these pictures, the ankle appears to be in equinus with the first metatarsal pointing downward (plantar flexion) [1]. The diagnosis is suggestive of congenital talipes equinovarus (club foot).

Examiner: What else could it be?
Candidate: Occasionally, a severe metatarsus varus can be confused with club foot. The heel is in a neutral position (unlike club foot) and there is no equinus. Positional calcaneovalgus in which there is dorsiflexion of the whole foot such that it may touch the tibia can sometimes be mistaken for a club foot deformity. (See Chapter 5 for more detail.)

Examiner: What are the deformities in this condition?
Candidate: The deformities in this condition can be remembered by the mnemonic CAVE: cavus (midfoot), abductus (forefoot), varus (hindfoot) and equinus (hindfoot). From proximal to distal, there is usually wasting of the calf muscles; the hindfoot is in equinus and varus, the talar head points laterally and downward (causing a bump on the outside of the foot, which is visible in the photograph). Although X-rays are not necessary in managing club feet, they would show that the talus and the calcaneum are parallel instead of at

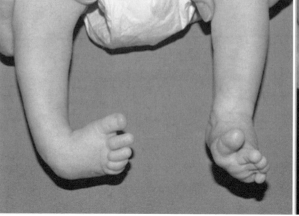
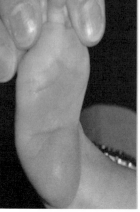

Figure 19.1 Club foot.

Postgraduate Paediatric Orthopaedics, ed. Sattar Alshryda, Stan Jones and Paul A. Banaszkiewicz. Published by Cambridge University Press.
© Cambridge University Press 2014.

Table 19.1 Diméglio scoring system

Rating	4	3	2	1	0	Scores
Equinus	45–90° Plantar flexion	20°–45° Plantar flexion	20°–0° Plantar flexion	0°–20° Dorsiflexion	>+20° Dorsiflexion	
Varus	45–90 Varus	20°–45° Varus	20°–0° Varus	0°–20° Valgus	>20° Valgus	
Supination	45–90 Supination	20°–45 Supination	20°–0° Supination	0°–20° Supination	>−20° Supination	
Adductus	45–90° Adduction	20°–45° Adduction	20°–0° Adduction	0°–20° Abduction	>20° Abduction	
Posterior crease				Yes	No	
Medial crease				Yes	No	
Cavus				Yes	No	
Deviant muscle function				Yes	No	
					Total	

an angle (the talocalcaneal angle of Kite is 20°–40°). The midfoot is deviated toward the midline (adductus), and the first metatarsal points downward (plantar flexion).

Examiner: How are you going to treat this patient?
Candidate: I would take a full history and examination. I would want to know if there has been a family history of club foot. There is a genetic component but not a recognizable pattern of inheritance. If one child has club foot, the risk of club foot in a subsequent child is increased 20-fold. With examination I would want to exclude any associated conditions, such as spina bifida (4.4% of children with club foot), cerebral palsy (1.9%) or arthrogryposis (0.9%). I would want to access the severity of the condition. Deep creases behind the heel or on the medial side of the foot tend to be associated with a more severe condition.

Examiner: How are the deformities usually corrected, and in what order?
Candidate: The disorder is normally corrected by the Ponseti method of cast manipulation using the head of the talus as a fulcrum. Cavus is corrected first by dorsiflexing the first ray and unlocking the forefoot and midfoot. With the cavus corrected, the forefoot is abducted and the heel goes into valgus by the coupling on the subtalar joint. Finally, the equinus is corrected. Serial above-knee casts (with the knee at 90°) are changed weekly with the old cast removed, the deformity scored and the new cast applied. Residual equinus (or less than 20° of dorsiflexion) requires Achilles tendon release in the majority of patients. This can be performed under local or general anaesthetic and a final cast is applied for a further 3 weeks while the tenotomy heals.

Examiner: What do we want to achieve?
Candidate: The aim of treatment is to achieve a painless, plantigrade foot with good mobility, with no need for special or modified shoes.

Examiner: What should we tell the parents?
Candidate: Club foot is a common problem and affects about 1 in 1000 babies. In most cases, there are no obvious causes although it can run in families. Treatment has changed dramatically in the last 10 years and instead of extensive surgical correction, most babies are treated with serial casting and bracing.

Examiner: How do you access the severity of foot deformity?
Candidate: Two grading systems are used: the Pirani score (see Chapter 5 for more detail) and the Diméglio score. I am familiar with the Diméglio score. It consists of eight items. Scorings for four of the items range from 0–4 (best to worst). The other four items only score 0 or 1. The total score ranges between 0 and 20: very severe, 16–20; severe, 11–15; moderate, 6–10, and postural 0–5) (Table 19.1).

Examiner: The parents want to know if everything will be fine.
Candidate: I would tell the parents that treatment with the Ponseti technique for an idiopathic club foot deformity usually has a good result; 90% of children will have painless feet with good functions. However, the foot and the calf will not be as normal as the other side. The affected foot and calf are usually smaller in size and the child may need different sized shoes. Extensive surgery is rarely needed, but minor surgery is often required (tendo Achillis tenotomy in 85% of patients and tibialis anterior transfer in about 15%). The child should wear Denis Browne boots with a bar on a full-time basis for 3 months after finishing serial casting, then at night and nap times for 3–4 years. This holds the affected foot externally rotated at around 70°. Compliance and tolerance of treatment is essential for success and avoidance of recurrence. Most children tolerate treatment very well and avoid the need for extensive surgery. Recurrence or persistence of a small degree of the deformity is not

uncommon; most children can be treated with a repeat of serial casting; however, some may need further surgery.

Examiner: What are the published results for the Ponseti method?

Candidate: Jowett *et al.*, in a recent systematic review, found that the Ponseti method provides excellent results, with an initial correction rate of around 90% in idiopathic feet. Non-compliance with bracing is the most common cause of relapse; this occurs in about 15% of patients [2].

Examiner: What are the complications of the Ponseti technique?

Candidate: Complications include recurrence of deformity, pressure damage due to casting, neurovascular injury with Achilles tendon release and overcorrection of deformity.

Clinical practice 1

This is a potentially difficult short case; possibly an intermediate case in an adult, especially if there is co-existing LLD.

The child is likely to be about 5 years old. In a paper by Lampasi *et al.* [3], the mean age for revision surgery was 4.8 years (2 to 10.1). As the Ponseti method continues to gain acceptance across the world, relapsing deformity after initial complete correction is becoming more prevalent. This could also be an adult intermediate or short clinical case with post club foot syndrome. There would be a hypoplastic limb with a short leg gait, possibly several scars in the foot from previous

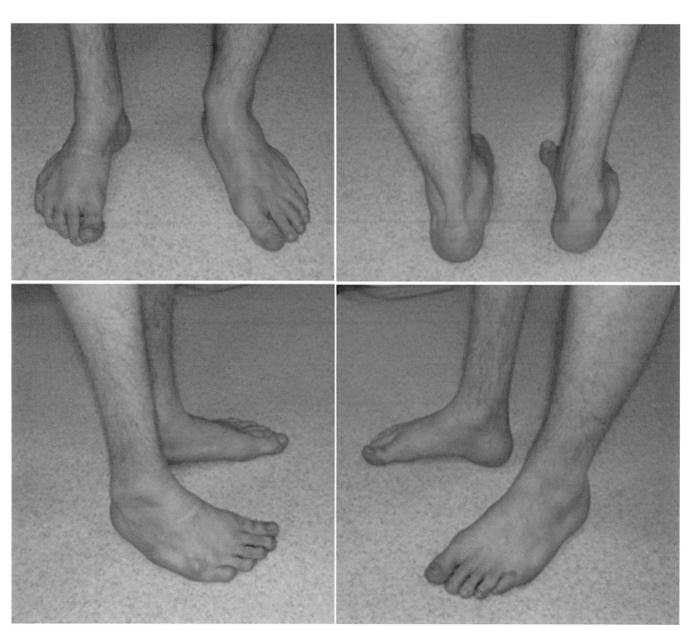

Figure 19.2 Relapsed club foot.

surgery and an LLD with shortening present in both the tibia and femur.

History

- Age at initial presentation,
- Treatment before relapse,
- Number of casts and tenotomies,
- Length of brace wear,
- Shoe wear.

Clinical examination

The appearance of the feet at follow-up can be classified according to Garceau and Palmer [4]. The paper is old – it was published in 1967 – but it does provide a framework that you can use. Not all components of the club foot tend to relapse to the same degree.

The relapse of the cavus deformity is rare and usually mild. The most important relapses occur in the hindfoot, first in the equinus, and then in the heel varus. In some relapsed club feet, the heel varus is very severe, while in others it is mild. Rarely, the heel in equinus may go into valgus, resulting in a calcaneovalgus deformity. This is a frequent occurrence in surgically treated club feet and is often referred to as over-corrected club foot. The following framework is useful:

- Describe the residue deformity to the examiner and in particular look for residual metatarsus adductus, heel varus and equinus. You can use Pirani or Diméglio scores to structure your description. Is it a correctable deformity?
- The affected foot may have several scars from previous surgery.
- Tendons: the strength of the peroneal and tibialis anterior tendons needs to be assessed. The direction of pull is important. If the tibialis anterior tendon pulls the foot into dorsiflexion and supination, it may need to be transferred to the midfoot.

- Check for LLD on the affected side (if unilateral).
- There have been several complicated residue club foot cases where epiphyseodesis of the normal contralateral femur and tibia at the knee has been performed.
- Gait:
  - No visible gait deformity,
  - Simultaneous heel-toe strike or mild genu recurvatum (due to equinus deformity),
  - Moderate genu recurvatum or lateral instability of the ankle,
  - Marked limp, failure of the heel to touch the floor, severe recurvatum or pivoting of the foot during step off.

Investigations

Weight-bearing AP, lateral and Saltzman's views of the foot (see Chapter 5 for more detail).

Management

The surgical technique for relapsed congenital club feet can be divided into three broad categories: namely soft-tissue releases, bony procedures and tendon transfers.

Surgical options for the correction of relapsed club foot could include:

- Medial release (almost every medial structure can be released or lengthened but avoid damaging the deltoid ligament),
- Posterior release (Achilles tendon and ankle posterior capsule),
- Tendon transfer,
- Bony procedures to correct alignment:
  - Calcaneum slide (lateral to correct varus, or medial to correct excessive valgus).
  - Cuboid osteotomy (to swing the forefoot around the talonavicular joint): a closing wedge corrects forefoot

Figure 19.3 Cuboid osteotomy.

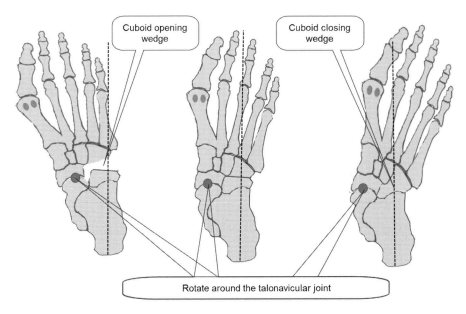

Cuboid opening wedge

Cuboid closing wedge

Rotate around the talonavicular joint

adduction, while an opening wedge corrects forefoot abduction.

- Dorsal closing wedge of the first metatarsal to elevate the first ray.
- Triple arthrodesis (or selective fusion) as a salvage for advanced and uncorrectable deformity.

The one thing to avoid with relapsed club foot surgery is overcorrection. Whereas a small degree of undercorrection is often well tolerated in adulthood, overcorrection is less acceptable and difficult to treat.

Topic 2: Limb length discrepancy
Viva practice 2

Examiner: A boy 12 years and 7 months old with Beckwith–Wiedemann syndrome was reviewed in the orthopaedic clinic with a LLD. His current height is 146.5 cm. These are his long leg alignment views taken in 2009, 2011 and 2012. Can you calculate his height at skeletal maturity?

Candidate: Several methods have been recommend to predict height and limb length and hence differences at maturity. All have some limitations and are based on certain assumptions, which in clinical practice are not always fulfilled. I use the multiplier methods (either using the pocket tables or more recently the multiplier phone apps) to predict height, limb lengths and LLD at maturity.

The child is a boy of 12 years and 7 months. The corresponding multiplier (from published tables) is 1.156.

$$\begin{aligned} \text{Height at maturity} &= \text{current height} \times \text{multiplier} \\ &= 146.5 \times 1.156 \\ &= 169.35 \text{ cm.} \end{aligned}$$

Examiner: Show me how you calculate his LLD in 2009, 2011 and 2012?

Candidate: I prefer to measure and tabulate each segment separately, as per Figure 19.5 and Table 19.2.

Examiner: Can you estimate his LLD at skeletal maturity?

Candidate: As with estimating height at skeletal maturity, there are various methods: none is perfect. The appropriate lower-limb multiplier is 1.16 (slightly different from that of height). The formula is:

$$\begin{aligned} \text{LLD at maturity} &= \text{current LLD} \times \text{the age and sex matched} \\ &\quad \text{multiplier} \\ &= 4.9 \text{ cm} \times 1.16 \\ &= 5.6 \text{ cm.} \end{aligned}$$

However, I prefer the Moseley straight-line graph when I have three previous readings, as it is more specific to the particular patient. The chart is based on skeletal age, with boys' age at the bottom and girls' at the top of the chart. The boys' age ranges from 3 to 16 while the girls' age ranges from 4 to 14. As the child grows, the age lines are closer, indicating less remaining growth. There is a diagonal line called 'long leg' that runs from bottom left to top right. The long leg measurement should be marked on this line corresponding to the skeletal age of the measurement. The short leg measurement is marked as well. This solid line represents the prediction of growth in the short leg.

Figure 19.4 Limb length discrepancy.

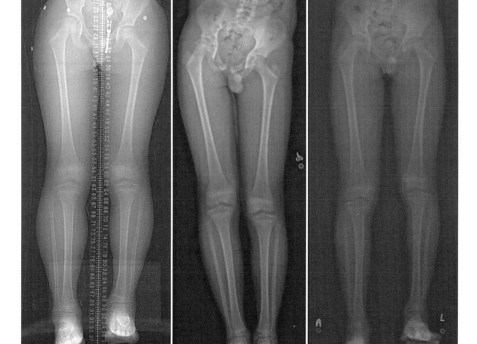

2009 **2011** **2012**

Table 19.2 Limb length discrepancy measurements

Year		Right	Left	LLD	Notes
2012	Femur	42.3	39.5	2.8	
	Tibia	33.2	31.1	2.1	
	Total	75.5	70.6	4.9	
2011	Femur	40.4	37.7	2.7	No blocks under the left leg
	Tibia	31.4	29.7	1.7	
	Total	71.8	67.4	4.4	
2009	Femur	37.2	34.6	2.6	
	Tibia	29.1	27.3	2.2	
	Total	66.3	61.9	4.8	

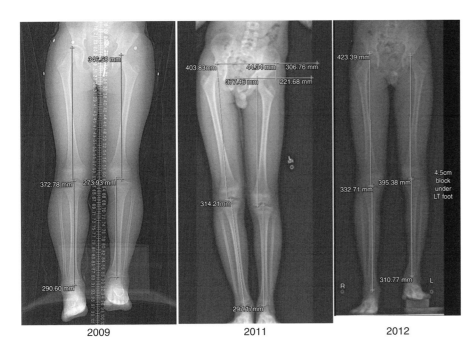

2009   2011   2012

Figure 19.5 Limb length discrepancy measurements.

To predict the LLD at a desired age, we need to draw a line that best fits the previous skeletal ages of measurement. From the intersection of this line with the desired age line, another line is drawn parallel to the side of the chart; its intersections with the long leg and short leg lines represent the length of these legs, respectively. The difference is the LLD at that desired age. In this example, the desired age is skeletal maturity; 5.5 cm.

Examiner: What about that small square called 'reference slope'?
Candidate: This helps predict the correct timing of the epiphysiodesis to treat LLD, as per Figure 19.7.

Topic 3: Paediatric spine
Viva practice 3

Examiner: This is a 15-year-old girl with adolescent idiopathic scoliosis. How would you describe her radiographs?
Candidate: These radiographs are a scoliosis series for this patient with a standing PA and lateral views on the top and right and left bending films (the right and left parts,

respectively) at the bottom. From the standing PA and lateral views, I can see that she has a thoracic curve, which is convex to the left side, and a thoracolumbar curve, which is convex to the right side. Both curves appear to be structural as they do not correct completely in the bending films. (However, I would measure the Cobb angles and see if they are correcting to less than 25° or not, according to Lenke [5].) The lateral X-radiographs show some increased thoracolumbar kyphosis; however, I should again measure the Cobb angle to know exactly how much. Triradiate cartilages are closed on both sides; regarding iliac apophysis, it is Risser grade 3 to 4.

Examiner: What are the main steps in your clinical assessment of such cases?
Candidate:

- History:
  - Main concern (pain or cosmesis),
  - Family history,
  - Growth and developmental history,
  - Onset of menses,
  - Review of systems and other work-ups.

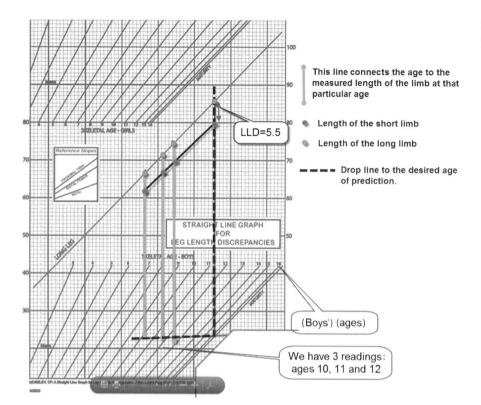

Figure 19.6 Moseley chart for estimation of LLD at maturity.

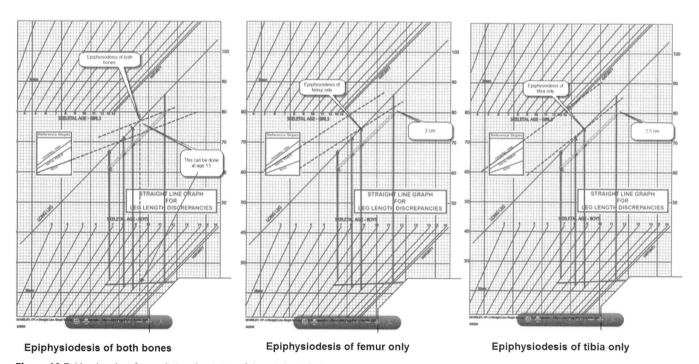

Epiphysiodesis of both bones **Epiphysiodesis of femur only** **Epiphysiodesis of tibia only**

Figure 19.7 Moseley chart for predicting the timing of the epiphysiodesis.

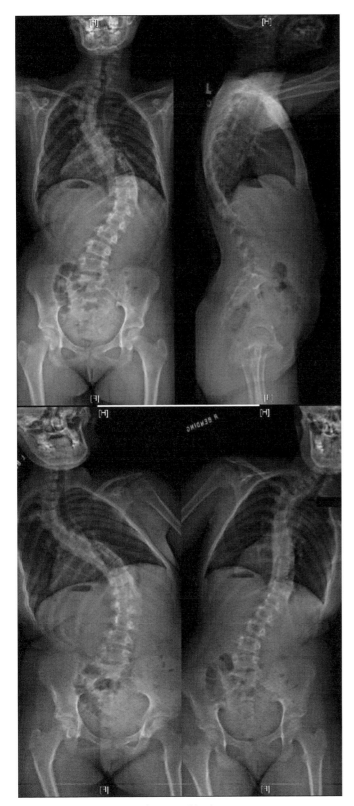

Figure 19.8 Scoliosis series of 15-year-old girl.

- Physical examination:
  · Height and weight growth chart,
  · Arm span to height ratio,
  · Limb length discrepancy,

- Shoulder heights,
- Rib prominence, waist asymmetry and lumbar prominence,
- Angle of trunk rotation as measured by scoliometer on Adam's forward bending test both in the thoracic and lumbar areas (Figure 6.6),
- Flexibility or laxity – Beighton scale,
- Skin examination and presence of café au lait spots,
- Complete neurological examination, including abdominal reflexes.

Examiner: How can you define different curve types?
Candidate: Each curve can be defined mainly by its apical vertebra or disc.
The apical vertebra or disc is the vertebra or disc with the greatest rotation and the farthest lateral deviation from the centre of the vertebral column and the horizontal (the least tilted in the curve).
The end vertebrae on both sides of a curve are those with the maximum tilt toward the concavity of the curve.
Neutral vertebrae are those that show no evidence of rotation on standing PA radiographs.
Curve types are mainly described according to the location of the apex of the curve (Scoliosis Research Society definitions) and then according to the direction of the convexity, either convex to the left or to the right.

Examiner: How do you measure the Cobb angle?
Candidate: The Cobb angle is the angle formed by the intersection of two lines, one parallel to the superior endplate of the superior end vertebra and the other parallel to the inferior endplate of the inferior end vertebra. If the endplates are obscured, the pedicles can be used instead. (See Chapter 6 for more detail.)

Examiner: What are the main limitations in measuring the Cobb angle?
Candidate: The main limitations are [6]:

- A diurnal variation of 5° has been observed in Cobb angle measurements of the same curve over the course of a single day, with an angular increase occurring in the afternoon.
- Because of the vertebral rotation associated with scoliosis, it may be difficult to position the patient so as to obtain an accurate frontal view, and the actual Cobb angle might be 20% greater than that plotted on radiographs.
- The Cobb angle varies with supine, prone (including during surgery), sitting and standing views.
- A total error of 2°–7° in Cobb angle assessment has been reported to result from variations in radiographic acquisitions and measurement error. Because the measurement error is smaller when end vertebrae are consistently defined, the same endpoints should be used at follow-up as at the initial curve assessment.
- An intra-observer variation of 5°–10° in Cobb angle measurement has been reported, and the inter-observer variation may be even greater.

Table 19.3 Lenke classification system

Curve type	Description	Proximal thoracic	Main thoracic	Thoracolumbar, lumbar
1	Main thoracic (MT)	Non-structural	Structural	Non-structural
2	Double thoracic (DT)	Structural	Structural (major)	Non-structural
3	Double major (DM)	Non-structural	Structural (major)	Structural
4	Triple major (TM)	Structural	Structural (major)	Structural
5	Thoracolumbar/lumbar (TL/L-M)	Non-structural	Non-structural	Structural
6	Thoracolumbar/lumbar – main thoracic (TL/L-MT)	Non-structural	Structural	Structural (major)

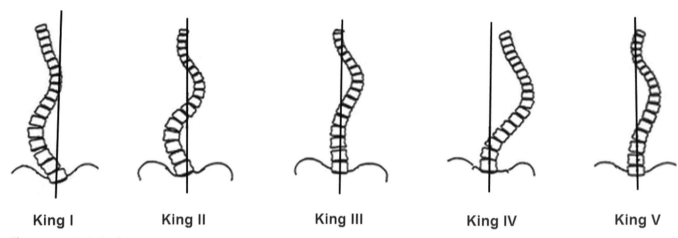

King I **King II** **King III** **King IV** **King V**

Figure 19.9 King's classification.

Examiner: How can you assess the vertebral alignment and balance on radiographs?

Candidate: The plumb line is a vertical line drawn downward from the centre of the C7 vertebral body, parallel to the lateral edges of the radiograph.

It is used to evaluate coronal balance on standing frontal radiographs and sagittal balance on standing lateral radiographs. Coronal balance is evaluated by measuring the distance between the CSL (central sacral vertical line) and the plumb line, and sagittal balance is evaluated by measuring the distance between the posterosuperior aspect of the S1 vertebral body and the plumb line. For both coronal and sagittal measurements, balance is considered abnormal if the distance is greater than 2 cm.

Examiner: Which classification system would you use for adolescent idiopathic scoliosis?

Candidate: There are two common classification systems. King and Moe described Types I to V, depending on the shape of the curve.

Type I: S-shaped double curve, where the lumbar curve is larger or less flexible,

Type II: S-shaped double curve, where the thoracic curve is larger or less flexible,

Type III: Single thoracic curve,

Type IV: Long thoracic curves, where L4 is tilted into the curve,

Type V: Double thoracic curve, where T1 is tilted into the thoracic curve.

The other widely used classification system for adolescent idiopathic scoliosis is the Lenke classification system. It is more sophisticated and complicated. According to Lenke, there are four types of curve pattern:

1. Proximal thoracic (apical vertebra located at T3–5),
2. Main thoracic (apical vertebra located at T6–11),
3. Thoracolumbar (apical vertebra located at T12–L1),
4. Lumbar (apical vertebra located at L2–4).

Each curve is further classified into a major curve (the curve segment with the larger Cobb angle) and a minor curve (the curve segment with the smaller Cobb angle). Major curves are always considered structural, while minor curves can be structural if they meet the following criteria:

- Minimal residual coronal curve on bending film of at least 25°,
- Kyphosis of at least 20°.

There are six curve types, corresponding to different combinations of structural and non-structural curve patterns (Table 19.3).

Lenke further proposed two modifiers.

A lumbar modifier to emphasize the importance of deformities in the lumbar region, as this affects spinal balance as well as proximal curves. The lumbar modifier could be A, B or C:

A: Central sacral vertical line (CSL) passes between pedicles up to the stable vertebra,

B: CSL touches the apical body up to the stable vertebra,

C: CSL passes medial to apical body up to the stable vertebra.

A thoracic spine sagittal modifier to introduce a three-dimensional analysis to the classification system. The thoracic spine sagittal modifier is denoted by −, N or +, based on the sagittal Cobb angle (between T5 and T12):

−: Hypo <10°,

N: Normal 10–40°,

+: Hyper >40°.

Examiner: So what type of curve does this patient have?
Candidate: To define this curve accurately, I need to measure the Cobb angle of the curves in the frontal and sagittal as well as bending films.

Examiner: The thoracolumbar curve Cobb angle is 65°, the thoracic curve is 54°, the thoracic T5–T12 kyphosis is 37°

and the thoracolumbar kyphosis (T10–L2) is 24°. In side bending films, the thoracic curve corrects to 46° and the thoracolumbar curve to 29°. How would you classify this deformity?
Candidate:

1. We have here two curves, a thoracic curve and a thoracolumbar curve. Both of them are structural and the thoracolumbar curve is the major curve, therefore it is Type 6 (thoracolumbar/lumbar – main thoracic).

2. If we draw the CSL, it would run outside the pedicles of the lumbar vertebrae, therefore the lumbar spine modifier is C.

3. Then, the thoracic spine sagittal modifier will be N because T5–T12 kyphosis is within the normal range (10°–40°).

4. The final classification of this curve would be Lenke type 6CN.

Examiner: How would you manage this patient's spinal deformity?
Candidate: The main lines of treatment of scoliosis deformity are observation, bracing and surgical treatment. Usually, the threshold for surgical treatment would be a thoracic curve >50° or a lumbar curve >40°. So this patient is already within the surgical indication and in such cases, we would do an instrumented posterior spinal fusion for the structural curves, which are the thoracic and thoracolumbar curves. Regarding the exact fusion levels, it is always a controversial subject but many surgeons would include both the upper and lower end vertebrae of the structural curves.

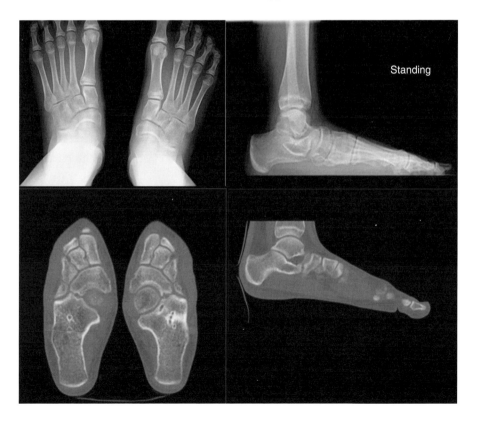

Figure 19.10 Child with bilateral foot pain.

Topic 4: Rigid flat foot

Viva practice 4

Examiner: These are the radiographs of a 9-year-old boy who came to the clinic complaining of foot pain.

Candidate: These are plain AP and lateral radiographs of the feet and coronal and sagittal CT scans. They demonstrate a calcaneonavicular coalition. This is the most common tarsal coalition. It occurs in approximately two-thirds of cases. There is usually an elongated anterior process of the calcaneum (the anteater nose sign).

Examiner: What do you mean by a coalition?

Candidate: A coalition is a fusion between tarsal bones caused by an embryological failure of segmentation of mesenchymal tissue in the hind and midfoot. The fusion could be fibrous, cartilaginous or osseous. A solitary coalition can range from a minimal fibrosis to complete bony synostosis.

Examiner: How do patients present?

Candidate: A large number of coalitions can be asymptomatic and never present to an orthopaedic surgeon. Symptoms usually appear by the age of 10–12 years, when the coalition ossifies or becomes stiffer. These include calf pain due to peroneal spasticity, flatfoot and limited subtalar motion. A child with a stiff hind foot may give a history of recurrent ankle sprains or fractures. Lateral heel pain is a common finding from fibular impingement on the valgus calcaneum. Subtalar movement is grossly reduced or absent.

Examiner: What investigations would you order?

Candidate: Computed tomography (CT) and magnetic resonance imaging (MRI) are generally not necessary to make the diagnosis of calcaneonavicular coalition. Most surgeons would prefer to order these image modalities to identify multiple coalitions and to assess coalition location and percentage of joint involvement. A talocalcaneal coalition can be difficult to diagnose on plain radiographs.

Examiner: What are the aims of management?

Candidate: These would be relief of pain, improvement of joint motion, correction of deformity and avoidance of degenerative joint disease.

Examiner: So what would you offer this patient?

Candidate: My initial treatment is to control symptoms using pain killers, shoe modifications and maybe a short period of immobilization (casting) or orthoses.
Persistence of symptoms is an indication for resection. The extensor digitorum brevis muscle is interposed between the resected bar to prevent recurrence. Raw bone areas are also covered with bone wax to further reduce the risk of recurrence.

Examiner: How successful is resection?

Candidate: This depends on the size of the coalition and whether degenerative joint disease is present.

Examiner: So what figure would you tell the patient?

Candidate: Cohen reported a series of 17 adult patients with symptomatic tarsal coalition in which three patients improved with conservative measures. Twelve patients had symptoms severe enough to require surgery. Of these patients, 10 of the 12 obtained pain relief at 3-year follow-up [7].

Examiner: Are any other options available?

Candidate: A subtalar arthrodesis or triple arthrodesis is usually reserved for failed resections with persistent pain and deformity.

Clinical practice 2

A GP letter refers an 8-year-old boy to the orthopaedic clinic; there is several months' history of left foot pain.

Examiner: Would you examine this young man's left foot please?

Candidate: On inspection, I note a planovalgus attitude of the left foot. The forefoot is abducted relative to the hindfoot. From behind, the lateral toes are more visible but it is not a too-many-toes sign, as more than two toes should be seen outside the heel for this sign to be positive.

Can you stand up on your tiptoe for me please?

The patient is unable to perform a double heel raise. The medial longitudinal arch does not form and is absent. There is failure to reconstitute the medial longitudinal arch when the patient attempts to adopt a weight-bearing equinus position. The heels fail to go into varus. The feet appear to be as a rigid flat foot. I am thinking about tarsal coalition as a diagnosis.

Examiner: What test would you like to perform to confirm your diagnosis?

Candidate: I would like to perform the Coleman block test.

I have no idea why I said this. This was the wrong test. The examiner quickly moved me onto a new case. I still, however, passed that particular short case.

I cannot remember if I asked the patient whether the foot was painful or not.

This condition is sometimes referred to as peroneal spastic flatfoot but the peroneal muscles are not truly in spasm. Equinovarus deformity or forefoot inversion might occur in some forms of massive and multiple tarsal coalitions.
With the 5-minute format, a candidate would have only used up about 3 minutes worth of time and so would be expected to perform a more detailed examination of the foot.

Examiner: Would you like to examine the range of movement of the feet?

The severity and limitation of joint movement depends on the site and extent of the tarsal coalition. A talocalcaneal coalition causes a marked restriction of subtalar movement, while a calcaneonavicular coalition causes some restriction of both subtalar and midtarsal joint movement. Children with multiple tarsal coalitions have no movement at all in the subtalar and midtarsal joint [8].

Therefore, as a candidate, you would need to slickly examine the range of movement of the ankle, subtalar and midfoot joints and pick up a reduction in movement of the subtalar or midfoot joints.

Remember examination of subtalar joint movement; this is a differentiator between candidates. It is quite obvious to examiners if you are well practised in examining foot and ankle movements with this test or have just learnt it for the exam.

Examiner: What are the causes of a rigid flat foot?
Candidate: Causes include:

1. Congenital vertical talus: this can occur in association with other congenital anomalies such as myelomeningocele, arthrogryposis, DDH.
2. Neuromuscular foot: this can occur in association with other neuromuscular conditions, such as cerebral palsy, Duchenne muscular dystrophy and poliomyelitis.

3. Skew foot: this is known as Z foot, serpentine foot. There is hindfoot valgus, midfoot valgus (often called lateral shift) and forefoot adduction (metatarsus adductus).
4. Trauma.
5. Seronegative arthritis.
6. Iatrogenic to treatment, such as club foot.

Examiner: These are the patient's radiographs. What do you see?
Candidate: The radiograph is a lateral weight-bearing X-ray of the left foot, which confirms the presence of a calcaneonavicular coalition. The anteater sign is present and I can see talar beaking.

> It is unlikely that you will be shown a young patient with secondary degenerative arthritis, but in this case there would be clinical features of reduced painful range of movement in the foot, possibly with secondary deformity.

References

1. Bridgens J and Kiely N (2010) Current management of clubfoot (congenital talipes equinovarus). *BMJ* **340**:c355.

2. Jowett C, Morcuende J and Ramachandran M (2011) Management of congenital talipes equinovarus using the Ponseti method: a systematic review. *J Bone Joint Surg Br* **93**(9):1160–4.

3. Lampasi M, Bettuzzi C, Palmonari M and Donzelli O (2010) Transfer of the tendon of tibialis anterior in relapsed congenital clubfoot: long-term results in 38 feet. *J Bone Joint Surg Br* **92**(2):277–83.

4. Garceau GJ and Palmer RM (1967) Transfer of the anterior tibial tendon for recurrent club foot. A long-term follow-up. *J Bone Joint Surg Am* **49**(2):207–31.

5. Lenke LG, Betz RR, Harms J *et al.* (2001) Adolescent idiopathic scoliosis: a new classification to determine extent of spinal arthrodesis. *J Bone Joint Surg Am* **83**-A(8):1169–81.

6. Kim H, Kim HS, Moon ES *et al.* (2010) Scoliosis imaging: what radiologists should know. *Radiographics* **30**(7):1823–42.

7. Cohen B, Davis W and Anderson R (1996) Success of calcaneonavicular coalition resection in the adult population. *Foot & Ankle International* **17**(9):569.

8. Loder R (2009) Tarsal coalition. In *Paediatric Orthopaedics: A System of Decision-Making*, ed. Joseph B, Nayagam S, Loder R and Torode I. Boca Raton, FL: CRC Press, p. 343.

Index

Entries in bold typeface refer to figures or tables.